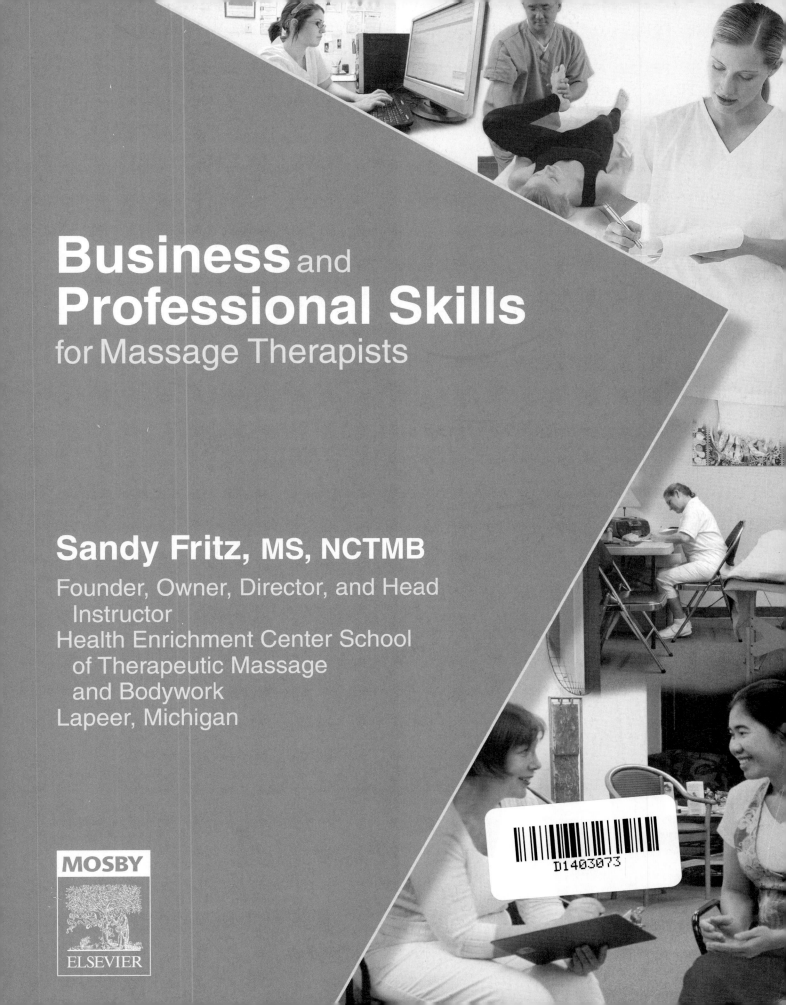

Business and Professional Skills
for Massage Therapists

Sandy Fritz, MS, NCTMB

Founder, Owner, Director, and Head
 Instructor
Health Enrichment Center School
 of Therapeutic Massage
 and Bodywork
Lapeer, Michigan

MOSBY

ELSEVIER

MOSBY
ELSEVIER

3251 Riverport Lane
Maryland Heights, Missouri 63043

Notices

Knowledge and best practice in this field are constantly changing. As new research and experience broaden our understanding, changes in research methods, professional practices, or medical treatment may become necessary.

Practitioners and researchers must always rely on their own experience and knowledge in evaluating and using any information, methods, compounds, or experiments described herein. In using such information or methods they should be mindful of their own safety and the safety of others, including parties for whom they have a professional responsibility.

With respect to any drug or pharmaceutical products identified, readers are advised to check the most current information provided (i) on procedures featured or (ii) by the manufacturer of each product to be administered, to verify the recommended dose or formula, the method and duration of administration, and contraindications. It is the responsibility of practitioners, relying on their own experience and knowledge of their patients, to make diagnoses, to determine dosages and the best treatment for each individual patient, and to take all appropriate safety precautions.

To the fullest extent of the law, neither the Publisher nor the authors, contributors, or editors, assume any liability for any injury and/or damage to persons or property as a matter of products liability, negligence or otherwise, or from any use or operation of any methods, products, instructions, or ideas contained in the material herein.

Library of Congress Cataloging-in-Publication Data
Fritz, Sandy, MS.
  Business and professional skills for massage therapists / Sandy Fritz. — 1st ed.
      p. ; cm.
  Includes bibliographical references and index.
  ISBN 978-0-323-05718-9 (pbk. : alk. paper) 1. Massage therapy—Practice. I. Title.
  [DNLM: 1. Massage—organization & administration. 2. Massage—economics. 3. Office
Management. WB 537 F9195 2010]
  RM722.F75 2010
  615.8'2—dc22

2009039287

Vice President and Publisher: Linda Duncan
Senior Editor: Kellie White
Senior Developmental Editor: Jennifer Watrous
Publishing Services Manager: Hemamalini Rajendrababu
Project Manager: K. Anand Kumar
Book and cover designer: Charles Seibel

Printed in the United States of America

Last digit is the print number: 9 8 7 6 5 4 3 2 1

This textbook is dedicated to the success of all who use it.

✍

Special thanks are offered to Amy Husted for all of her hard work.

Boundless appreciation goes to Betty Ladley Finkbeiner and Charles Allan Finkbeiner,
authors of *Practice Management for the Dental Team* (Elsevier, 2006),
which was a major source of information and inspiration for this textbook.

Thank you to The Gathering Place in St. Louis for opening its massage school and
practice for us to take some of the photos in this book.

And my sincere gratitude is extended to all of the individuals
on my support team at Elsevier—especially Kellie White, Jennifer Watrous,
April Falast, Linda Duncan, Joy Moore, Anand Kumar,
Charlie Seibel, Allison Wyffels, and Julie Burchett.

✍

Reviewers

Liz Halat, LMT
Owner, Zenza Spa & Massage
Instructor, Academy of Massage Therapy
Englewood, New Jersey

Bridget C. Healy, MFA (Creative Writing)
St. Louis, Missouri

David MacDougall, MA, LMT
Associate Professor/Director, Massage Therapy Program
North Country Community College
Saranac Lake, New York

Scott G. Rayburn, CMT, LMT
D.B.A Waterock Massage Therapy
Massage Therapy Instructor
Central State Massage Academy
Oklahoma City, Oklahoma

Jonelle Thomas, BBA, CMT, NCTMB
President
Half Moon Wellness
Member
International Association of Yoga Therapists (IAYT)
Registered Yoga Teacher, as a member of Yoga Alliance
 (RYT)
Atlanta, Georgia

Howard Weingarten, NCTMB
Massage Therapist
Integrative Therapies
Warrenton, Virginia

Special Contributors

David K. Anderson, LMT, NCTMB
Co-Owner
Tucson Touch Therapies
Tucson, Arizona

Sandra K. Anderson, BA, LMT, NCTMB
Co-Owner
Tucson Touch Therapies
Tucson, Arizona

Bruce Froelich, JD, NCTMB
Member, American Massage Therapy Association
Adjunct Instructor
Owosso Campus, Baker College
Auburn Hills, Michigan

C. G. Funk, LMT
Vice President of Industry Relations and Product
 Development
Massage Envy Limited
Arizona and California

W. Randy Snyder, DC, MS, NCTMB, CHCQM
Owner/Director
College of Integrative Medicine
Oceanside, California

Every field has its giants–individuals whose influence and contributions stand far above those of others. In massage therapy, perhaps no one over the last half century better fits this description than Sandy Fritz.

With the publication of this book, *Business and Professional Skills for Massage Therapists,* Sandy has given massage training programs a blueprint that, if followed, will increase the success rates of their graduates, and hence, the schools and the industry as a whole.

Although most other books devote a chapter to business, Sandy has expanded the concept to an entire book on the subject, allowing her the freedom to delve into the subject in great detail specific to a massage practice. Sandy explores all the basics such as scope of practice, documentation, ethics, trends in the profession, communication, setting up an office, appointment management systems, marketing, inventory and supplies, safety and sanitation, and planning your career path. She examines the office from both the employee and the employer point of view.

One of my favorite chapters is "Technology in the Massage Practice." Sandy provides the reader with a basic understanding of computer hardware; software such as word processing, spreadsheets, and databases; and the value of the internet as a communication tool for both gathering and disseminating information.

Then stepping beyond the basics, she tackles what many consider to be the most complicated parts of a massage practice: insurance reimbursement, basic accounting, and money management. The chapter on money management is a "how-to" that should be required reading not just for prospective massage therapists, but for every high school student.

Other important features of this book include:

- Good Stuff from the Government: contains Web links or addresses for free government publications on a variety of topics.
- Evolve Annotated Web links: contain internet references for extended study of different business subjects.
- Self-Reflection: a question box designed to be a "devil's advocate" for provoking readers to question their own abilities, insights, motives, and liabilities.
- Dozens of charts, letters, screen snapshots from the accompanying software, and other practical examples that can be used in setting up a practice.

Over the last few decades, as a therapist, teacher, and author, I have observed the turnover rate in our field and have come to a few conclusions about it. I know many college graduates who are not working in their degreed field, and that seems like a tremendous waste. Although the turnover rate among massage therapists is probably no higher than in other professions, I still believe it could, and should, be lower.

Massage therapists are good at what they do. Their technical skills are superior, and their clients love them. When massage therapists do not succeed, one of two reasons is to blame. Either the therapist is not taking care of himself or herself physically and cannot keep up with the pace of the work, or the therapist is lacking in business skills. I believe that the latter reason is the most common explanation for attrition from our field. If you cannot balance a checkbook, how can you run your own business? Logically then, better education in the area of business practices can increase therapist longevity and employee retention by the industry.

This book will be one that will be used beyond graduation from massage school. It is a perfect desk reference for the established therapist, whether working as an employee at a day spa, as a self-employed therapist in a small private practice, or as the owner/operator of a large practice with a dozen or more employees.

I have had the pleasure of working with Sandy on numerous projects, and my admiration and respect for her grows and grows. Her warmth and compassion comes through every aspect of her life and her work. She loves what she does, and it shows. Furthermore, Sandy is the best hugger (I hope that is a real word)!

I felt honored when asked to write the Foreword to her latest book.

Everyone is familiar with Sandy Fritz as a visionary pioneer of the massage industry from her wealth of books. It is my hope that her latest contribution to the field, a business model, will indeed increase your professional life span by giving you the tools for success.

Susan G. Salvo
Lake Charles, Louisiana

Preface

The therapeutic massage profession is maturing and many changes have occurred as the profession has continued to gain respect and popularity. Massage therapists are expected to conduct themselves as professionals, and your success depends not only on your skills as a massage therapist but also on your business skills. This textbook can help you understand and develop the business and professional skills necessary for a successful massage therapy practice.

There are two distinct career pathways in massage therapy. You can be self-employed or be an employee. Both directions offer the opportunity for career success. This textbook explores these options and identifies overlapping professional skills.

BACKGROUND

The practice requirements for massage therapy continue to increase. In addition to working independently, massage therapists can work in a variety of environments such as spas, chiropractic offices, sports facilities, integrated medicine facilities, and massage franchises. Because of these changes, it became evident that a textbook that targeted professional and business skills was needed.

Excellent professional skills and behavior are comparable in many professions. As this textbook was being planned, Elsevier published a book for the dental profession called *Practice Management for the Dental Team*. Its content was very similar to the book being planned for the massage therapy community, and it became the framework for this textbook. You could say that it was massaged in the direction of professional skills for the massage therapist! As the content was developed for this unique textbook, it was polished after careful scrutiny of many reviewers.

Massage therapy research is proving that the multitude of massage methods and modalities influence the physiology of the human body in similar ways. There are many more similarities than differences. Similarly, the professional expertise, solid business practices, and interpersonal skills remain consistent throughout the service professions. This level of consistency indicates that massage therapy has indeed become a profession—and you are part of it.

WHO CAN BENEFIT FROM THIS TEXTBOOK?

This textbook is targeted to massage therapy students in entry-level training for professional practice. Topics explored range from the abstract ideas of intention, intuition, and inspiration to the concrete skills of how to file client records. The business tasks may be considered mundane, but ask anyone who has undergone a tax audit how important record keeping is. You will learn about communication, conflict management, and working as part of a professional team. You will also learn what is involved in being self-employed or becoming a business owner and employer.

Even though this text is targeted to the entry-level student, those who have been in practice also can benefit from the content. It is productive to revisit the basics and rethink current practices while planning for the future.

WHY THIS TEXTBOOK IS IMPORTANT TO THE PROFESSION

When I began a massage practice in the late 1970s, many of us were maturing hippies from the 1960s. We embraced the ideas of alternative, anti-establishment, and holistic living. Although massage is an ancient healing system, it had become relegated to the background of health services. The social revolution of the 1960s demanded changes in many areas, and health care systems could no longer ignore the benefits of methods such as massage therapy.

Massage therapy is still not totally integrated with other health services, but the trend indicates continued growth and acceptance. This development coincides with expectations of professional standards of conduct and business skills. Successful group practice, as demonstrated by the rapid growth and acceptance of franchises, such as Massage Envy and Elements, requires learning how to work with others and following business protocols.

Your future as a massage therapist will be very different from my past experience. For example, advances in technology can manage many of the tedious tasks necessary for any business professional. The content in this textbook can prepare you to become part of the future of massage therapy.

CONCEPTUAL APPROACH

Massage therapy has been and will always be a compassionate service profession. The wholeness of the interaction between practitioner and client, combined with the knowledgeable application of massage skills and the understanding of their mechanisms of benefit, will continue to be the foundation of our professional path of service. The heartfelt passion to serve others in a humble and simple way by using skilled touch will not be replaced by technology. The ethical expectation of respect and mindfulness of the client's best interests constitute a thread that runs through the entire textbook.

The textbook also is written as a guide to self-discovery, critical thinking, and decision making. There is no specific protocol for business skills. Just like massage, you need to assess the situation, research information, brainstorm, evaluate, and implement. The textbook embraces this concept by supporting your ability to be your own teacher.

ORGANIZATION

Each of the 18 chapters describes a segment of professional practice. The chapter topics have two main themes: people and processes. People topics, such as ethics, professional relationships, and career motivation, are interwoven with process topics. Processes are activities such as documentation, filing, purchasing, accounting, cleaning, and maintaining equipment. Interspersing the important process information with the interesting and insightful people information should help you remain interested and focused.

The material is organized so that it moves from exploring the business professional topic of massage in Chapters 1 and 2 to a focus on client service and ethical and legal practices in Chapters 3 and 4. A shift occurs to processes involving the use of technology and office design in Chapters 5 and 6. In Chapters 7 and 8, documentation and maintenance of records are described. Various forms of communication are addressed in Chapters 9 and 10, and scheduling is targeted in Chapter 11.

At this point, you should have enough information to begin to seriously investigate marketing, which is the topic of Chapter 12. Chapter 13 is very process oriented and provides points to consider in the daily management of business operations and the costs involved. Chapters 14, 15, and 16 discuss the flow of money. Chapter 17 combines people and process information to describe the components of an interpersonal and environmentally safe environment. Chapter 18 reviews earlier content and lays down the platform for launching your career.

DISTINCTIVE FEATURES

The content of this book is progressive and future focused. As the massage profession changes, our approach to professional development also must change. In the past, a massage therapist often opened his or her own small business. Today, a massage therapist is more likely to work as an employee. Pursuing a career as an employee is quite different from being self-employed. This textbook is the first to equally explore both options for career development.

Professionalism is emphasized, and professionalism is more than just business practices. Most textbooks on the market are focused on the nuts and bolts of business management and marketing as a self-employed practitioner. This textbook both includes and goes beyond this content to address the more nuanced approaches to professional behavior required in massage therapy practice.

I have been in an active massage practice for 30 years. I also own, manage, and teach in a unique and highly respected, single-owner massage therapy school in the United States. Because I function as an employer and educator of future massage therapists and teachers, the approach I bring to the content is practical, based on experience, adaptive to the changing world of economics, massage therapy practice, and small business ownership. In other words, I am still in the trenches—working, transporting the massage table, making appointments, and doing laundry.

One of the most valuable features of the textbook guides you to resources for your professional development. The Good Stuff from the Government feature at the end of each chapter opens the virtual doorway to almost endless sources of online information from U.S. and Canadian governmental agencies and from colleges and universities. Most material is free and in the public domain. The recommended sites have been chosen as starting points, and I hope that they will provide an ongoing source of support. All of the links are also provided on the Evolve site that accompanies the textbook, which allows you to easily access the information.

The Self-Reflection feature leads you through a series of questions to help you explore your feelings, values, and beliefs about the topics in each chapter.

Activities involve content integration. Marked by the icon of a brain plugged in, they are easy to identify. Space is provided to complete the activities and to personalize the text as one you will review often as your career progresses.

Each chapter begins with defined key terms and learning objectives and concludes with learning exercises. Figures, boxes, and tables highlight content for easy location and ongoing reference.

ANCILLARIES

The student Evolve Website features exercises, case studies, additional activities, annotated Web links, a glossary of key terms from the textbook, and a comprehensive bank of templates for building items such as resumes, letters, advertisements, forms for documentation, client histories, schedules, and budgets. These samples are customizable, providing an excellent collection of templates for students to try out during the course and to take with them as they go into practice. Evolve icons throughout the text indicate when online resources apply.

For the instructor, there also are many resources on the Evolve site:

- A test bank in ExamView® format
- An instructor manual and lesson plans for a professional development course
- An image collection to use for lectures

Bound into the back of the textbook is a CD-ROM containing practice management software from leading massage office software provider, Island Software. The software is provided in a demonstration program for student practice. Utilities on the CD include the following: Client Contact Record, Documentation, Business Contact Record, Appointment Scheduling, and more. Activities in the textbook include interaction with this practice management software, with icons directing students to open the software and use it.

NOTE TO THE STUDENT

This textbook can become a useful resource as you pursue your massage career. According to the Bureau of Labor Statistics and the Department of Labor, continuing employment growth is projected in the service-providing sector of the economy. Service-providing industries, such as massage, will generate almost all of the employment gain from 2006 to 2016 and will provide more than three fourths of all jobs in 2016. Professional and business services, health care, and social assistance are expected to experience the largest growth in employment. Massage therapy can be classified in all of these categories. What they have in common is professional service—one of the main themes of this textbook. Another commonality is expectation of occupational education. Massage therapy educational requirements are listed as postsecondary vocational awards. These programs lead to a certificate or diploma but not a degree. Some of these programs last only a few weeks, but others may require more than a year of study. Massage therapy education is typically at the high end of the training requirements. Occupations in this category usually require the completion of a specific vocational training program and require individuals to pass a licensing or certification examination after completion of the program before they can work.

In most states, massage therapy is a licensed occupation. It is expected that massage therapists have graduated from high school and have formal training in an educational setting (i.e., school rather than on-the-job training). Some areas of this formal training are the same regardless of the occupation chosen, and one of those areas is professionalism. To achieve success as a massage therapist, you are expected to meet the educational criteria and to achieve professional excellence. This text can act as a map as you embark on your learning journey.

Sandy Fritz

Contents

THE BUSINESS OF MASSAGE THERAPY

KEY TERMS

Business
Communication

Massage therapy
Leadership

Management
Service

LEARNING OUTCOMES

Mastery of the content in this chapter will enable the reader to:

- Explain the concept of massage therapy as a business
- Describe the service concept
- Define communication
- Differentiate between various styles of management
- List characteristics necessary for establishing relationships

e Guidelines for the Learning Activities and answers to the Workbook questions are located on Evolve at http://evolve.elsevier.com/Fritz/business.

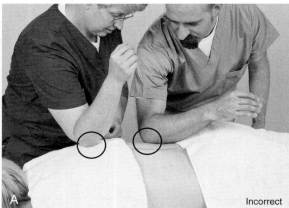 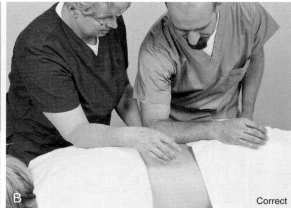

FIGURE 1-1. Mentoring and teaching require experience and wisdom.

What is it like to be a massage therapist? What does it take to have a successful massage career? What skills are necessary for success other than providing excellent massage services? What makes massage therapy a profession? What is professional behavior? These and more questions need to be answered for the massage profession as a whole and for individual massage therapists. The learning system presented in this textbook does not have the answers to all of the questions, but it does have much of the information you need to answer many of these questions for yourself, and it provides the foundation necessary for you to learn how to ask your own questions. Intelligent questions, not answers, lead to discovery. If you know how to research, listen, engage others in conversation, observe, and model (i.e., do what you see others do), you can find answers. The answers often depend on the circumstances; the questions typically are more of a constant guiding force. Success is built on questions and how you find your answers.

Certain traits and behaviors can support success in your massage business. Being genuine, honest, enthusiastic, compassionate, knowledgeable, and polite will support success. A mentor is a wise and trusted counselor or teacher, especially in occupational settings. As a mentor (Fig. 1-1) and teacher, my task in writing this textbook is to provide you with information that is valid, time tested, and accepted as beneficial. Sometimes, the instructions sound like a parent telling you what to do. Statements such as "do this," "you must," or "you should" can seem commanding and bossy, but some things are best learned from the experience and likely mistakes of others. Your classroom teacher occasionally also may be directive. Think of these "just do it this way" statements as shortcuts. Although you can learn from your own mistakes and successes, it is also wise to not make the same mistakes of those who have gone before you.

A learning system is a multifaceted portal to understanding. This learning system includes the textbook and accompanying Evolve Web site. The Evolve Web site is your gateway to many resources. This learning system can lead you on this journey of discovery. It is based on information from many experts that constitute an advisory board.

An advisory board is a collection of individuals who provide unique knowledge and skills. An effective advisory board provides informed guidance, but it is you who will make and implement decisions. Efficient and effective decision making involves the following:

- Facts and information
- Ideas and inspiration
- Practicality and resources
- People's feelings and perceptions

If we are going to succeed, we need hope for the future, people willing to help behind the scenes, and those who can lend a helping hand (Fig. 1-2).

LEARNING ACTIVITY

Identify three important factors that contribute to your learning process, and attach a name or symbol to them. For example,

1. Bumble bee—nothing is impossible. Be your own best teacher.

   List your three factors below:
   1. _____
   2. _____
   3. _____

SELF-REFLECTION

It is important that you sift and sort all of the information yourself. Successful individuals make their own decisions and take responsibility for those decisions. They seek information and guidance but do not necessarily do what others say they should. When you see the mirror icon, you will find a list of questions to guide this internal dialog.

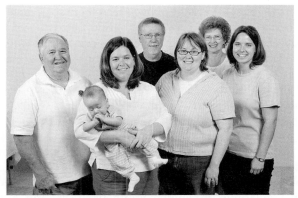

FIGURE 1-2. Example of an advisory board in someone's life, built up of family and friends. *(From Fritz S:* Mosby's Fundamentals of Therapeutic Massage, *ed 4, St. Louis, 2009, Mosby.)*

BOX 1-1   What Employers Are Looking For

Besides excellent massage skills, employers are looking for the following:
- Communication skills
- Computer (documentation) skills
- Flexibility and adaptability
- Interpersonal abilities
- Research skills
- Leadership and management skills
- Planning and organization skills
- Problem solving and creativity skills
- Teamwork ability

Data from Hansen RS, Hansen K: What Do Employers Really Want? Top Skills and Values Employers Seek from Job Seekers; http://www.quintcareers.com/job_skills_values.html

This learning system has been designed to provide information and guidance, act as a trusted mentor, and provide a platform for an expert advisory board. It can help you find your path to success, but you have to walk it. This chapter furnishes an overview of the massage profession, and more detail is provided in subsequent chapters.

PROFESSIONAL TRENDS IN MASSAGE THERAPY

During the past 30 years, most massage therapists worked alone in private practice. Recent surveys and data from various professional groups serving the massage community indicate that although this is still the case, there is a significant and steady increase in massage therapists working with other professionals in multidisciplinary environments from full-service spas to hospitals. The spa industry and chiropractic practices show the largest gains. Web links that pertain to this section are given at the end of this chapter.

These trends indicate an increasing need for massage professionals to be able to interface with people and systems in a professional manner, including how information about shared clients is exchanged, electronic office and documentation systems, and how to answer the phone, dress, display work ethics, and maintain finances. Massage therapy is also subject to various licensing rules and regulations, which must be understood and attended to.

There are two avenues in the massage profession for career development: self-employment or employment by another person or business. If you plan to be self-employed, you must be knowledgeable about every aspect of the business end of the professional practice. It is not good enough to be excellent at giving a massage. You also have to be a savvy businessperson.

It is easier to be an employee, because many of the business office responsibilities are taken care of by others, such as an office manager, receptionist, or accountant. More energy can be directed to being an excellent massage therapist. Being employed as a massage therapist is the increasing trend for career development. Because many of the management and marketing responsibilities are taken care of by the employer, it is important to support the organization by being a great employee.

What Employers Want

Employers have basic expectations of their employees (Box 1-1). They want an employee who is well trained, with a good appearance that fits the professional environment. A massage therapist must be dependable and have the skills to do the job for which he or she was hired.

Employers seek three types of skill strengths. Job skills are those used to perform a job: being able to give a beneficial massage based on outcomes. Self-management skills are usually a part of your personality and include honesty, dependability, sense of humor, tolerance, and flexibility. Transferable skills are those that can be taken from one job to another or used on any job. Examples include the ability to maintain appropriate business records, communicate effectively, and be a team player and a leader (Fig. 1-3).

As more massage therapists are employed by larger systems, such as spas, massage franchises, sports organizations, and health care establishments, it is important for massage professionals to learn communication skills, conflict management skills, and record-keeping skills and to understand the nature and demands of complex business structures, even though they may not be responsible for the actual business operations. It is sometimes difficult to balance the compassionate nature of massage and the one-on-one interaction with clients with the more concrete and less sympathetic business and professional practices, such as collecting fees, making appointments, and enforcing policies. An employee can maintain a separation between the massage interaction and the business interaction. A self-employed person must play both roles.

Whether you are self-employed or an employee, you have to understand the business end of a professional practice. When self-employed, you need do all the tasks or supervise

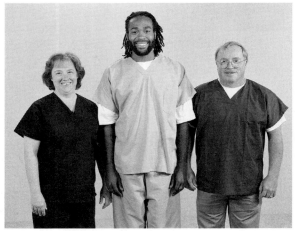

FIGURE 1-3. Professional massage therapists. *(From Fritz S: Mosby's Fundamentals of Therapeutic Massage, ed 4, St. Louis, 2009, Mosby.)*

those you hire to take care of the responsibility. When you are an employee, you can better support those involved in the business operation and have an appreciation of the complexities of their careers and related tasks.

Service Business

The massage professional's role in the therapeutic massage practice of the 21st century is changing and challenging. Massage therapy is immerging as a health profession with a twofold role: to provide health and service and to make a profit as a small business. As a health service, massage therapy provides quality care for the client, following standards of care established by governmental agencies and the profession itself. As a health and service profession, massage therapy embraces the following objectives:

- Supporting wellness, prevention, and healing
- Managing pain with massage therapy
- Supporting function and performance
- Helping clients manage stress
- Providing safe and beneficial massage services

Massage therapy as an evolving business must face the same issues as other health service and business systems, including diversity in the ethnicity, gender, and age of clients and the workforce. The therapeutic massage practice is a business engaged in to achieve a livelihood. To do this, the enterprise must accomplish the following:

- Operate efficiently
- Operate safely
- Make use of technology
- Create a profit

This learning system targets the necessary professional and business skills for a successful career. Business activities are often referred to as the *front office*. A more accurate term is the *business office*, because all business activities of the practice take place there, including financial transactions, client and staff communication, appointment management, and records maintenance.

The traditional education of the massage therapist has placed great emphasis on developing a highly competent clinician but has often left a noticeable void in the area of professional practice management. Massage therapy in the 21st century faces an ever-changing population, a culturally diverse workforce and clientele, heightened awareness of consumer rights, increased state and federal regulations, expanding group practices, and multiple career paths, including massage franchises, the spa industry, sports and fitness organizations, and health care institutions.

Forward-thinking massage practitioners embrace change as a lifelong process. Successful massage practices are led by individuals who look at all situations as opportunities to employ excitement and enthusiasm in meeting new challenges while remembering and respecting our rich history.

THE KEYS OF SERVICE

Massage therapy is a health profession and a personal service profession. Massage treatment may be the objective for a client, but the massage professional must be aware the client also is seeking the most important product—service, an intangible product in the form of care and compassion. Service can be considered a method of accommodating or providing assistance for another person.

Competence, thoughtfulness, dedication to a client's needs, and meticulous attention to detail are key elements of professional service. Top-quality massage skills, ongoing skill development, integrity, compassion, empathy, and commitment to ethical behavior are necessary to provide quality service.

 SELF-REFLECTION

Consider a time when you received great service. It might have been when you were shopping for clothes or at a restaurant. Perhaps it was from the housekeeping staff at a hotel, the attendant at a drive-through car wash, an emergency room nurse, an excellent tour guide, or a plumber who was available for an emergency on the weekend. Assess the experience and behavior of the individual, and identify the key components of service. Perform the same assessment about a time when you received poor service. What made the service poor? Which of the components of quality service were missing? Recall times when you gave excellent service and poor service. What were the factors that made the difference (Box 1-2)?

BOX 1-2	Activities That Promote Service

- Maintaining regularly scheduled business hours
- Providing a flexible schedule for unusual circumstances
- Maintaining the appointment schedule without delays
- Maintaining professional ethics
- Practicing quality care
- Recognizing the client's needs
- Taking time to listen to the client's concerns
- Respecting the client's right to choice
- Informing clients about alternative treatment plans
- Allaying fears and educating about massage therapy
- Hiring qualified and compassionate support staff
- Encouraging an environment of caring
- Maintaining a clean and pleasant environment
- Maintaining professional skills routinely
- Operating safely
- Participating in community services
- Being genuine and honest

MASSAGE THERAPY AS A SERVICE PROFESSION

Message therapists touch with skill, compassion, intention, integrity, and respect with an expected result and are compensated monetarily for the service. Massage is a service profession. The massage therapist develops professional relationships with the client. A relationship involves mutual dealings between people, parties, or countries and the types of expectations that each has of the other. Professional relationships are different from friendship, family, or romantic relationships. Friendships are freely chosen associations with others that are mutually beneficial. Family relationships are based on a parental, sibling, or extended family connections, communication patterns, and cultural roles. Romantic or life partner relationships share passion, commitment, and emotional, physical, and spiritual intimacy. A professional relationship is also based on a mutually beneficial association, but the exchange for service is typically money, not personal connection.

Certain factors contribute to a successful professional relationship. Some of the most important are reliability, listening to understand, honesty, effective conflict management, and providing more than expected.

Reliability is necessary for good customer service. Listening more than talking is a vital professional skill. A massage therapist lets the client talk and indicates listening by making the appropriate responses using reflective listening skills. This topic is discussed in greater detail later. Honesty is a professional skill.

Honesty means correctly stating facts and views, and it includes being honest with others and yourself. Honesty sometimes has the ability to harm, and some things that may be hurtful can remain unsaid because they have no relevance to the professional relationship. If something is

relevant to the professional interaction, it is important to be honest even if the potential for hurt feelings or conflict exists. For example, if a client arrives for the massage in very ugly high heel shoes, it is not necessary to say, "Honestly, those are ugly high heels." If, however, the client has recently sprained an ankle and is unsteady on the shoes because of the high heel, it is important to state something such as, "Based on your recent history of a sprained ankle and because high-heeled shoes cause the ankle and knee to be unstable, it would be best if you did not wear this type of shoe."

Conflict is unpleasant, but it is important to deal with difficult situations and complaints. No one likes hearing complaints, and although it is true that you cannot please all the people all the time, if you are going to develop a strong and loyal massage client base, it is necessary to listen to complaints and deal with difficult situations with an objective and open mind. Interpret complaints in an impersonal way. Find the concrete process. What happened? What was done? What went wrong? What could be different?

Provide more than is expected. People love to get more than they anticipated. The gesture does not need to be large or extravagant to be effective, but it must be sincere. Throw in something extra, such as a coupon for a future discount, additional information on self-help, a genuine smile, or a sincere compliment. Small things that are given freely are appreciated.

Massage is a service profession that has a long and rich history. Originally part of the healing traditions of most cultures, massage has experienced many developments and is now regaining its rightful place in the health care and wellness environments. Professional service is more than clinical and cognitive skills; it comprises attitudinal skills that evolve into a commitment to the welfare of others. "No one cares how much you know until they know how much you care" is a statement that summarizes the service concept.

Retention

Clients will remain with the massage practice only if they are satisfied with the services rendered. Figure 1-4 illustrates the many "ifs" the massage therapist encounters in the retention of a client in the massage practice. Clients have choices. If clients choose someone as their massage therapist from a recommendation or by random selection and if they are satisfied with the treatment and care, they may return. If clients are satisfied with the return visit, they may continue to return. However, if there is dissatisfaction at any stage of the service, clients may choose to go elsewhere for massage therapy services. Massage is a service, and success is based on client satisfaction, client benefit, and long-term professional relationships in the form of client retention and regularly scheduled appointments.

If clients do not return after receiving the first massage, there was some sort of dissatisfaction on their part, and you

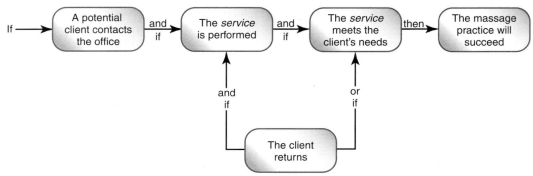

FIGURE 1-4. The service concept. *(Modified from Finkbeiner BL, Finkbeiner CA: Practice Management for the Dental Team, ed 6, St. Louis, 2006, Mosby.)*

need to seriously evaluate how you are responsible. There are factors related to an individual client's expectations that affect retention, but you cannot change someone else—only yourself. It is unlikely that you will be able to build a sustained business if you do not figure out what happened and seek to correct the situation for future clients. For instance, a client came in and told you he wanted a relaxation massage, but you perform a massage that is more rehabilitation focused, or he told you the pressure was too light or too heavy, but you did not adjust. Issues such as these may keep you from retaining clients. There are exceptions. For example, the massage was a gift, and the individual was not a "massage person," or there were extenuating circumstances, such as a massage on a vacation that was meant to be a one-time treat.

Despite a few exceptions, if retention is a problem, it must have something to do with factors such as the massage application; the personality, appearance, smell, or mannerisms of the massage therapist; the fee charged; the location; or the facility. Marketing, advertising, and location are all important for the initial exposure to be able to find the first few clients. However, if a client does not return for massage on a regular basis—even once each year for a "birthday massage"—the problem is about how you are providing massage services. Service professions are built on relationships. People must be comfortable with you. You have to give an expert massage uniquely designed each time to achieve the client's goals. You have to be pleasant, happy, flexible, clean, professional looking, and engaging, and you must eliminate any weird quirks that can make people uncomfortable. The massage may be very good, but behavior, eye contact, voice tone, gender, age, hairstyle, how the environment is decorated, or some smell in the office can put people off. Honest self-evaluation about how others perceive you is absolutely necessary.

Clients and their family members and friends must be comfortable with you. If a spouse does not like the massage therapist, the client will be unable to continue to see the massage therapist without conflict. Sometimes, it is too difficult to make a client comfortable. When this occurs, refer him or her.

The basis for client retention is quality care and clear communication—the ability to understand and be understood. Other factors influence retention, including volume, cost, and the client base. These issues are explored in the following sections.

 SELF-REFLECTION

How am I going to self-evaluate? Who can help me figure out what displeased the client? How am I going to honestly seek to change behaviors that keep clients from getting regular massages from me? How do I maintain a healthy self-concept while evaluating client retention problems? What do others do differently from what I do to retain clients? What would my mentor say? What guidance would the advisory board provide?

VOLUME

You need to know how many massage sessions you can provide and maintain quality. Are you are able to give a very good massage, and can you give five massage sessions per day at least 5 days a week? It is amazing how many of those who have graduated from massage school do not commit to increasing expertise through practice and ongoing education. Your skills must be excellent.

COST

This is a service business even if insurance of some type is paying. The cost-benefit ratio is a huge issue in successful client retention. A massage can cost just so much before people determine that the benefit is not worth the cost. I often ask a student to determine how much she could afford to pay for massage weekly, every other week, or monthly. It is a real eye opener. How much could you afford?

The fee must be balanced by how much the massage therapist needs to make to be able to meet her financial needs. If the cost of the massage is prohibitive, the client will not be able to justify the cost to regularly receive a massage. However, the message therapist must have a sense of financial stability. Each geographic and socioeconomic area has a slightly different cost-benefit ratio. Typically, white-collar workers in urban settings pay more than rural blue-collar workers. In the United States, on the coasts, the fees are higher, and in the middle of the country, the fees are lower.

You should be able to average 20 to 25 massage sessions each week. Based on this projection, how much do you need to feel financially secure? For example, assume the yearly net income desired is $30,000. If self-employed, you need to gross about $60,000 per year to net $30,000. If you work 50 weeks each year (assuming 2 weeks' vacation time), multiply 25 massage sessions/week by 50 weeks and divide the result into $60,000 to determine how much you need to charge per massage In this case, it is 1,250 massage sessions per year, or about $50 per session.

These calculations also apply to the client. If a client wants to see you each week, he or she must budget about $200 per month or $2,400 per year (assuming 48 weeks per year). If the client sees you only twice each month, the cost burden is $1,200 per year, and if once each month, the cost burden is $600 per year.

Several questions must be answered. Are the services provided worth this much to the client? How realistic is it that I will see the same 25 clients every week? How do I keep them coming for massage so that I can meet the cost-benefit structure of the business?

The same type of formula is applicable if you are employed, but the employer must generate at least $60,000 of gross income to pay you $30,000. Because employers usually have to gross more income because of employment taxes and additional expenses, $70,000 is more reasonable.

How much can an employer pay per hour and remain viable? If you desire to become an employer of massage therapists, how much would you pay? Let's do the math. Based on $70,000 of gross income, the cost to the employer for providing all overhead costs, marketing, advertising, payroll, and benefits (e.g., paid vacation, medical insurance) is about 57% of the gross intake. That is about $40,000, leaving $30,000 for you. If the employer has more than one massage therapist working for her or him, some of the overhead can be dispersed, decreasing the needed gross income somewhat. In any case, to have an income of $30,000 per year as a self-employed or employed massage therapist, you must do 25 massage sessions per week and charge approximately $50 per session. With some minor variations, this is a reasonable expectation. Clients in urban areas may be able to bear a fee of more that $50 per session, whereas clients in less affluent areas may need fees set at about $40 per session.

CLIENT BASE

You typically do not have the same 25 clients each week. It is more likely that your schedule (based on the 1-hour massage) looks like this: 5 weekly clients (take really good care of regular clients!); 20 clients who get a massage every other week (i.e., 10 during one week and 10 the next); and 20 clients who come once each month (5 each week). This schedule includes a total of 20 clients per week who are regulars,

the sustaining base of a successful professional practice. This leaves five sessions per week open for referrals, the occasional client, and the first-time client.

These people are your future, and it is important to impress them the first time you see them with your professional behavior and massage expertise. These individuals may become regulars or tell people about the excellent massages they had. If you are excellent and provide a safe and neutral environment, you will eventually fill the remaining five appointments. The base of clients to support a massage practice (self-employed or employee) requires between 75 and 100 solid contacts. That is not very many compared with other service professionals.

Ultimately, all business is service. It does not matter if you are an internationally known entertainer, political figure, hometown dentist, professional athlete, high school teacher, nurse, or food service provider—it is all about service.

SELF-REFLECTION

Retention is influenced by your desire to be a massage therapist. Who do you want to serve? You may make more money working at a high-end spa, but if your heart is with food service workers, there is a disconnect. Maybe you have waited tables, and you know how hard of a job it is. How long do you think you will be satisfied in the spa-based job? How motivated will you be to encourage retention?

If you have a professional dream that includes making more money than the example previously described, what are you going to do about it? You could charge more per massage. This is possible if your services are worth it. Would you pay what you want to charge for a massage? You can expand income by creating an environment in which you can earn income by being an employer. Supplementing income with more passive services such as hydrotherapy (e.g., hot tub, sauna) or through product sales is a possibility.

What is your career dream? What is your ultimate professional goal, and how are you going to achieve it? Is your dream to have a spalike massage profession? If so, do you have the education needed to achieve this? If not, you need a plan to get it. If money is the issue, preplanning and self-education are beginning points. Go to the library, and read some books or magazines on spas. The Internet is a vast information resource.

What will it take to get retention commitment from clients so that your appointment schedule is consistently full? You have to want to do massage to be successful. It is like anything else; you can do well for a while even if you do not like it, but eventually, your clients will be able to tell that you do not want to be there, and you will not have the motivation to persevere. When considering career options, it is important to ask what aspect of a massage career motivates you to achieve success.

LEADERSHIP

Leadership is vital to the success and growth of a massage practice. Leadership is not about being the boss or being a good manager. According to Hastings and Potter in the leadership management textbook *Trust Me*, leadership is not what we do; it is who we are: "Simply put, leadership is influence. Leadership involves influencing others for good, rousing others to action, and inspiring them to become the best they can be, as we work together toward common goals."

A leader worth researching is Randy Pausch (http://download.srv.cs.cmu.edu/~pausch). He had his TV debut after giving his "Last Lecture," which was broadcast on the program *60 Minutes*. He was terminally ill, and his goal was to leave a record of his wisdom and advice for his children. He died of pancreatic cancer on July 18, 2008. He had been a professor at Carnegie Mellon University, and in his lecture, he mentions that he achieved most of his childhood dreams and helped others pursue theirs. He said, "We cannot change the cards we are dealt, just how we play the hand." He lived life to the fullest. In terms of *Winnie-the-Pooh* characters, he was a Tigger personality, not an Eeyore.

SELF-REFLECTION

Think about the persons who have influenced or motivated you to make major decisions. They were leaders because they caused you to take action. How did they influence you? Was it by example? Did they share their experiences of failure and success? Did others talk about them? Did you read their biographies or autobiographies?

Leaders in therapeutic massage practice must be able to motivate themselves and others to pursue excellence and to be forward thinkers by paying attention to the historical past, considering the current moment, and preparing for the future. As massage therapy continues to expand into many environments, such as sports and fitness facilities, chiropractor offices, multidisciplinary health care practices, massage clinic franchises, and the popular spa industry, it will be increasingly important for massage therapists to develop leadership skills to meet the changes in the profession that will inevitably occur.

LEARNING ACTIVITY

For a brainstorming exercise, list all of the changes that may occur in the massage therapy profession within the next 5 years.

_____

_____

_____

Leadership can be defined as doing the right thing, whereas management is defined as doing things right. Participatory leadership is considered to have the greatest advantages for a massage practice. This form of management is a team effort and recognizes each member of the staff as a person whose skills are necessary in obtaining the ultimate goals of the practice. Participatory management requires that all staff members have a part in making decisions. This system provides an opportunity for communication. Each person seeks to understand the others, and staff members are encouraged to express their ideas.

There can be many forms of leadership in the therapeutic massage practice. Self-employed massage therapists with their own small businesses may be responsible for all business functions and for providing massage. Self-employed massage therapists must be their own leaders. In a large, multistaffed, and multidisciplinary practice, such as a freestanding massage clinic franchise, a privately owned spa, or medical office, the massage professional may be accountable to the office manager, who is the leader in the business area. The medical professional (i.e., nurse, physician's assistant, or physician) may be the leader in the clinical practice. Massage therapists may find themselves responding to two leaders—one in the business office and one for massage delivery. In massage clinics, the clinic owner or massage supervisor may be the leader, or you may find yourself becoming the leader in the massage clinic practice.

The leader in a therapeutic massage practice must embrace trust, a willingness to understand change, humility, commitment, focus, compassion, integrity, peacemaking, and endurance (Box 1-3). As a businessperson, the massage leader of the 21st century must strive to achieve practice goals by

- Considering long-term results over short-term results
- Stressing effectiveness over efficiency alone
- Thinking strategically rather than operationally
- Being proactive rather than reactive to situations
- Being driven by plans rather than problems

LEARNING ACTIVITY

Write down what these words or phrases mean to you.
1. Long term _____
2. Short term _____
3. Effectiveness _____
4. Efficiency _____
5. Strategically _____
6. Operationally _____
7. Proactive _____
8. Reactive _____
9. Plans _____
10. Problems _____
11. Solutions _____

BOX 1-3	Elements That Build Effective Leadership

- Trust promotes good relationships and confidence.
- A leader who understands change recognizes that disruptions are inevitable and is willing to shift gears to pave the way for change.
- Humility is a focus on being open, teachable, and flexible.
- Commitment seeks to develop vision and values in a leader and moves leaders to stand for something greater.
- Focus gives leaders the ability to achieve and direct their time and energy to important objectives.
- Compassion is the desire to understand and care for others, such as staff, family, clients, and people in the community.
- Integrity demands that leaders be responsible for seeking to create quality assurance in their service for clients and in all their relationships.
- Leaders who are peacemakers ensure calmness by listening to and learning from others, and they seek sound solutions rather than making quick decisions.
- Endurance refers to courage, perseverance, and strength when situations, people, or the environment become chaotic or difficult.

Even if self-employed, the effective therapeutic massage practitioner cannot think and act independently. Marketing a service such as massage means considering human, financial, and technical resources in a worldwide market. Clients seen in the therapeutic massage practice come from diverse backgrounds and present complex and diverse treatment options. The therapeutic massage practice must also embrace a virtual office concept that serves the local community and the client base. Technology allows for appointment booking and changes, educational services, and networking with other like-minded professionals and businesses. For example, the virtual office may provide links to other forms of bodywork or types of health care, such as acupuncture, Ayurveda, chiropractic, osteopathy, mental health, nutrition, or yoga. This form of research and referral creates a mutually beneficial network that connects many providers, even if they are located in separate locations.

Characteristics of an Effective Leader

Typically, the first contact a client has sets the stage for the rest of the professional interaction. It is difficult to find any job or career today in which communication is not important, and it has been found that 80% of the people who fail in professional practice do so not because of a lack of technical skills, but because they do not relate well with people.

Your attitude can give the client a positive impression or convince the client to seek massage care elsewhere. Whether communicating with clients, staff, or friends, you must develop basic people skills for successful communication. In addition to the elements found in a leader (discussed earlier), the massage therapist must have skills that include

self-confidence, genuineness, enthusiasm, assertiveness, honesty, acceptance or tolerance of others, the ability to be a good listener, and willingness to be a team player.

SELF-CONFIDENCE

Self-confidence is the ability to believe you can do a job well. To have self-confidence, you must accept yourself. You must have a healthy mental picture of yourself and learn to accentuate your positive attributes. Having self-confidence includes identifying your strengths and building on them and accepting your weaknesses, not dwelling on them, and providing necessary strategies to overcome them. This may take the form of using support staff such as a receptionist or assistant to handle activities (e.g., schedule organization and paperwork, facility management, and cleaning services or other professional services, such as bookkeeping and tax preparation). It will take more time and energy to attempt activities that you are not good at (and will likely never be good at) than it will to generate enough income to pay others to help.

A massage professional with self-confidence assumes responsibility, adapts to change, accepts challenges, and is an effective decision maker. For instance, massage professionals who are self-confident research and gather relevant data and then confidently make suggestions for changes and implement new procedures without hesitancy because they know what is going on. They are willing to take risks and are able to recommend changes in a routine or procedure with confidence that the idea is worthwhile and merits consideration.

GENUINENESS

Being genuine means being sincere and straightforward. This is important when dealing with people in a service profession. A genuine, caring person is not afraid to reach out, demonstrate a caring attitude, and display a genuine concern for another person's feelings. Put yourself in the client's place, and show the kind of concern you would like to receive. As a massage professional, you can be genuine and maintain professional boundaries by remembering that in professional practice, the energy flows toward the client (i.e., it is about them, not about you).

Clients feel comfortable with a genuinely caring massage professional and are likely to open up and share their innermost feelings. This sharing is sacred space that belongs to the client, and the massage professional needs to be respectful and compassionate but not intrusive. Being intrusive means that the massage therapist offers suggestions and advice by sharing personal stories and does not listen to the client. Clients may simply need a person to listen, a friendly smile, or a comforting pat on the shoulder.

ACCEPTANCE OF A CULTURALLY DIVERSE POPULATION

Massage professionals must communicate with people who speak English as a second language. It may be necessary to use another dictionary or reference if an interpreter is not available. Electronic dictionaries are available, and such references can aid in communicating with clients to determine basic information for informed consent and assessment procedures.

You will find that each person's values are established from his or her background and previous experience. You must be willing to accept others as worthy human beings without a desire to change them to fit into your value system. Accept them as they are, not for what you think they ought to be. Communication is often difficult when a person acts or appears "different" from what is perceived as the norm. For instance, when a client with a prosthesis replacing his or her right arm visits the office, the prosthesis may attract your attention, and you may even stare at the device. Your focus is on the disability and not on the client. In the therapeutic massage profession, it is important to concentrate on seeing the person, not the disability.

ENTHUSIASM

Being enthusiastic means you are interested in your work, you are expressive, and you leave your problems at home. To be enthusiastic does not mean you are a phony or a constant chatterbox; it means that you have a sincere interest in your work and the world around you. Massage therapists who are enthusiastic about their work are likely to read professional journals, seek knowledge about new technology or specific areas of interest, participate in community activities or professional organizations, and become an involved professional. To be enthusiastic you must act enthusiastic.

An enthusiastic massage therapist takes time to learn about the clients and their interests, and when the clients ask questions, the therapist seeks to find the answers. An enthusiastic person is happy to get to work, enjoys sharing others' experiences, appreciates good humor, and is not totally exhausted at the end of the day. An enthusiastic person has a positive outlook on life.

ASSERTIVENESS

Being assertive does not mean being aggressive. An assertive person is bold and enterprising in a nonhostile manner. To be assertive often requires tact, initiative, and willingness to take a risk. Assertiveness is not an emotional response. It is a very logical process that requires research and planning. If you work in a spa, for example, and want to suggest a change in the services offered, it is important to do your homework first. Before suggesting change, prepare an alternative and justify it. If a client or coworker is not behaving appropriately in the environment (e.g., constantly being late, not attending to hygiene, telling offending jokes), it can be difficult to assertively discuss the matter. These types of issues can feel personal to the massage professional and be taken personally by the client or coworker. Being assertive is a logical process, and the avoidance or confrontation is based on feelings.

RECOGNITION OF OTHERS' NEEDS

All people need some form of recognition. In the professional setting, it means that you should be willing to work cooperatively with others to accomplish the objectives of the practice. Ignoring another person's needs does not facilitate good interpersonal relations.

SENSE OF HUMOR

A therapeutic massage practice can provide opportunity for some unique occurrences. After all, you are working with people's bodies. Look at the situation with a sense of humor, but be careful to laugh at the situation and not at the person. Your clients and colleagues should not be made the brunt of a joke.

Consider adding humor to the office with cartoons on the bulletin board. Humor lessens conflict and eases tension, and it is perhaps the best stress management strategy in any therapeutic massage practice.

WILLINGNESS TO BE A TEAM PLAYER

Massage therapy is increasingly a team-oriented business. There is no "I" in the word *team*. Building a team is a simple concept when you realize that teams are made up of individuals with diverse skills and talents. Each team member must have clearly defined skills that need to be identified and measured against the skills of other team members. After a person realizes his or her role on the team and how best to accomplish specific tasks, achieving team goals can be accomplished and eagerly anticipated.

The anatomy and physiology of the body is a great metaphor for a team. The little toe is confident and contributes to walking. It does not aspire to be a liver but does depend on the liver for a clean environment. The liver does not think it is more important than the kidney; instead, the liver and kidney cooperate. Cells that are not team players and consider only themselves become tumors. They can get out of control and use resources selfishly. None of us wants to be a tumor, which can become malignant, spread, and destroy. Health and homeostasis is a team effort.

Effective Listening

Listening is more than hearing. A good listener hears the facts and perceives the feeling behind the stated facts. Good listening is a combination of hearing what a person says and becoming involved with the person who is talking. Sometimes, hearing loss or a preoccupation with your problems, goals, or feelings can make it difficult for you to hear what is communicated. In a busy therapeutic massage practice, you may ignore what a person is saying because you are too preoccupied with your work, deadlines, or future activities to listen effectively to a client's needs. Often, you hear only what you want to hear or have time to hear. Listening to understand is a very important skill and much more important than talking.

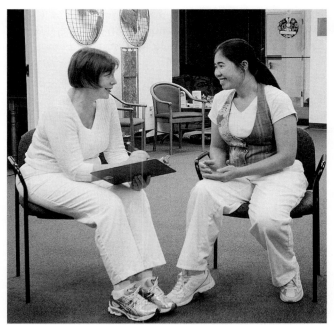

FIGURE 1-5. A massage therapist "listens with her eyes" during an intake interview with a client.

BOX 1-4   Principles of Reflective Listening

- More listening than talking—ears and mind open but mouth shut
- Restating and clarifying what the other has said; not asking questions, interpreting, or telling what the listener feels, believes, or wants
- Trying to understand the feelings contained in what the other is saying, not just the facts or ideas
- Responding with acceptance and empathy, not with indifference, cold objectivity, or fake concern or discounting the importance (i.e., Don't worry; it will work out.)
- Avoid why questions. The question "Why?" can be particularly damaging, because it defies the other to find a justification or logical explanation. Instead ask, "Can you tell me more about it?"
- Respond to feelings, not just to content. Feelings, such as anger, disappointment, discouragement, fear, joy, elation, or surprise emerge in the emotional tone that the speaker expresses. Content refers to ideas, reasons, theories, assumptions, and descriptions. Especially initially in the conversation, people want understanding, not solutions. Carl Rogers observed that a person who receives a response at the emotional level has "the satisfaction of being deeply understood."

From Active Listening (drawn from Communication in Organizations by Dalmar Fisher), http://www.analytictech.com/mb119/reflect:htm *and* http://www.archindy.org/family/files/marriage/reflective%20listening.pdf

Sometimes, you forget pay attention with your eyes. You need to see what the person is saying; you need to look at the speaker when he or she is talking (Fig. 1-5). When you observe a person's body language, you observe facial expressions, gestures, and posture that can give you clues to that person's feelings. Consequently, you understand what people are saying by observing the emotions they display.

In reflective listening, the listener absorbs what has been said, reflects on it, and restates or paraphrases the feeling or content of the message in a way that demonstrates understanding and acceptance. Often in Western culture, listening is considered to be the passive part of a conversation, and speaking is seen as active. Reflective listening practices require focus, intent, and very active participation. The term *reflective listening* stems from work done by psychologist Carl Rogers, who developed client-centered therapy. Rogers believed that by listening intently to the client, a therapist could determine best what the client needed. This type of listening is beneficial because the parties interact to create a better understanding of the situation. A scenario in a therapeutic massage practice might look like this:

Client: I just don't know whether to schedule a massage weekly when finances are so tight.
Massage therapist: You feel as if you benefit by weekly massage but are not sure you can justify the cost. Is that right?
Client: Uh, huh.

The massage therapist has restated the basic statement of the client. The statement was in her own words and was not judgmental. When correctly paraphrased, the speaker usually responds in the affirmative. If not, the paraphrase needs to be restated until the message is received clearly.

At first, using these active listening techniques may seem cumbersome or artificial. After practicing them, you soon will realize the benefits of reflective listening. Good listening skills require that you understand a person before you speak. In reflection, the listener tries to clarify and restate what the other person is saying. This can have a threefold advantage: (1) it can increase the listener's understanding of the other person; (2) it can help the other to clarify his or her thoughts; and (3) it can reassure the other that someone is willing to attend to his or her point of view and wants to help. Such action can result in improved relations with clients and coworkers and may result in fewer conflicts (Box 1-4).

METHODS OF REFLECTIVE LISTENING

When using reflective listening, Carl Rogers and others who have refined the system indicate it contains four components: empathy, acceptance, congruence, and concreteness.

Empathy

The empathic listener tries to get inside the other's thoughts and feelings with the intention of understanding the situation. Phrases such as "I understand" or "I get what you're saying" indicate empathy. Empathy may seem easy, but it is difficult to achieve. It is hard to switch from the view point of "me" to "them." People tend to advise, tell, agree, or disagree from their own point of view.

Acceptance

Acceptance means having respect for a person just as they are. Acceptance should be as unconditional as possible. The listener does not agree or disagree (even silently). Just listen. This is hard. People naturally want to make sense of something based on their own experiences.

Congruence

Congruence refers to openness, frankness, and genuineness on the part of the listener. The listener is willing to acknowledge when his or her ability to listen is being altered by his or her own issues. For example, if angry or irritated, the congruent person admits to having this feeling rather than pretending not to have it. In some cases, the principle of congruence can be at odds with the principles of empathy and acceptance. For example, if the listener is annoyed with the other person, he or she probably has to suspend empathy and acceptance until things are sorted out.

Concreteness

Concreteness means focusing on specifics rather than vague generalities. The listener can encourage concreteness by asking the speaker to be more specific.

Although the ability to be empathic, accepting, congruent, and concrete is valuable, the listener must be prepared to deviate from the four principles if that is what the other person wants. For example, if the other person asks for an opinion, the listener should give it but make sure that it is acknowledged (i.e., "This is just my opinion.").

LEARNING ACTIVITY

This quiz is intended to build your skill in applying the concepts previously discussed.

A fellow massage therapist says, "Why do you get more clients than I do?" Which of the possible responses listed represent reflective listening, and which do not?

- I'll talk to your clients for you to see what they like and don't like.
- It sounds as if this is really getting you down.
- You sound as if you think I am doing something wrong.
- It's difficult getting those first clients.
- Have you discussed it with the receptionist?
- Do you feel you are struggling to understand people?
- If you are doing a good job, the client will rebook.
- You sound interested in discussing how to build your practice.

INEFFECTIVE LISTENING

Just as some things make communication effective, there are common things we do that make communication more difficult:

- *Stereotyped reactions*: Constantly repeating a phrase such as "you feel that …" or "you're saying that …"
- *Pretending understanding*: If you get lost, say, "Sorry, I didn't get that. What are you saying?"
- *Discounting*: Missing the feelings or making responses that understate them
- *Long-windedness*: Giving very long or complex responses that emphasize the listener's massive effort to understand more than they clarify the other person's point of view. Short, simple responses are more effective.
- *Not paying attention to nonverbal cues.* Facing or leaning away from the other, not maintaining eye contact, looking tense, sighing, looking at your watch, or presenting a "closed" posture by crossing the arms
- *Problem solving*: Telling people what to do instead of listening, making suggestions about how you solved a similar situation
- *Planning your response*: If you want to get 100% of what a speaker is saying to you, you cannot give him or her 25% or 50% of your attention. It means not letting your mind wander to irrelevant topics and not letting your attention wander to your own (relevant) thoughts while the speaker is talking.
- *Defending yourself*: A related problem is allowing yourself to become defensive in the face of comments that can be interpreted as antagonistic. Defensiveness, even when it is justified by a speaker's attack, is a major barrier to understanding. It is a natural reaction.
- *Interrupting*: Interrupting the person is counterproductive. Even if the person seems to be rambling on, it may be his or her way of sorting information. Listen first; take a moment, and then respond.
- *Telling your story*: A common misuse of reflective listening, especially of empathy statements, is trying to "top" the speaker's story by relating it to one of your own. "I know just how you feel. I had the same thing happen to me." Then the "listener" goes off on a tangent, talking about him or herself. Clients do not like this. They will be polite, but remember that the session is about them, not you. Limit discussion about yourself to professional topics that relate to the client. Do not discuss your personal life.

Several phrases can be used when effectively listening (Box 1-5):

- I understand the problem as …
- I'm sensing …
- I wonder if …
- I get the impression that …
- Correct me if I'm wrong, but …
- From your point of view …

- In your experience …
- As you see it …
- You believe …
- I'm picking up that you …
- Where you're coming from …
- You mean …
- You feel …
- What I hear you saying is …
- Let me see if I understand. You …

Other phrases can be used when you have difficulty understanding:

- I'm not sure if I'm with you, but I …
- This is what I think I hear you saying …
- I somehow sense that you feel …
- Maybe you feel …
- Maybe this is a long shot, but …
- I'm not certain I understand; you're feeling …
- As I hear it, you …
- Is that what you mean?
- Let me see if I understand you; you …
- Is that the way it is?
- Is that the way you feel?
- Let me see if I'm with you; you …

SELF-REFLECTION

What are my conversational downfalls? Do I interrupt? Do I speak too loudly or too softly? Am I hard to understand? Am I bossy or overbearing? Do I come across as a know-it-all? When I am honest with myself, what do I do that annoys others? What do others do to annoys me? Do I nitpick, tease, gossip, criticize, complain, and whine?

What are my conversational strengths? Am I really a good listener? Do I listen more than I talk? Do I really listen or just pretend to? How do I let others know that I really do understand? How do I support a team effort? Do I laugh good-heartedly? How to I recognize when someone else needs my support? Do I provide effective feedback and suggestions that are logical and valid? How do I do that? How do I express my opinions and feelings?

SCOPE OF PRACTICE AND PROFESSIONAL RESPECT

The scope of practice defines the knowledge base and practice parameters of a profession. Each health and service profession has a unique information or knowledge base, but members of many professions share common knowledge and methodology. Because of this shared information, the lines defining a profession's scope of practice are not always clear, and overlap can occur.

Each member of a particular profession acquires a specific knowledge base and must define her personal scope of practice. A professional must be able to evaluate her acquired body of knowledge and skills realistically to determine the parameters of ethical practice within the scope of practice. True professionals understand the limits of their technical skills and scopes of practice and choose to work with other professionals for the best possible outcome for the client.

Much of the literature defines the scope of practice of massage by what cannot be done to avoid infringing on the scope of practice of other health and service professions (Box 1-6). The scope of practice authorized by a medical or surgical degree is broad and extensive. It authorizes the physician to use drugs and medical preparations and the surgeon to sever and penetrate human tissue during treatment. It further authorizes them to use other methods to treat disease, injuries, deformities, and other physical and mental conditions. The law grants such a broad authorization to physicians because the education and testing requirements for a physician's license ensure that the individual is qualified to act as a healer.

No one but the physician has the legal right to perform any act that falls within the parameters of a medical license. The principle underlying this is simple: a person may not dispense therapeutic or medicinal advice about the effect of his or her services on a specific disease, ailment, or condition unless that person has adequate training, knowledge, and experience to ensure that the advice given is sound and reliable.

All the professionals listed in Box 1-6 must meet educational standards that far exceed the current accepted requirements for massage in most areas. Professionals with more education are allowed to do more within their specialized fields. Those with less education work under supervision or within a limited scope of practice. The scope of practice for therapeutic massage should complement but not infringe on the boundaries of the work of these professionals. It is hoped that more flexibility and overlap of professional practice will be allowed in the future for the benefit of clients. The trend

BOX 1-6	Occupational Definitions and Scope of Practice

The following are typical regulations governing scope of practice. Most of these regulations have been taken from the administrative rules of the Michigan Department of Licensing and Regulation and the Occupational Regulations section of the Michigan Public Health Code. The information on acupuncture and Asian medicine is based on Florida legislation and the book *Planning Your Career in Alternative Medicine,* by Dianne J. B. Lyons. Each state has slightly different regulations, but they are consistent enough to provide a sense of uniformity across the United States. More specific information on occupational regulations and health codes can be obtained from the department responsible for licensing and regulation in each state.

ACUPUNCTURE

Acupuncture is a form of primary health care based on traditional Chinese medical concepts. Acupuncture is employed in diagnosis and treatment, as are adjunctive therapies and diagnostic techniques, to promote, maintain, and restore health and prevent disease. Acupuncture includes the insertion of acupuncture needles and the application of moxibustion (medicinal herbs burned on or near the skin) to specific areas of the human body.

ATHLETIC TRAINING

Athletic training is the study of athletic performance, injury prevention, and rehabilitation. It includes training regimens; evaluation and assessment of injury; treatment, rehabilitation, and reconditioning of athlete injury; therapeutic exercise; and use of therapeutic modalities.

CHIROPRACTIC

Chiropractic is the discipline within the healing arts that deals with the nervous system, its relationship to the spinal column, and its interrelationship with the other body systems. Chiropractic uses radiography to detect spinal subluxation and misalignment and adjusts related bones and tissues to establish neural integrity through techniques that use the inherent recuperative powers of the body to restore and maintain health. Examples of these techniques include the use of analytic instruments, the provision of nutritional advice, and the prescription of rehabilitative exercise. Chiropractic does not include the performance of incisive surgical procedures or any invasive procedure that requires instrumentation or the dispensing or prescription of drugs or medicine.

COSMETOLOGY

Cosmetology is a service provided to enhance the health, condition, and appearance of the skin, hair, and nails through the use of external preparations designed to cleanse and beautify. It includes the application of beautification processes, such as makeup and skin grooming.

DENTISTRY

Dentistry is the discipline of diagnosis, treatment, prescription, and surgery for disease, pain, deformity, deficiency, or injury of human teeth, alveolar processes, gums, jaws, and dependent tissues. Dentistry is also concerned with preventative care and the maintenance of good oral health.

ESTHETICS

An esthetician is one who works to clean and beautify the skin.

MEDICINE

Medicine is the diagnosis, treatment, prevention, cure, or relief of human disease, ailment, defect, complaint, or other physical or mental condition by attendance, advice, device, diagnostic test, or other means.

NATUROPATHY

Naturopathy is the combination of clinical nutrition, herbology, homeopathy, acupuncture, manipulation, hydrotherapy, massage, exercise, and psychologic methods, including hypnotherapy and biofeedback, to maintain health. Naturopathic physicians use radiography, ultrasound, and other forms of diagnostic testing but do not perform major surgery or prescribe synthetic drugs.

NURSING

Nursing is the systematic application of substantial specialized knowledge and skill derived from the biologic, physical, and behavioral sciences to the care, treatment, counsel, and health education of individuals who are experiencing changes in the normal health process or who require assistance in the maintenance of health and the prevention or management of illness, injury, and disability.

OSTEOPATHIC MEDICINE

Osteopathic medicine is an independent school of medicine and surgery using full methods of diagnosis and treatment in physical and mental health and disease, including the prescription and administration of drugs and vitamins, operative surgery, obstetrics, and radiologic and electromagnetic diagnostics. Osteopathy emphasizes the interrelationship of the musculoskeletal system with other body systems.

PHYSICAL THERAPY

Physical therapy is the evaluation or treatment of an individual by the use of effective physical measures, therapeutic exercise, and rehabilitative procedures, with or without devices, to prevent, correct, or alleviate a physical or mental disability. It includes treatment planning, performance of tests and measurements, interpretation of referrals, instruction, consultative services, and supervision of personnel. Physical measures include massage, mobilization, and the application of heat, cold, air, light, water, electricity, and sound.

BOX 1-6	Occupational Definitions and Scope of Practice—cont'd

PODIATRIC MEDICINE

Podiatric medicine is the examination, diagnosis, and treatment of abnormal nails and superficial excrescences (abnormal outgrowths or enlargements) on the human feet, including corns, warts, callosities, bunions, and arch problems. It also includes the medical, surgical, or mechanical treatment and physiotherapy of ailments that affect the condition of the feet. It does not include amputation of the feet or the use or administration of general anesthetics.

PSYCHOLOGY

Psychology is the rendering to individuals, groups, organizations, or the public service involving the application of principles, methods, and procedures of understanding, predicting, and influencing behavior for the purpose of diagnosis, assessment, prevention, amelioration, or treatment of mental or emotional disorders, disabilities, and behavioral adjustment problems. Treatment includes psychotherapy, counseling, behavior modification, hypnosis, biofeedback techniques, psychologic tests, and other verbal or behavioral methods. Psychology does not include the prescription of drugs, performance of surgery, or administration of electroconvulsive therapy.

Modified from Fritz S: *Mosby's Fundamentals of Therapeutic Massage,* ed 4, St. Louis, 2009, Mosby.

toward integrated health care appears to support cooperation in health care delivery.

Unique Practice Parameters for Therapeutic Massage

Therapeutic massage is unique in that it can be used in two distinct professional worlds: wellness and personal services and health care services. Massage professionals are involved in various levels of care and support, each requiring more education and increased levels of competence.

According to Associated Bodywork and Massage Professionals, massage, bodywork, and somatic therapies are defined as the application of various techniques to the muscular structure and soft tissues of the human body:

- *Massage:* The application of soft tissue manipulation techniques to the body, generally intended to reduce stress and fatigue while improving circulation. The many variations of massage account for several different techniques.
- *Bodywork:* Various forms of touch therapies that may use manipulation, movement, or repatterning to affect structural changes to the body
- *Somatic:* Technically, somatic (of the body) work does not unify body and mind because no separation is assumed. Often, this term is used to denote a body-mind or whole-body approach as distinguished from a physiology-only or environmental perspective.

There are more than 200 variations of massage, bodywork, and somatic therapies, and many practitioners use multiple techniques. The application of these techniques may include stroking, kneading, tapping, compression, vibration, rocking, friction, and pressure to the muscular structure or soft tissues of the human body. This may also include nonforceful, passive or active movement and application of techniques intended to affect the energetic systems of the body. The use of oils, lotions, and powders may also be included to reduce friction on the skin (http://www.massagetherapy.com/learnmore/index.php).

The American Massage Therapy Association provides two definitions of massage:

- *Massage therapy:* A profession in which the practitioner applies manual techniques and may apply adjunctive therapies with the intention of positively affecting the health and well-being of the client
- *Massage:* A manual soft tissue manipulation that includes holding, causing movement, or applying pressure to the body

The terms *massage,* *bodywork,* and *somatic therapies* specifically exclude diagnosis, prescription, manipulation or adjustments of the human skeletal structure or any other service, procedure, or therapy that requires a license to practice orthopedics, physical therapy, podiatry, chiropractic, osteopathy, psychotherapy, acupuncture, or any other profession or branch of medicine.

The student of therapeutic massage must be able to define therapeutic massage, identify the types of professional services a massage practitioner legally and ethically can provide, and establish guidelines for conduct in the professional setting. This chapter cannot provide specifics for all of these issues because the massage community itself is unclear in many areas, and professionalism in many ways evolves as a profession evolves. This chapter is intended to encourage the student to develop the level of professionalism essential to the successful practice of therapeutic massage.

There will always be opportunity for the sole-practice massage professional, but the sophistication of professional practice mandates massage therapists to obtain more sophisticated education. The entrepreneurial vision for massage practice will falter if not built on solid business practice and effective interpersonal skills. That is the focus of the next chapter.

Good Stuff from the Government

Some may laugh at the title of this segment in the book, but there are excellent resources available from various government organizations. The most helpful are the Small Business Association and the Internal Revenue Service. At the end of every chapter, this section will provide information from government Web sites and links on how to find out more. Most Government information is in the public domain. It is there for our benefit, and it is freely available. The information in the book may be enough to pique your interest, and there is so much more on the listed sites. A synopsis of the information is provided to give you an idea of the content found at the site. Take advantage of our tax dollars, and explore and use the information, classes, and services provided.

The links to these sites are conveniently available on the Evolve site and are listed by chapter in the textbook. From the Evolve site, you can link directly. Be aware that Web addresses can change, and they may not be active in the future. Search programs can help you find the main pages by using search terms such as *Small Business Association*, *US Gov*, or *Internal Revenue Service*.

e Sign on to the Evolve website at http://evolve. elsevier.com/Fritz/business, set up your account, and explore the resources for this chapter.

The U.S. Small Business Association (SBA) is a great resource (http://www.sba.gov/). Since its founding on July 30, 1953, the SBA has delivered about 20 million loans, loan guarantees, contracts, counseling sessions, and other forms of assistance to small businesses. After you are on the SBA main page, look for the small business planner feature and then explore these topics (which have been edited for those most relevant to massage):

Success tools
Online business planning course
Local SBA resources
Forms
Small Business Training Network
Library
10 Steps to start a business
Business matchmaking online network
Training and counseling resources

STARTUP GUIDE AND MANAGING YOUR BUSINESS

The small business guide is intended to serve as a roadmap for starting a business. It is comprehensive and easy to use. It includes numerous electronic links for additional information. Use this powerful interactive tool with its many supporting resources to help you start a successful business. Topics covered at this site (http://www.sba.gov/smallbusinessplanner/plan/getready/index.html) include the following:

How to start a small business
Types of business organizations
Sole proprietorship
Partnership
Corporation
Business plan outline
Marketing
Financial management
Operations
Concluding statement
To lease or not to lease: things to know
Learn the lingo

SMALL BUSINESS TRAINING NETWORK

The Small Business Training Network (SBTN) is a virtual campus that provides quality and targeted free and online training to meet the information needs of prospective and existing small business owners. The SBTN operates like an electronic umbrella under which many SBA and agency resource training programs are captured, aggregated, sorted by content, and made available in multiple formats (http://www.sba.gov/training/index.html).

FORECASTING GROWTH: STRATEGIC THINKING

Strategic thinking is a process whereby you learn how to make your business vision a reality by developing your abilities in team work, problem solving, and critical thinking. Strategic thinking requires you to envision what you want your ideal outcome to be for your career and then to work backward by focusing on the story of how you will be able to reach your vision. Overall, you can apply strategic thinking skills to any area of your life, but by making a concerted effort to apply them specifically to your career as a massage therapist, you will have a much better chance of bringing your vision to life. And isn't that what you want?

SUMMARY

The massage profession is many things and has many unique features. Most vocational and professional training is targeted to one professional practice arena. For example, if someone trains to be a nurse, employment typically occurs in some sort of health care environment. If an individual is an athletic trainer, the primary focus is on sports and fitness.

This is not so with therapeutic massage. The realm of career possibilities is limited only by the imagination. Massage therapists can work in one environment, such as a spa or chiropractor's office, and can work full time or part time as employees, independent contractors, or partners in the business. They can specialize, such as with the geriatric population or with a specific approach (e.g., myofascial massage). Massage therapy is provided in multiple venues, from very formal office settings to resorts where massage is given on the beach. Massage is found in offices, hospitals, cruise ships, all types of spas, rehabilitation clinics, wellness care, horse stables, veterinary clinics, long-term care facilities, various festivals and events, malls, airports, sport arenas, sports training facilities, and wedding showers. The application of massage is limited only by the imagination.

The SBA is an outstanding resource for information, guidance, and training. Each chapter in this text will direct you to the SBA Web site. The site is a portal into a vast pool of information. Use it to the fullest.

Bibliography

Abrams R: *Wear Clean Underwear: Business Wisdom from Mom*, New York, 1999, Villard.

Fulton-Calkins PJ: *General Office Procedures for Colleges*, ed 12, Cincinnati, 2003, South-Western.

Hastings W, Potter R: *Trust Me*, Colorado Springs, CO, 2004, WaterBrook.

Mosby: *Spanish Terminology for the Dental Team*, St. Louis, 2004, Mosby.

Thill JV, Bovée CL: *Excellence in Business Communication*, ed 5, Upper Saddle River, NJ, 2002, Prentice-Hall.

Evolve Annotated Web Links

http://evolve.elsevier.com/Fritz/business

Massagetherapy.com (http://www.massagetherapy.com/)

National Certification Board for Therapeutic Massage and Bodywork, Survey for massage therapists/bodyworkers who have practiced 5+ years (http://www.ncbtmb.org/survey_results/industry_changes/SurveySummary.html)

American Massage Therapy Association, 2009 Massage Therapy Industry Fact Sheet (http://www.amtamassage.org/news/MTIndustryFactSheet.html#1)

Massagetherapy.com, practitioner characteristics and professional membership patterns (http://www.massagetherapy.com/media/)

U.S. Small Business Administration (SBA) (http://www.sba.gov/)

SBA, about SBA, overview and history (http://www.sba.gov/aboutsba/)

SBA, small business planner, manage your business, forecast (http://www.sba.gov/smallbusinessplanner/)

SBA, online training (http://www.sba.gov/services/training/)

SBA, free online courses (http://www.sba.gov/services/training/)

Workbook

1. List the qualities of a leader that you respect. Assess you own strengths and weaknesses and identify your leadership qualities.

_____

_____

_____

_____

_____

_____

_____

_____

2. Practice paraphrasing the following statements in a reflective listening manner:

Last time I got a massage, I did not get very much attention on my feet.

_____

_____

_____

You know we share a massage room, and it was a mess this morning.

_____

_____

_____

_____

Someone needs to talk to Tina about her breath odor.

_____
_____
_____

The receptionist seems to be playing favorites by booking Roger more than Tasha.

_____
_____
_____

I really like it when you give me a massage. Others just don't understand me like you do.

_____
_____
_____

I love coming here for massage, but it is more expensive than the spa on the next block.

_____
_____
_____

2

BEING A PROFESSIONAL

OUTLINE

KEY TERMS

Administrative skills
Anomaly
Closure
Communication
Conceptual skills
Conflict
Continuation
Cultural diversity
Etiquette
Evaluating
Gestalt

Horizontal communication
Human relations skills
Implementing
Inspiration
Intention
Intuition
Organizing
Planning
Professional etiquette
Proximity
Rapport

Recognition
Remuneration
Respect
Responsibility
Similarity
Standard
Standards of practice
Task
Technical skills
Time management

e Guidelines for the Learning Activities and answers to the Workbook questions are located on Evolve at http://evolve.elsevier.com/Fritz/business.

LEARNING OUTCOMES

Mastery of the content in this chapter will enable the reader to:

- Define glossary terms
- Determine goals and objectives for a massage therapy practice
- Demonstrate professional etiquette
- Identify the five Rs of good management
- Manage interpersonal communications in the professional setting
- Explain employee empowerment
- Discuss procedures for conducting a staff meeting
- Define time management
- Describe how to manage time efficiently

- Explain the purpose of an office procedural manual
- Identify components of an office procedural manual
- Describe recruitment and hiring practices
- Describe the contents of a personnel policy in an office procedural manual
- Explain the use of pre-employment testing
- Describe new employee orientation
- Access and use information available from U.S. government Web sites, such as the Small Business Administration (SBA).

PROFESSIONALISM: INSPIRATION, INTENTION, AND INTUITION

Inspiration, intention, and intuition provide the foundation for a successful massage career. These three intangibles create the motivation and desire to become a professional. They also are the basis of management decision making.

Inspiration

Inspiration can direct you to the right path. The source of this direction takes many forms, but the outcome is the same: motivation. Inspiration typically takes the form of a vision of the totality of an end result.

Gestalt describes a structure, configuration, or pattern of physical, biologic, or psychological phenomena that are integrated to constitute a functional unit, with properties not derived by the sum of its parts. The *whole* of inspiration that is experienced is more structured and cohesive than the separate components. In this context, *gestalt* means a "unified whole." Initially, gestalt referred to theories of visual perception developed by German psychologists in the 1920s. The theories attempted to describe how people tend to organize separate visual elements into groups or unified wholes by applying certain principles. Over the years, the term has taken on a more abstract meaning and is used to indicate a philosophy of the nature of wholeness. For example, a sugar cookie takes on its own existence separate from its components of butter, flour, and sugar. Anatomy and physiology provide an example relevant to massage. Anatomy consists of the various parts of the body, but each human being has a unique physiology, with functional integration of all the parts.

Structure and chaos coexist simultaneously. This concept is important for being successful in business. Moreover, this is how the mind seems to work. The complex behavior of the brain seems to be random and chaotic, but it does have

order. Freeman (1991) thinks this is the very property that makes perception possible. He speculates, "Chaos underlies the ability of the brain to respond flexibly to the outside world and to generate novel activity patterns, including those that are experienced as fresh ideas." As you consider your unique abilities and professional goals, your ability to generate fresh ideas comes into play as you seek to market your massage business.

Actions often result from inspiration. Where, who, or what does inspiration come from? Because inspiration is related to perceptual processes in the brain, it is useful to better understand how we perceive and process information. Perceptual elements include the following:

Similarity: When objects look similar to one another, people can perceive them as a group or pattern. In Figure 2-1, the example, 10 distinct objects appear as a single unit because all of the shapes have similarity. Unity exists because the triangular shapes at the bottom of the eagle symbol look similar to the shapes that form the sunburst pattern.

Anomaly: When similarity occurs, an object may be emphasized or considered anomalous if it is dissimilar to the others (Fig. 2-2).

Continuation: Continuation occurs when the eye is compelled to move through one object and continue to another object. Continuation occurs because the viewer's eye naturally follows a line or curve (Fig. 2-2).

Closure: Closure occurs when an object is incomplete or a space is not completely enclosed. If enough of the shape is indicated, people perceive the whole by filling in the missing information (Fig. 2-3).

Proximity: When objects are placed a distance apart without pattern, they are perceived as separate (Fig. 2-4). When elements are placed close together, they tend to be perceived as a group (Fig. 2-5).

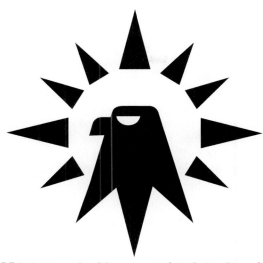

FIGURE 2-1. Example of the concept of similarity. *(From http://graphicdesign.spokanefalls.edu/tutorials/process/gestaltprinciples/gestaltprinc.htm)*

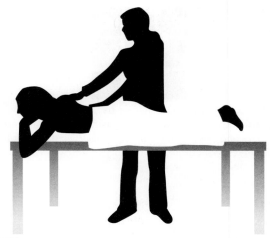

FIGURE 2-3. Example of the concept of closure. Although the client on the massage table is not complete, enough is present for the eye to complete the shape. When the viewer's perception completes a shape, closure occurs. *(Courtesy Clipart.com [28610/ KJ Pargeter])*

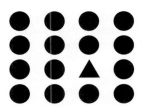

FIGURE 2-2. Example of the concept of anomaly. The triangle becomes a focal point because it is dissimilar to the other shapes—anomaly. *(Courtesy of John Smith, Graphic Design, Spokane Falls.)*

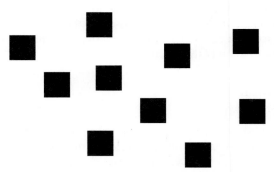

FIGURE 2-4. Example of the concept of proximity. The 10 squares are placed without proximity, and they are perceived as separate shapes. *(From http://graphicdesign.spokanefalls.edu/tutorials/process/gestaltprinciples/gestaltprinc.htm)*

Inspiration occurs when a certain combination of ideas suddenly reveals a simple underlying pattern. When this occurs, you typically have an intellectual, emotional, and physical response that often results in clarity and in motivation to bring ideas into tangible form. People seem to be wired to see a pattern and make sense of it.

Inspiration is difficult to explain but easy to recognize because it enlivens us and creates passion and energy. Inspiration is the big picture, and in its simplicity, the complicated becomes uncomplicated. It is like a cookie. The cookie is the whole, and the flour, sugar, eggs, butter, and vanilla are the pieces. They do not form a cookie until combined and baked.

Being inspired can be likened to a spiritual experience, including the moment of clear understanding resulting in a deep sense of peace. More than the "aha" moment or gut feeling of intuition, being inspired is the beginning of purpose.

SELF-REFLECTION

At some level, you were inspired to learn to be a massage therapist. How did that process occur? How did all the pieces come together?

For example, you might have watched a family member or a friend rub her neck at the end of a long day. Perhaps you noticed the security of a puppy being licked and groomed by its mother. Someone might have rubbed your shoulders after you carried boxes for him. You begin to recognize that touching is everywhere. It relieves pain, creates comfort, and provides connection, and these effects are important.

You realize that this is something you can do to make life better. In thinking about how to achieve this goal, you have an inspiration—you can be a massage therapist.

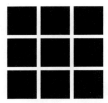

FIGURE 2-5. When the nine squares are set with proximity, unity occurs. Although they continue to be separate shapes, they are perceived as one group. *(From http://graphicdesign.spokanefalls.edu/ tutorials/process/gestaltprinciples/gestaltprinc.htm)*

Intention

Intention is knowing what you want and knowing comes from inspiration. For example, if you are looking for a red ribbon, you will eventually find it because you are focused on it. We have all experienced a moment when we find what we are looking for, but we have to know what it is we seek. If you have been inspired to be a massage therapist, you will seek skills and knowledge and will find a teacher and a school. The same process occurs when building a massage clientele. If you are inspired to work for a specific group, such as the military, first responders, or the elderly, you will seek what you need to build the practice.

Intuition

Intuition is the conscious awareness of the collected and integrated subconscious information that is processed through the environment, experience, and circumstances. We have all experienced an intuitive thought to give someone a call, and when we do, the person says, "I was hoping you would call." Intuition, sometimes called gut instinct, is an important guide, and the intuitive process is more concrete than it appears. Although science does not totally understand the phenomenon, there is little doubt that intuition is an aspect of survival mechanisms. With development, intuition can become a valuable source of information for important personal and professional decision making.

You may experience intuition as a feeling, a gut reaction, images that reoccur, a dream, or an internal voice with a message. You need to figure out how your inner self communicates with your conscious self. You can get in touch with your intuition in several ways:

1. Ask the question: What is the next step I need to take to expand my massage skills? At some level of consciousness, you already know what you need to do. Trust yourself. Gather factual information about the area you are exploring, and then let the process happen. Intuition cannot be forced; you need to be patient. You can do several things to build a factual database, including reading, asking people questions, and talking to experts.

2. Be quiet, and perform repetitive mundane tasks, such as weeding the garden, folding massage linens, meditating, knitting, doing dishes, soaking in a tub, or going for a walk. Let the thoughts flow.

3. Be aware of the thoughts and dreams that come to you. For example, how did you decide on which massage training program to attend? Did you research the various schools? What criteria influenced your choice—cost, location, schedule, reputation? How did the final decision moment feel? Was it solid or iffy? As you develop your massage career, the same process may occur in deciding on what location to rent or which position to take.

As you learn to recognize and trust inspiration, intention, and intuition you will achieve a level of confidence with professional decision making. Although these concepts appear abstract, they are not. We all have these abilities that evolved from basic survival mechanisms. To survive, we need to have an instinct about what is safe, what path to take, and who to build relationships with for mutual benefit. The gut instinct, new idea, and aha moment are manifestations of the gestalt whole of knowing. All it takes is a little practice, increased awareness, and observation of the results. These internal mechanisms of self-awareness become powerful tools for professional development.

PROFESSIONALISM AND THERAPEUTIC MASSAGE

The subjects of ethics and professionalism are important for the therapeutic massage profession. In any professional practice, the ambiguity of ethics and the concreteness of professionalism and standards of practice converge to form the basis for ethical decision making. A profession is different from a job, and a professional does more than go to work. A professional has the following:

- A specialized body of knowledge
- Extensive training
- An orientation toward service
- A commonly accepted code of ethics
- Legal recognition through certification or licensure by a professional association
- A professional association

Elements of Professionalism
SPECIALIZED BODY OF KNOWLEDGE
Massage therapy methods are grounded in a specialized body of knowledge (some of this knowledge base is presented in this textbook). Historical foundations and current research validate this body of knowledge.

EXTENSIVE TRAINING

Questions have arisen about the duration of massage training and the information and technical skills to be included in the training. The area of professional development for therapeutic massage requires elements of some standardization to allow continued progress toward professionalism. No agreement has been reached on the difference between a wellness orientation to massage and a medical or rehabilitative orientation. Three distinct career tracts for massage are emerging: spa; sport and fitness; and medical, clinical, and rehabilitative paths.

The evolving spa environment encompasses a range of massage services for wellness- and pleasure-based massage that overlaps with sports and fitness. Massage is directly related to health care in the so-called medical spa.

The sport and fitness career tract encompasses a range from wellness to medical intervention that is typically based on issues related to the environment (i.e., exercise and sport performance). The importance of exercise in the management of most lifestyle-related diseases (e.g., diabetes, weight management, cardiovascular care, mental health) is well documented. Massage can support physical changes related to exercise and manage the discomfort related to physical activity and injury for those beginning an exercise program and the extensive performance demands of entertainers and professional athletes.

The medical, clinical, and rehabilitative career paths have a common thread of integration with health care systems, which include stress management and prevention, chronic disease and pain management, acute care palliation before and after surgery, prenatal care, elder care, and hospice care.

The current standard for massage therapy education of 500 to 750 contact hours (i.e., 15 to 20 credit hours) appears to be sufficient for entry-level massage practice. Although 350-hour programs exist, the trend is toward a higher amount. Judging from data collected from actual job duties and current trends in licensing requirements, 1000 contact hours (i.e., 30 to 40 credit hours) probably is more appropriate for supporting professional development in the future. It does not seem reasonable to expect that programs of 500 to 1000 contact hours provide sufficient time for integration of clinical reasoning methods, extensive physical assessment procedures, and the study of pathophysiology, pharmacology, psychology, and other information. These topics must be integrated into the programs so the massage professional can work effectively with other health care professionals and with complicated, multifaceted health concerns. The same can be said for sports massage or working with athletes. To work effectively with athletes, the professional must have an in-depth education in the dynamics of sports activity, the injury process, and rehabilitation.

Trends in employment education focus on the development of two professional tracks in therapeutic massage: (1) vocationally trained wellness massage service professionals and paraprofessionals in the health care area and (2) degree-holding professionals in the allied health care system.

The model for service professionals (e.g., those in the field of cosmetology) and paraprofessionals (e.g., those trained to assist a professional) in health care and in sports and fitness calls for 300 to 1800 contact hours (i.e., 7 to 40 credit hours) of vocational training in technically based programs, after which the student is granted a certificate or diploma. There is wide variation in training standards.

A professional usually is considered to be one who has a degree; it may be an associate's degree (usually requiring 64 credits), a bachelor's degree (usually requiring 124 credits), or a master's or doctoral degrees, such as those held by teachers, physicians, athletic trainers, and mental health professionals.

Most educational models for therapeutic massage in the United States fall into realm of the vocational services professional or paraprofessional. However, more massage programs have begun offering programs leading to an associate's or higher degree. Some Canadian provinces, Australia, England, New Zealand, Poland, Russia, and other countries require or offer training that meets the current definition of a professional degree. Individuals who already have professional degrees are obtaining massage therapy training and combining the two skills to function effectively in the health and athletic worlds. Examples of these combinations are nurse plus massage therapist, athletic trainer plus massage therapist, respiratory therapist plus massage therapist, physical therapy assistant plus massage therapist, occupational therapist plus massage therapist, and social worker or psychologist plus massage therapist. Career options are increasing in the areas of medical and specialty massage (e.g., sports massage).

ORIENTATION TOWARD SERVICE

For this discussion, *service* is best defined as meeting a need. Although reimbursement is expected for services rendered, the desire to meet a need takes precedence over financial return in a service orientation. Observation of those who practice massage professionally and of the attitudes of students indicates that providers of therapeutic massage definitely have an orientation toward service, sometimes to the detriment of sound business practices. Although it is important to care for the people we serve, it is just as important to generate the necessary and appropriate income base to support the professional practice and a reasonably comfortable lifestyle for the professional.

ACCEPTED CODE OF ETHICS, CERTIFICATION, AND PROFESSIONAL ASSOCIATIONS

Although general agreement exists about what a code of ethics for massage therapy entails, no agreement has been reached on a specific code of ethics to serve the entire massage profession. Legal recognition through certification and licensure by a professional association are important parts of the ethical development of the profession.

About two thirds of the United States and one half of the Canadian provinces have formal licensing or legislated certification for massage professionals. Legal recognition in various other countries ranges from extensive licensing requirements to no legal control. The trend is for licensure. It is just a matter of time before there are regulations in all 50 states in the United States and in other countries.

Several organizations attempt to represent the therapeutic massage profession, and each of the various bodywork methods (e.g., reflexology, shiatsu, polarity) has its own professional organization. Although diversity is good for a profession and supports professional development, the lack of coherence in the field of therapeutic massage confuses the public, the massage therapists, and other professionals.

SELF-REFLECTION

Does massage therapy meet all the criteria of a profession? If not, what needs to take place? How will the process influence my own professional development? What can I do to help the transition? How would I want the process to evolve?

Therapeutic Massage Standards of Practice

The *standards of practice* for a profession describe what and how well a professional is expected to perform and therefore become the foundation of competency-based education. The massage therapy community does not agree on a unified standard of practice. There is ongoing discussion about this situation but no agreement. When the massage profession as a whole agrees on standards of practice, it will form a dynamic document that can evolve as changes in practice evolve.

A *standard* is a description of a minimum level of performance required to demonstrate achievement of a task. A *task* is a description of what a therapist is expected to accomplish. A standard is stated in observable and measurable terms. It must be precise and clear to the individual who is held accountable for accomplishing it. It must also be clear to the clients and the public, who assess the therapist's ability to accomplish a task as measured by the required standard.

When formally developed, the standards of practice will serve as a tool to determine whether a massage therapist can do the job at an acceptable level. These standards serve as a reference tool for many people and procedures:

- Therapists, to better understand their job requirements
- Educators, to address as objectives in curriculum design
- Regulation in the form of licensing or certification
- Investigation of complaints
- Discipline hearings
- Fitness to practice
- Quality assurance

- Client relations
- Protection of the public by providing objective standards for assessing the quality of treatment

Role of the Massage Therapist

Massage professional roles vary based on job expectations at the spa, wellness clinics, sport and fitness facilities, and various health care settings. Massage therapists can specialize in more than 80 types of massage, called *modalities*. Swedish massage, deep tissue massage, reflexology, acupressure, sports massage, and neuromuscular massage are a few of the many approaches to massage therapy. Most massage therapists specialize in several modalities that require different techniques. The vast number of styles is confusing, and a trend in the profession is beginning to consolidate massage application based on the effects of mechanical force and the physiologic response of the body. In this approach, massage application is based on client outcomes instead of massage methodology.

Massage therapists work by appointment. Before beginning a massage therapy session, therapists conduct an interview with the client to determine the person's medical history and desired results from the massage. This gives therapists a chance to discuss which techniques could be beneficial to the client and which could be harmful. Based on the person's goals, ailments, medical history, and stress- or pain-related problem areas, a massage therapist concludes whether a massage would be harmful, if the client should be referred, and if the session should move forward by implementing necessary adaptation in application based on cautions for massage while concentrating on any areas of particular discomfort to the client.

Most massage therapists, particularly those who are self-employed, supply their own table or chair, sheets, pillows, and body lotions or oils. Most modalities of massage require clients to be covered in a sheet or blanket, and they require clients to be undressed (typically underclothing is left on to cover the groin area) or to wear loose-fitting clothing. The therapist exposes only the body part that he or she is massaging, and the groin area is never exposed. Some types of massage are done without oils or lotions, and they can be performed with the client fully clothed.

Massage therapists work in an array of private and public settings, including private offices, studios, hospitals, nursing homes, fitness centers, sports medicine facilities, airports, and shopping malls. Some massage therapists also travel to clients' homes or offices to provide a massage. It is not uncommon for full-time massage therapists to divide their time among several different settings, depending on the clients and locations scheduled.

Because massage is physically demanding, massage therapists can succumb to injury if efficient body mechanics are not used. Repetitive motion problems and fatigue from standing for extended periods are common. This risk can be limited by the use of good technique, proper spacing between sessions, exercise, and in many cases, by the therapists themselves receiving a massage on a regular basis. With proper training, a massage therapist should be able to work a typical 40-hour work week and provide 25 massage hours. Because the massage application can vary from 10 minutes to 90 minutes, the number of people seen each week can vary. A typical 8-hour day consists of 6 hours of massage.

Employment Opportunities

According to the U.S. Bureau of Labor statistics (http://www.bls.gov/oes/2008/may/oes319011.htm), employment for massage therapists is expected to increase faster than average until 2014 as more people learn about the benefits of massage therapy. In states that regulate massage therapy, therapists who complete formal training programs and pass the required licensing examination are likely to have very good job opportunities. In states that do not require licensing, the most commonly used outcome measure for professional practice is the National Certification Examination.

Massage therapists must develop a rapport with clients to support retention. Because those who seek a massage therapist tend to make regular visits, developing a loyal clientele is an important part of becoming successful. Referrals are an important source of work for massage therapists, and networking therefore can increase the number of job opportunities. Joining a state or local chapter of a professional association can also help build strong contacts and further increase the likelihood of steady work.

Massage is an increasingly popular technique for relaxation and reduction of stress. As workplaces try to distinguish themselves as employee-friendly, providing professional in-office, seated massages for employees is becoming a popular on-the-job benefit.

Increased interest in alternative medicine and holistic healing means increased opportunities for those skilled in massage therapy. Health care providers and medical insurance companies are beginning to recognize massage therapy as a legitimate treatment and preventative measure for several types of injuries and illnesses. The health care industry is using massage therapy more often as a supplement to conventional medical techniques for ailments such as muscle problems, some diseases, and stress-related health problems. Massage therapy's growing acceptance as a medical tool, particularly by the medical provider and insurance industries, will greatly increase employment opportunities.

Older citizens who are in nursing homes or assisted living homes are finding benefits from massage, such as increased energy levels and reduced health problems. Demand for massage therapy should grow among older age groups because they increasingly enjoy longer, more active lives. Persons 55 years old or older are projected to be the most rapidly growing segment of the U.S. population over the next decade. However, demand for massage therapy is greatest among young adults, and they are likely to continue to enjoy the benefits of massage therapy as they age.

Income Potential

It is important to be realistic when anticipating income. You can expect to earn $25,000 to $30,000 per year at full-time, entry-level employment or in the first couple of years of self-employment. Current wage information is provided on the Internet by the Bureau of Labor Statistics, U.S. Department of Labor, Occupational Outlook Handbook, 2008-2009 edition, Massage Therapists (http://www.bls.gov/oco/ocos295.htm).

ESTABLISHING PRACTICE GOALS AND OBJECTIVES

It is time to decide how you want to develop your massage career. You will benefit from putting thought in planning a professional philosophy and establishing specific objectives for the career plan. A lack of goals and objectives results in lack of direction in professional development. As you mature in the massage profession, these goals and objectives will evolve. A common sequence for establishing objectives includes the following steps:

1. *Develop a practice philosophy.* The massage therapist identifies in a broad statement the basic concepts about client focus, business management, and continuing education for the practice. This is sometimes called a mission statement. For example, *massage outreach will be targeted to the military, police, fire fighters, and first responders.*
2. *Develop practice objectives.* Each broad goal is broken into a series of specific objectives for the career plan. These objectives should be specific, positive action statements that indicate the expected results. For example, *the massage practice will be located near Selfridge Air National Guard base.*
3. *Develop business policies.* These are statements of basic policy that will affect the massage therapist, staff, and clients. For example, *payment for massage services will be made at the time of service by cash or credit card.* These statements may be covered by broad headings (e.g., fees) and followed by specific policies.
4. *Develop procedural policies.* Each broad statement can be broken down again into specific objectives and further defined as specific tasks for all of the common office procedures. For example, *to ensure sanitation, all surfaces will be wiped down with disinfectant every day.* This effort should result in a formal procedural manual.
5. *Develop business principles.* These objectives place emphasis on the business activities of the office. The massage therapist outlines in numeric terms the budget process for the practice and procedures for managing business activities. For example, *the gross income will support one massage therapist at $35,000 and one staff member at $25,000.*
6. *Develop practice standards.* It is necessary for the massage therapist to identify quality standards that define a self-performance level and a performance level expected of the

staff. The massage therapist should provide for the staff an explanation of how these standards are to be maintained. For example, *clients who schedule massage every other week will constitute 60% of the massage appointment schedule.*

As you work through the development of objectives for the practice, these objectives become rules by which the office is managed and the basis of policy and procedure statements. If you plan to seek employment, you can evaluate the integrity and stability of the business by reviewing these policies. As the massage practice expands and matures, it will be necessary to review and revise these goals and objectives.

LEARNING ACTIVITY

Using the six steps previously described, develop a sample outline for a policy and procedure statement.

_____

_____

_____

_____

_____

PROFESSIONAL ETIQUETTE

Professional etiquette refers to business manners. *Etiquette* is the proper mode of conduct or procedure within a certain social realm. Being aware of business manners gives you a professional and attractive look. Rules that applied to social graces 25 or 10 years ago may no longer work in our society. Many former rules of etiquette were formal and rigid and often do not apply to the more casual lifestyles of modern society. However, in a professional world, your actions and behavior will be observed by clients, coworkers, and those who have the potential to promote your professional development. Although practicing good etiquette alone will not move you up the business ladder, it can give you a boost. Good manners can lead to promotions over equally qualified persons with less poise; create a self-confident, successful, professional person; help professionals handle their superiors; and lessen awkwardness among people. They are essential to building good relationships.

For a massage therapist who is also an employer, the potential for practice growth and client acceptance depends on the etiquette of the staff and her or his own behavior. Specific applications of etiquette are applied to different types of business activities. A good point to remember is that everyone should be treated with equal courtesy and respect (Box 2-1).

Developing Professional Etiquette

Several points are important to consider in developing professional etiquette.

| **BOX 2-1** | Suggestions for Improving Staff Etiquette |

- Determine the office code of behavior.
- Extend a friendly greeting to coworkers each day.
- Make introductions when individuals are not acquainted.
- Extend friendly greetings to people who enter the office; stand when you greet the person, and introduce yourself.
- Extend a cordial "thank you" or "good-bye" when someone leaves the office for the day.
- Maintain good relations with your peers.
- Learn how to handle your rivals with tact.
- Be a team player.
- Avoid becoming a do-gooder who seeks constant recognition.
- When conflict exists, learn to mend fences.
- Dress and act professionally when representing the office at conferences or seminars.

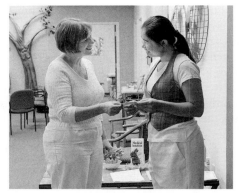

FIGURE 2-6. Greeting, handshake, and introductions.

GREETING

When meeting someone, rise if you are seated, smile, extend your hand, and repeat the other person's name in your greeting. A good handshake is important; it should be firm and held for 3 to 4 seconds. In the business world, it is not necessary to wait for a woman to initiate the handshake. Men and women should be ready to initiate the handshake (Fig. 2-6).

INTRODUCTIONS

Introducing people is one of the most important acts in business life, but few people know how to do it. Introduce a younger person to an older person; introduce a nonofficial person to an official person; and in business, introduce the junior to the senior. Be sure to explain who people are and use their full names. Do not assume that everyone wants to be called by his or her first name; wait until you are told to use a first name.

TELEPHONE

Telephone or cell phone manners are very important (Fig. 2-7). Have a definite purpose for calling someone, because telephone calls are an intrusion into a busy day. Identify yourself, and speak clearly into the phone. Never chew gum, eat, drink, or smoke while using the telephone.

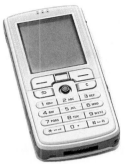

FIGURE 2-7. Cell phone with text and instant messaging. *(2005 ©Gustava Fadel. Image from BigStockPhoto.com.)*

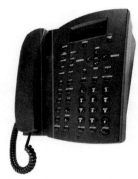

FIGURE 2-8. Telephone with an answering machine and voicemail. *(From Finkbeiner BL, Finkbeiner CA:* Practice Management for the Dental Team, *ed 6, St. Louis, 2006, Mosby.)*

VOICEMAIL AND ANSWERING MACHINES

When leaving a message on voicemail, state your name, organization, and reason for calling; slowly give your telephone number; and then slowly repeat the number (Fig. 2-8). Voicemail is most efficient if you leave a concise but detailed message. Many times, the person receiving the call will be able to get the information you need and leave it in the return call or message to you. Place a concise, professional greeting on your answering machine or voicemail system.

TEXTING AND INSTANT MESSAGING

This area of business communication is evolving, and the manners for business texting are ambiguous. It is convenient to use texting to relay basic data such as appointments, schedules, time changes, and reminders. Some prefer text messaging to a phone call for the exchange of this type of information. Suggestions include keeping the message brief and spelling out all words because many do not understand the abbreviations and do not text during conversations (see Fig. 2-7).

E-MAIL

E-mail can be a quick and effective means of business communication (Fig. 2-9). Always put identifying information in the subject line to help the individual receiving the message know what it is in reference to. The text box of the e-mail message should begin with a salutation such as "Dear Ms. Jones" or "Hello Larry," depending on the relationship. After the salutation, drop down to the next line to begin the message. Use complete sentences and appropriate capitalization and punctuation, as you would use in a business letter. The casual e-mail exchange that occurs with family and friends is not appropriate for business. Do not use all caps

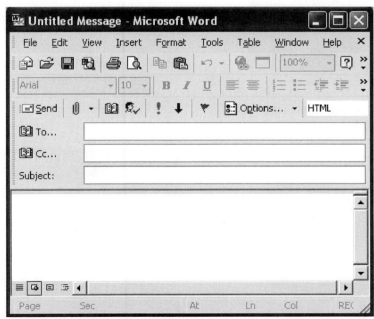

FIGURE 2-9. E-mail. *(Microsoft product screen shot reprinted with permission from Microsoft Corporation.)*

or the symbols for happy faces in the message. Even if you have automatic signature on your e-mail, you should still close the message (e.g., "Thank you, Eli Stone"). Remember to read your message through after you have written it and to run spell check before you click on the send button.

PUNCTUALITY

Be on time. No one wants to be kept waiting (Fig. 2-10). If it is an unavoidable delay, try to contact the person.

SMOKING

Be aware of smoking policies (Fig. 2-11). You should never smoke during an interview, at a meal, or when you are aware that the other person's pleasure does not include tobacco smoke. Nonsmokers can smell smoke on clothing and hair, and it is offensive.

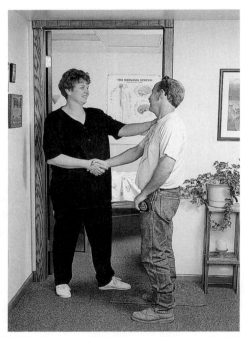

FIGURE 2-10. Example of the concept of punctuality. The client is pleased to be greeted professionally and on time by the massage therapist. *(From Fritz S:* Mosby's Fundamentals of Therapeutic Massage, *ed 4, St. Louis, 2009, Mosby.)*

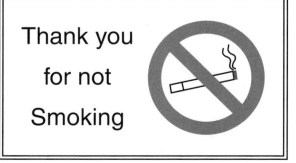

FIGURE 2-11. No smoking sign.

HYGIENE

It is necessary to maintain excellent hygiene, meaning that you must bathe regularly, maintain dental health, and prevent breath or body odor (Fig. 2-12). Do not use perfumes or after shave or other strong-smelling products. Clothing and shoes must be clean, modest, and appropriate to the environment. Always wash hands after using the restroom, and make sure you leave the facilities neat. Clean up after yourself after eating. Do not chew gum. Do not clip nails or perform other personal care activities in the work setting. Do not wear jewelry, including piercings, that can be a safety or sanitation hazard.

APPEARANCE

Professional appearance is necessary, including modest hair, makeup, and jewelry if allowed (Fig. 2-13). If you do not have tattoos, avoid getting any on areas of the body that would be exposed in typical business attire. If you do have visible tattoos, develop a strategy for camouflage during business operations. Avoid wearing jewelry and piercings.

Respect for Diversity

Diversity issues relate to race, gender, age, disabilities, religion, job title, physical appearance, sexual orientation, nationality, multiculturalism, competency, training, experience, and personal habits. Success in life and in business is based on valuing diversity. The U.S. Equal Employment Opportunity Commission (EEOC; http://www.eeoc.gov/) provides information related to diversity issues in the workplace. Box 2-2 lists available publications. Reading through the topics in the box provides an overview of the many aspects of diversity in the business setting.

Cultural diversity encompasses the cultural differences that exist between people, such as language, dress, and traditions, and the way societies organize themselves, their conception of morality and religion, and the way they interact with the environment. Cultural courtesy is becoming very important as the world becomes a global community. You should always be aware of these cultural differences. Be sensitive to others' rules of etiquette. Research the customs and culture of those you interact with.

SELF-REFLECTION

What comes to mind as I read Box 2-2? How comfortable with diversity am I? What has been my experience with a diverse population? How could I expand my understanding of different cultures? Based on the definition of diversity, where do I fit? In one area or more? How does it feel to be categorized? How will diversity increase or interfere with my path to career success?

Remember to say please, thank you, excuse me, nice job, and well done.

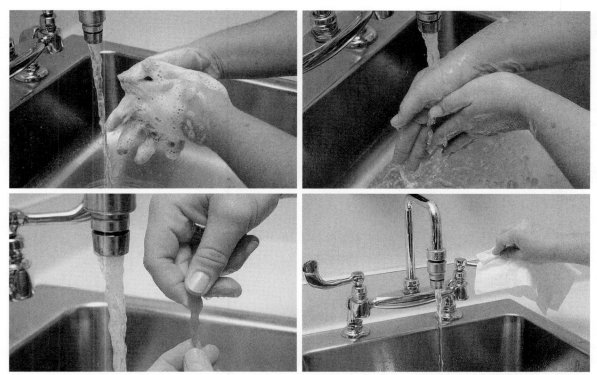

FIGURE 2-12. Examples of hygienic practices. *(Modified from Zakus SM:* Mosby's Clinical Skills for Medical Assistants, *ed 4, St. Louis, 2001, Mosby.)*

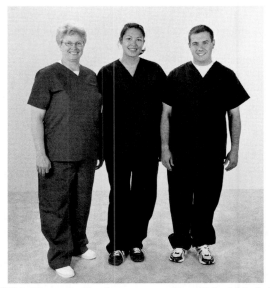

FIGURE 2-13. Professional appearance. *(From Fritz S:* Mosby's Fundamentals of Therapeutic Massage, *ed 4, St. Louis, Mosby, 2009.)*

PROFESSIONAL MANAGEMENT

The term *management* has many definitions. For our purposes, it is the process of getting things accomplished in the business environment though self-discipline and with other people by guiding and motivating efforts toward common objectives.

Some people say that managers are born, not made. However, individuals can nurture their natural skills into sound management skills through experience, effort, and learning. If the skills and discipline required to provide effective business management in the self-employed career path fall into your weakness category, it may be a wise decision to pursue a career as an employee and to target your energy into being a solid team member. You will make mistakes, but you can learn from mistakes as well as successes. If you are choosing to be an employee, your palace of employment needs to be well managed for you to achieve your career goals.

The Five Rs of Management

Successful management can be attributed to five Rs: responsibility, respect, rapport, recognition, and remuneration.

Responsibility denotes duty or obligation. It also denotes follow-through and completion of a project. If you are delegated responsibility, it is important to focus energy to meet the obligations of the responsibility. If you delegate responsibility to another person, make sure he or she has the skills and resources to be able to complete the project.

Respect is consideration or esteem given to another person. Respect is earned. If an individual is not honest, ethical, responsible, and motivated to excellence, he or she is not working on being respected.

BOX 2-2	Publications You May Wish to Order from the U.S. Employment Opportunity Commission

General information on all statutes, in the form of fact sheets and various other documents, are available at http://www.eeoc.gov. Following is a list of the publications you will find available on that site to order:

- Equal Employment is the Law (poster)
  Federal laws prohibiting job discrimination: questions and answers
  Policy statement on mandatory binding arbitration of employment discrimination disputes as a condition of employment
- Employment rights of immigrants under federal antidiscrimination laws
  Equal Employment Opportunity Commission (EEOC) enforcement guidance: vicarious employer liability for unlawful harassment by supervisors
  Questions and answers for small employers on employer liability for harassment by supervisors
  Compliance manual on retaliation (section 8)
  Fact sheet on national origin discrimination
  Fact sheet on age discrimination
  Fact sheet on pregnancy discrimination
- Fact sheets on religious discrimination
  Fact sheet on race or color discrimination
  Get the Facts series on mediation
- Get the Facts series on small business information
  Fact sheet on Americans with Disabilities Act (ADA) discrimination:
  Fact sheet on disability-related tax provisions
  Facts about compensation discrimination
- Age discrimination in the Employment Act
  Fact sheet on age discrimination
- Job advertising and pre-employment inquiries under the Age Discrimination in Employment Act (ADEA)
  ADA: questions and answers
  ADA: your responsibilities as an employer
  ADA: your employment rights as an individual with a disability
- ADA resource list
  Enforcement guidance on pre-employment disability related inquiries and medical examinations
  Compliance manual definition of the term *disability* (section 902)
  Questions and answers: enforcement guidance on disability-related inquiries and medical examinations of employees under the Americans with Disabilities Act
  EEOC enforcement guidance on disability-related inquiries and medical examinations of employees under the ADA
  ADA enforcement guidance: the Americans with Disabilities Act and psychiatric disabilities
  EEOC enforcement guidance on the effect of representations made in applications for benefits on the determination of whether a person is a qualified individual with a disability under the ADA of 1990
  EEOC enforcement guidance: reasonable accommodation and undue hardship under the ADA
  Small employers and reasonable accommodations
  ADA: a primer for small business
  Fact sheet on the ADA
  Fact sheet on disability-related tax provisions
- ADA guide for people with disabilities seeking employment
  EEOC enforcement guidance on workers' compensation and the ADA
  Fact sheet on the Family and Medical Leave Act, Americans with Disabilities Act, and Title VII of the Civil Rights Act of 1964
  Federal Register Part V: 29 CFR Part 1630; EEOC for Individuals with Disabilities; Final Rule 29 CFR Parts 1602 and 1627 Recordkeeping and Reporting Under Title VII of the Civil Rights Act of 1964 and the ADA, Final Rule
- National origin
  Fact sheet on employment discrimination based on religion, ethnicity, or country of origin
  Fact sheet on questions and answers about the workplace rights of Muslims, Arabs, South Asians, and Sikhs under the EEOC laws
  Fact sheet on questions and answers about employer responsibilities concerning the employment of Muslims, Arabs, South Asians, and Sikhs
- Harassment
  Fact sheet on sexual harassment discrimination
  EEOC enforcement guidance: vicarious employer liability for unlawful harassment by supervisors
  Policy guidance on current issues of sexual harassment

Rapport is a mutual trust or emotional relationship with clients, peers, and coworkers. The massage therapist sets the tone for the rapport in professional setting. Good rapport generates the energy that draws and retains clients and supports team members working together to enjoy each other's professional friendship.

Recognition of achievement is important. A person can be recognized for a task well done, for special achievements, and for loyalty. Recognition can come in the form of verbal praise or other forms of acknowledgment, such as personalized notes and rewards. Clients can be recognized for progress made in the management of their stress or for their loyalty as long-term clients. Staff and coworkers can be recognized for a job well done or for going the extra mile for you by helping beyond the scope of their job description.

Remuneration is a monetary recognition of achievement. Most employees say that they are willing to work hard if they are compensated for their efforts. Remuneration should be based on education, merit performance, longevity, and cost of living. Employers who affirm that their employees have worked with them for many years with repeated job satisfaction reviews are those who delegate responsibility; create good rapport in the office; respect, trust, and recognize their employees; and provide compensation similar to other small massage therapy businesses.

If you are the employee, you deserve fair remuneration if you have worked for the employer for many years, received repeated job satisfaction reviews, increased and perfected your massage skills, continually created good rapport in the business, earned respect and trust, have been loyal and willing to go the extra mile, and have been compassionate, understanding, and a team player.

More and more massage therapists are pursuing their careers as part of a team and are employees. Bob Adams, in his book *Streetwise Managing People: Lead Your Staff to Peak Performance*, declares, "Empowered employees attempt to work above and beyond their anticipated capabilities." If you expect to be an empowered employee, you need to act like one:

- Behave as an owner of the job and company.
- Behave in a responsible manner.
- See the consequences of the work done.
- Know how other employees are doing and how they are valued in the practice.
- Strive to be included in determining solutions to problems.
- Seek to have direct input into the way in which the work is done.
- Spend much time smiling.
- Ask others if they need help.

Many concepts that Adams introduces seem to show common sense. When applied to a massage practice, these concepts seem to fit like a glove. Box 2-3 lists concepts that can easily be adapted to any business setting to empower each member of the business to become a meaningful member of the team.

BOX 2-3 Management Skills

DEVELOPING MANAGEMENT SKILLS

- Individuals can nurture their natural skills into sound management skills through experience, effort, and learning.
- Develop human relations skills, which aid in understanding people and interacting with them.
- To be successful, the massage therapist must be able and willing to recognize the value that each employee brings to the office.
- The staff meeting provides an opportunity to define and review the goals for the practice.

CREATING POSITIVE STAFF INTERACTIONS

- Good manners begin with the staff.
- Help others to be right rather than criticizing them for being wrong.
- Whenever possible, have fun.
- Be enthusiastic.
- Seek ways for new ideas to work rather than reasons for why they cannot.
- Be bold and courageous; take chances.
- Help others achieve success.
- Maintain a positive mental attitude.
- Maintain confidentiality.
- Verify information given to you before you repeat what you hear; avoid gossip.
- Speak positively about others whenever the opportunity arises.
- Say "thank you" for kind gestures or a job well done.
- Express a happy attitude in your nonverbal communication.
- If you have nothing positive to say, do not say anything.

Management Planning, Organizing, Implementing, and Evaluating

Management requires several skills:

- *Planning* is identifying what should be done in the future. The goals and objectives discussed earlier are vital to planning.
- *Organizing* is determining how the work will be delegated and scheduled.
- *Implementing* involves putting the plan into action.
- *Evaluating* is a process of investigation to determine if the plan is achieving the intended outcomes. Evaluating occurs after the plan has been implemented for some period to see if it is accomplishing the intended goals.

Basic Skills for Business Success

At this point, you may be wondering what basic skills you need to function in the professional world successfully. You need conceptual skills, human relations skills, administrative skills, and technical skills.

Conceptual skills involve the ability to acquire, analyze, and interpret information in a logical manner. These skills allow you to put an idea or concept into perspective and to perceive how this idea would affect the whole practice.

Human relations skills aid you in understanding people and allow you to interact with them effectively. These skills are vital in a health profession and involve communication, motivation, and an ability to lead.

Administrative skills help you to use all of the other skills effectively in performing administrative functions. They include the ability to establish and follow policies and procedures, to process paperwork in an organized manner, and to coordinate business activities.

Technical skills include the ability to use of all of the knowledge of massage therapy plus business and technology skills that allow you to perform day-to-day operations. It is necessary to be able to use computer software programs. This textbook and Evolve site feature various screen shots of the software program on the CD provided with this text, which was developed by Island Software. The Web site is www.islandsoftwareco.com. There is a fully functioning massage office software program on the CD. Follow the instructions carefully because there is a time limit on how long access is allowed. You will be instructed to activate the CD in another chapter. Until then, visit Island Software's website for more information on the software.

SELF-REFLECTION

What are my strengths—planning, organizing, implementing, evaluating, conceptual skills, human relations skills, administrative skills, technical skills? What are my weak points? What can I do to maximize my strengths? What can I do to get help with the areas where I struggle? How do I find the help I need?

PROFESSIONAL COMMUNICATION

Communication is an essential element in management. It becomes a vital link in establishing a meaningful with other members of the staff and the client.

The definition of communication is to understand and to be understood by another person. In his book *Streetwise Managing People: Lead Your Staff to Peak Performance*, Bob Adams states, "Quality Communication Leads to Positive Interaction." When you are transmitting information to another person, a good relationship supports understanding. To support communication, consider the steps suggested in Box 2-4.

Channels of Communication

The pathway of communication is simple in a one-person massage practice. However, as soon as more than one person

---

BOX 2-4	Concepts to Empower Employees

- Create a communication process that is complete, consistent, and clearly understood by all members of the staff.
- Ensure that all employees understand what is expected of them in their respective job positions.
- Provide each employee with the appropriate training, information, and materials to successfully accomplish their job duties.
- Clearly define and establish evaluation instruments for the responsibilities for each job.
- Create controls that are guidelines that allow flexibility.
- Encourage and practice behaviors that promote encouragement, support, and clear feedback to employees.
- Encourage and promote a sense of responsibility in each employee.
- Encourage and promote continuing education and credentialing.
- Create opportunities for staff members to work together in teams.
- Make it easy for people to praise each other. Make the office an environment that recognizes and acknowledges praiseworthy actions.
- Listen to employees at all times, and make the office systems listen to the employees.
- Trust the employees.

---

is involved, the channels of communication become more complicated.

Communication may be formal or informal. A formal communication channel is dictated by the type of management that exists in the massage practice. Formal communication may be downward, upward, or horizontal.

Downward communication occurs when a massage therapist issues a mandate that is disseminated to the staff members at the next level. The basic channel is shown in Figure 2-14. A more complex system, as shown in Figure 2-15, illustrates an office as it increases in staff size, including several massage therapists and auxiliaries. Downward communication includes instructions, explanations, and communication that can aid the employee in performing work.

Upward channels of communication are vital in a formal setting. Employees should be free to express their attitudes and feelings. This type of communication reverses the flow of information (see Figs. 2-14 and 2-15) and is generally of a reporting nature. It may include suggestions, complaints, or grievances. A lack of upward communication may result in frustrated employees.

Horizontal communication is essential for a larger organization. This type of communication involves transmittal of information from one department to another, and it exists within large offices, clinics, and spas.

Informal channels of communication can also be referred to as the *grapevine*. Frequently, the grapevine carries rumors,

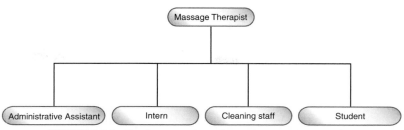

FIGURE 2-14. Employees and employers in a massage practice.

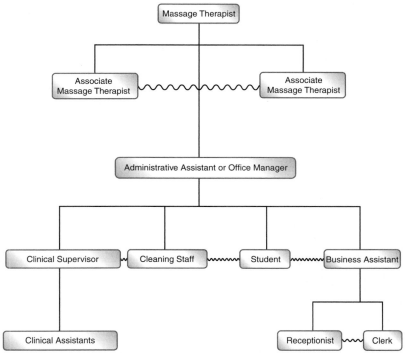

FIGURE 2-15. Employees and employers in a massage practice. Notice that the levels of the massage therapists may vary according to the organization of the practice.

personal interpretations, or distorted information. Fear often produces an active grapevine. If you are part of a group-type practice, do not feed the grapevine; there is nothing more damaging to a business than misinformation, gossip, and rumors (Fig. 2-16).

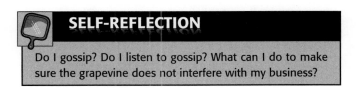
SELF-REFLECTION

Do I gossip? Do I listen to gossip? What can I do to make sure the grapevine does not interfere with my business?

Barriers to Communication

Barriers that exist in client communication are prejudice, poor listening, preoccupation, impatience, and impaired hearing. Additional barriers, such as status or position,

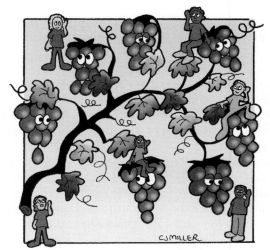

FIGURE 2-16. Do not feed or rely on the grapevine because it damages business. (Modified from Zerwekh J, Claborn JC: Nursing Today: Transition and Trends, ed 5, Philadelphia, 2006, WB Saunders.)

resistance to change and new ideas, or attitudes about work, compound communication difficulties in the professional world. Because these barriers exist, never assume that the message being sent will be received as it was intended. Be aware of potential misinterpretations, and work to overcome barriers to improve channels of communication.

CONFLICT AND CONFLICT RESOLUTION

Conflict is an expressed struggle between at least two interdependent parties who perceive incompatible goals, scarce resources, or interference from the other party in achieving goals. Conflict is common, and it arises from several sources:

- Varied perspectives on a situation
- Different belief systems and values, which have arisen from the involved parties' accumulated life experience and conditioning
- Different objectives and interests

Conflict and conflict resolution play important roles in individual development and social evolution. Many cultures value harmony, compatibility, satisfaction, and independence. Because of these values, there has been a tendency in the past to avoid conflict. Conflict arises when people view the current system as not working. At least one person is sufficiently dissatisfied with the status quo that he or she is willing to speak up in the hope of influencing the situation to arrive at an improved condition. Through conflict, we have opportunities to do things differently in the future.

Conflict exists at two levels. In addition to interpersonal disputes among individuals, some measure of intrapersonal conflict usually exists within us. This inner conflict may be evidenced by confusion, inconsistency, or lack of congruity.

People in conflict share common ground as well as differences. Areas of common ground include overlapping interests, interdependence, and points of agreement. The common ground can serve as the starting point for conflict resolution.

Conflict resolution does not necessarily resolve tensions between people. Conflict resolution may align matters sufficiently to allow each person to make progress toward his or her goals rather than stall in an uncertain and stressful state of disagreement.

Many people think that the best way to resolve conflict is to "do battle," and they believe that the one who "wins" ends the conflict. This approach is more about power and control than conflict resolution. Doing battle and winning or losing supports a corresponding belief that every situation involves a "right" and a "wrong." If we respond to conflict this way, we have limited our awareness and understanding of the nature of conflict and of alternative means of responding to conflict, such as mediation and negotiation. Factors and influences necessary for mediation and negotiation include the following:

- Concern about the impact of the dispute on the relationship
- Time concerns
- Expense
- Impact on others
- Lost opportunities
- Stress
- Lack of closure
- Uncertain compliance
- Areas of existing common ground

Types of Conflict

The decision-making process provides a format for mediated and negotiated types of conflict resolution. Various types of conflict exist, and if we can pinpoint the type of conflict, we are more likely to be able to resolve it.

RELATIONSHIP CONFLICTS

Relationship conflicts, often called personality conflicts, occur as a result of strong negative emotions, misperceptions or stereotypes, poor communication or miscommunication, or repetitive negative behaviors. Relationship problems often lead to an unnecessary escalation in destructive conflict. Conflict resolution supports the safe and balanced expression of the perspectives and emotions of each person involved, leading to acknowledgment and understanding of another person's point of view. Gaining a broader perspective of diversity of culture and individual operational style is very helpful.

Evaluations exist for identifying different personality styles, and using these evaluation tools can help conflict resolution. One of the most researched methods is the Myers-Briggs Type Indicator, which is a psychometric questionnaire designed to measure psychological preferences in how people perceive the world and make decisions. These evaluations help individuals with opposite perspectives to interact well, rather than allowing conflict to develop. The more we personalize another's operational style, the more likely it is that conflict will develop.

DATA CONFLICTS

Data conflicts occur when people lack information necessary to make wise decisions, are misinformed, disagree on which data are relevant, interpret information differently, or have collected data differently. Some data conflicts may be unnecessary because they are caused by poor communication between the people in conflict. Other data conflicts may be incompatibilities associated with data collection, interpretation, or communication. Most data conflicts have data solutions, and after the information has been corrected, the conflict can resolve, unless it has developed into a relationship conflict.

INTEREST CONFLICTS

Interest conflicts are caused by competition over perceived incompatible needs. Conflicts of interest result when one or more people believe that to satisfy their needs, the needs and interests of an opponent must be sacrificed. This often occurs during times of scarcity or when it is perceived that there is not enough to go around. Interest-based conflicts may occur over things such as money, physical resources, or time; over procedural issues, such as the way a dispute is to be resolved; or over psychological issues, such as perceptions of trust and fairness and the desire for participation and respect. For an interest-based dispute to be resolved, those involved need to define and express their individual interests so that all these interests may be addressed jointly. Interest-based conflict is best resolved through maximum integration of the parties' respective interests, positive intentions, and desired experiential outcomes. A third person, such as a mediator, is often necessary to successfully resolve this type of conflict.

VALUE CONFLICTS

Values give meaning to our lives. Values explain what is considered to be just or unjust. Different values need not cause conflict. People can live together in harmony with different value systems. Value disputes arise only when people attempt to force one set of values on others or lay claim to exclusive value systems that do not allow for divergent paths. It is useless to try to change values and systems during relatively short and strategic mediation interventions. However, supporting each participant's expression of his or her values and beliefs for acknowledgment by the other party can be helpful. Belief systems are more amiable to change than values. Values are like the ethical principles described earlier, whereas belief systems are like standards of practice. Belief systems are often superimposed on us during our childhood years. We are taught what is right or wrong, good or bad. Because we learn our belief systems, we can change them through education and a willingness to be open to new possibilities.

Dealing with Conflict

There are five common ways of dealing with conflict. Learning about the alternative means of handling conflict gives us a wider choice of actions to use in any given situation and makes us better able to respond to the situation. Although the following methods are common ways of increasing the chance of success, we use each of these ways of dealing with conflict at least some of the time. We approach conflict in the way we believe will be most helpful to us. Our style for dealing with conflict changes with the circumstances. Conflict-handling behavior is not a static procedure; rather, it is a process that requires flexibility and constant evaluation to be effective.

DENIAL OR WITHDRAWAL

With denial or withdrawal, a person attempts to eliminate conflict by denying that it exists and refusing to acknowledge it. Usually, however, the conflict does not go away; instead, it grows to the point that it becomes unmanageable. When the issue and the timing are not critical and the issue is short-lived and will resolve itself, denial may be a productive way to deal with conflict. The effectiveness of this approach depends on knowing when to use denial.

SUPPRESSION OR SMOOTHING OVER

A person using suppression plays down differences and does not recognize the positive aspects of handling the conflict openly. Instead, the situation is acknowledged (unlike with denial), but it is glossed over. The source of the conflict rarely goes away. However, suppression may be used when preserving a relationship is more important than dealing with a relatively insignificant issue.

POWER OR DOMINANCE

Power is often used to settle differences. Power may be inherent in a person's authority or position. Power may take the form of a majority (as in voting) or a persuasive minority. Power strategies result in winners and losers. The losers do not support a final decision in the same way the winners do. Future meetings of a group may be marred by the conscious or unconscious renewal of the struggle previously "settled" by the use of power. In some instances, especially when other forms of handling conflict are not effective, power strategies may be necessary. Parents often say to children, "Because I said so." This use of power works in the short term, but over time, it results in deeper relationship conflict.

COMPROMISE OR NEGOTIATION

Compromise (i.e., "You give a little, I'll give a little, and we'll meet each other half way.") has some serious drawbacks. Such bargaining often causes both sides to assume initial inflated positions, because they are aware that they are going to have to give up something and want to reduce the loss. The compromise solution may be watered down or weakened to the point that it cannot be effective. There may be little real commitment by any of the parties. However, compromise makes sense in some cases, such as when resources are limited or a speedy decision needs to be made.

INTEGRATION OR COLLABORATION

The integration or collaboration approach suggests that all parties to the conflict recognize the interests and abilities of the others. Each individual's interests, positive intentions, and desired outcomes are thoroughly explored in an effort to solve the problems in a maximizing way. Participants are expected to modify and develop their original views as work progresses. This sounds like the ideal way to manage and resolve conflict; however, for collaboration to be successful, those involved need a nonthreatening and collectively supportive system. This process takes time, openness, and energy.

Conflict Climate: Defensive or Supportive

A defensive climate reflects the type of atmosphere characteristic of competition—an atmosphere that inhibits the mutual trust required for effective conflict management. A supportive climate reflects collaboration—an environment that leads to mutual trust and to an atmosphere conducive to managing differences. Participants in conflict resolution hopefully come to appreciate that the apparent presenting problem does not need to limit their discussions. Participants are encouraged to express the full breadth and depth of their interests, with each participant seeking to identify a value that he or she can bring to the discussion and the maximized satisfaction of underlying interests and intentions.

Conflict is important. If managed well, it identifies and supports effective change. Conflict can foster avoidance, or it can expand our experiences. Making good decisions about managing and resolving conflict can pave the way for greater understanding and well-being.

During the process of resolving a conflict, written documentation should be maintained about the nature of the conflict, the type of resolution attempted, the success of the conflict resolution, and the outcome. Because conflict already exists, interpretation of the requirement for resolution can become confused. Objective documentation that is agreed on by the parties helps maintain clarity. If the conflict cannot be resolved independently, documentation of the nature of the conflict is essential in case the situation escalates to legal action.

Managing Conflict

Although it is common to react defensively and in an irritated manner when confronted with a complaint, it is a poor business strategy. Some people think that a complaint is a reflection on them personally. However, conflicts are common, and learning how to respond can change the distress of conflict into opportunity. Concern should be raised if numerous complaints arise, because this may indicate a serious problem.

Regardless of the nature of the complaint, it is important to review the details of the complaint and seek to resolve the problem quickly. Problem resolution can involve the following steps:

- Make time available as soon as possible to discuss the problem. A delay may result in additional conflict or may be interpreted as disinterest in the problem.
- Listen patiently to all of the issues, and keep an open mind.
- Determine the real issue. Frequently, a complaint is made about a problem, although a deeper concern is the real issue. For example, a person may be complaining about unfair work assignments, but the source of the problem is a personality clash between two staff members.

- Exercise self-control. Avoid arguments or expressions of personality conflicts between the complaining parties. Emotional outbursts do not lead to constructive resolution of the problem. If this results, it is wise to terminate the meeting until a future meeting can be scheduled and the problem can be discussed in a calm manner.
- Avoid a delay in decision making, but do not make rash decisions.
- Maintain a record. Documentation of meetings or discussions is helpful in case a conflict arises in the future about the same problem. It is impossible to recall all of the issues about an incident, and the documented information should be retained for future reference.

It is not easy to resolve conflict. Most of us wish to avoid it. However, conflict may arise whenever two or more people interact. You should try to be fair and objective. This can be difficult when you are one of the parties in the conflict situation. If you follow these suggestions, you will have at least attempted to resolve the complaint in a professional manner and will possibly avoid minor conflicts that can escalate into major crises.

Communicating When Dilemmas Arise

The following steps can be used to resolve ethical dilemmas:

1. Carefully examine the facts, possibilities, logical causes, effects, and your feelings about the situation.
2. Speak with a mentor, peer, or a supervisor about the situation in a peer review or support context.
3. Plan a time to talk about the situation with the other person or people involved.
4. Begin the conversation by identifying the problem as you see it.
5. Use the standard I-message format to provide information and professional disclosure about your inability to work with or be comfortable with the situation. Use reflective listen skills to make sure you understand the viewpoint of all parties concerned.

THE STAFF MEETING

A staff meeting is an effective means of keeping communication channels open. In a staff meeting, all members of a business staff get together to discuss business operations. The staff meeting provides an opportunity to define and review the goals for the practice. Although criticism may be part of a staff meeting, a meeting should not be designed as a gripe session. The time and length of a staff meeting varies according to the needs of the staff. Some offices schedule an hour per week, others close the office for a half or a full day for a retreat session, and still others find luncheon or breakfast meetings effective. Several suggestions for an effective staff meeting follow.

Begin with an agenda, which is a plan for how the meeting will proceed. An agenda is used in planning a staff meeting. Obtain suggestions for items to be placed on the agenda. Determine the priority of the agenda items. Distribute the agenda to the staff before the meeting.

- Notify each staff member of the time and place of the staff meeting.
- Request a return reply for attendance.
- During staff meetings, adhere to the agenda items.
- Review outcomes of the meeting, and provide keyboarded minutes to the staff.
- Maintain a strict meeting schedule.
- Do not allow one person to monopolize the meeting.
- Do not turn the meeting into a gripe session.

All of the business etiquette and communications skills previously discussed come into play in staff meetings.

LEARNING ACTIVITY

Develop a fictitious staff meeting agenda based on the following scenario. You are in charge of conducting a staff meeting to evaluate the past three in-service sessions for six massage therapists working in the sport and fitness center in your community. Because there is a cost for in-service presenters, it is necessary to have management personnel for the center in attendance along with the massage therapist. Efficiency is important. The goal is to find in-service content and presenters who will also benefit the four personal trainers on staff.

PROFESSIONAL TIME MANAGEMENT

A vital aspect of successful business practice is *time management*. There is more to working efficiently than just knowing how to perform a specific task. Understanding the relationship of time to production is also important. All of these concepts together make up time management.

Time management involves planning and scheduling your work and avoiding wasted time. Behaviors that waste time are failing to plan and budget time, giving in to interruptions, failing to follow through and complete a task, slowness in reading and making decisions, performing unnecessary work, and failure to delegate. Other time wasters are lack of privacy and desk clutter. Solutions to many common time wasters are suggested in Box 2-5.

To determine the effectiveness of your own time management, you must assess the way you are working. Determine ways to use your time more effectively, or confirm that you are already using your time efficiently. Evaluation of time management is an ongoing process and can

BOX 2-5	Solutions to Eliminate Time Wasters
TIME WASTER	**SOLUTION**
Lack of goals	Prepare a to-do list, and use it.
Telephone or e-mail interruptions	Use an answering machine or voicemail system during specified work times.
Procrastination	Do it first!
Feeling tired, stressed, or irritable	Schedule a thorough physical examination; develop a wellness plan; enroll in stress-management course; get a massage.
Lack of future plans	Develop short- and long-range plans.
Disorganized work area	Purchase organizers; put away work when finished; do not begin a new project until one is complete.
Accepting too many jobs	Learn to say no!
Waiting for information or return calls	Use an answering machine or voicemail system.
Incomplete work	Plan time to finish projects with no interruptions.
Socializing with coworkers	Avoid the situations; restrict others from too much socializing.
Unnecessary work	Analyze the task; eliminate it if not necessary.

be done routinely by recording the way you spend your time; analyzing how you spend your time; determining what activities can be adjusted to make you a more effective worker; scheduling your activities daily, weekly, monthly, and long-range; and adhering to the schedule. Efficient time management requires that you organize individual tasks, maintain daily schedules, analyze daily tasks, schedule major projects, establish deadlines, and organize workflow.

Maintaining Daily Schedules

To efficiently maintain a daily schedule, it is necessary to use a calendar of activities and tasks and a to-do list, determine priorities, show flexibility, use free time, and review the schedule with other members of the staff if you are the employer or with your supervisor if you are an employee.

The use of a calendar, personal appointment book, and the office appointment book is necessary in maintaining a daily schedule. A desk or electronic calendar provides a method for keeping track of your daily schedule, and it is used for short- and long-range scheduling. Make entries neatly if done manually, be consistent in making entries, and avoid making confidential entries if you use an electronic calendar that is accessible to others.

A to-do list should provide a summary of all pending tasks, not just those to be done on a specific day. This list need not include routine daily tasks, such as opening and closing the office or opening mail. Delete each task on completion, and transfer tasks not completed to a list for the following day.

Determine priorities by ranking each task on the list by its priority or its level of urgency and importance. Items on the list can be ranked by giving a 1 to tasks that must be completed immediately, 2 to tasks that must be completed that day, and 3 to tasks that must be done whenever you have time.

Be flexible in your plans for the day, because emergencies arise and new priority tasks will be identified. In addition to the routine to-do list, another list could be kept that details various tasks that should be completed when time permits. This list provides tasks to do during a slow period or when no clients are scheduled.

Do not overschedule or underestimate how long some tasks will take. It is better to underschedule than overschedule. Plan for the unexpected.

LEARNING ACTIVITY

Complete an analysis of your time management abilities. For one typical work or school day (24 hours), maintain an hour by hour log of what you did and how long it took. Include all time for travel, phone, text, computer, breaks, eating, and sleeping. Analyze the log for areas where time management could be improved. Identify at least three areas, then list improvements in the space provided:

1. _____
2. _____
3. _____

DESIGNING A PROFESSIONAL PROCEDURAL MANUAL

The procedural manual is a valuable instrument in maintaining maximum efficiency in the massage practice while providing a means of communication. A well-planned procedure manual prevents problems. It includes the massage therapist's philosophy of the business practice and defines the job responsibilities for each team member. If you are being hired for a position, you should read the procedure manual to make sure you are able to be in compliance with the rules and regulations of the business.

Guidelines for a Procedural Manual

The following list provides subjects to be included in an office procedural manual. You can purchase basic office manual formats and add inserts for the massage therapist's philosophy and specific duties relating to the practice.

I. Statement of purpose or objective of the manual
II. Statement of philosophy for the practice
III. Table of contents
IV. Office communications

    A. Vocabulary
    B. Telecommunications
    C. Reception techniques
    D. Written communication
    E. Client education

V. Staff policies

    A. Conduct
    B. Grooming and appearance
    C. Dress codes: clinical and business office attire
    D. Staff meetings

VI. Employment policies

    A. Probationary period
    B. Promotion
    C. Hours of work
    D. Overtime
    E. Holidays
    F. Vacations
    G. Absences and leaves
    H. Salaries
    I. Insurance
    J. Additional benefits
    K. Termination of employment
    L. Personal telephone calls and personal mail

VII. Safety and infection control

    A. Infection-control policy
    B. Occupational Safety and Health Administration (OSHA) guidelines
    C. Health risk categories
    D. Nomenclature (i.e., set or system of names or terms used in a particular science or art and used by an individual or community)
    E. Disinfection and sterilization guidelines
    F. Waste management
    G. Standard precautions

VIII. Office records

    A. Medical history procedures
    B. Client records
    C Employee records
    D. Transfer of records
    E. Accounts receivable
    F. Accounts payable
    G. Filing

IX. Massage practice procedures

    A. Health Insurance Portability and Accountability Act (HIPAA) compliance

X. Professional organizations

Writing a Personnel Policy

As part of the office procedure manual, a well-defined personnel policy must be established. A fair and equitable personnel policy may help to eliminate conflicts that could arise among team members. The material in Box 2-6 illustrates a suggested personnel policy. This policy may be altered to satisfy the needs of an individual office.

THE MASSAGE PROFESSIONAL AS AN EMPLOYER OR EMPLOYEE

Your career goals may include having employees. You may hire a receptionist or a staff of massage therapists. If you plan on working for someone, it is valuable to understand what to expect from the employment process. Whether you are the employer or employee, the process begins with the job description.

Job Description

A current, accurate job description should exist for each position in the business structure. These job descriptions aid employers in telling prospective employees what will be expected of them on the job and can aid in training new staff members.

To write a job description, you need to do a job analysis. A job analysis involves gathering information about the job and includes a list of the tasks that make up the job, and determining the skills, personality characteristics, and educational background needed for the employee to perform the job satisfactorily. Existing staff or a mentor then reviews the job description. It is revised as necessary and placed in the procedural manual. An outline for a job description is shown in Box 2-7.

If you are applying for a massage position, you need to be informed of the job description to determine employment expectations and duties. If you intend to employ massage therapists as an aspect of your business plan, it is necessary to concisely determine what will be expected of the employee.

EXPERT OUTLOOK

EMPLOYER PERSPECTIVE
C. G. Funk
Vice President of Industry Relations and Product Development, Massage Envy

The massage therapy profession has changed much in the past 10 years. One of the most visible changes has been the rapid increase in employment opportunities for massage therapists.

Historically, the massage profession was private practitioner driven, which means the majority of therapists in the country were self-employed. Massage therapists were in private practice either by choice as their desired path or by default from a lack of available job/career opportunities.

Currently, our profession is shifting to an employer-driven market. Today, there are more job opportunities than ever before because of the growth of the spa/resort industry, the spread of national franchise massage clinic businesses, and the integration of massage services into medical and holistic health facilities.

For massage therapists, being an employee varies greatly from being a private practitioner. A massage therapist employee is a member of the team as opposed to working solo. Employees must adhere to all the company's policies and procedures, and they are held accountable for their actions and behavior.

Similar to other service industry jobs, employees are hired based on their education, experience, and skill set. Employers will look to fill positions with individuals that present a professional demeanor, facilitate effective and safe hands-on sessions, and exhibit the ability to develop positive relationships with clients.

Although your hands-on talent will get you part of the way toward securing a position, showing your excellent customer service skills during the interview process is just as important.

As a representative of the largest employer of massage therapists in the United States, I can share with you some inside information on what employers look for in a massage therapist applicant. During the verbal interview, an employer will assess your resume, interest in the position, communication skills, and performance standards. Furthermore, during the practical interview the employer will observe not only your flow, techniques, draping, and body mechanics, but also your interaction with her or him as a client before, during, and after the massage session. This is the time where the employer experiences the level of service you are capable of offering.

As employees, therapists will find a different work environment than in a private practice. All employers have set expectations of their staff, and therapists will need to understand their role and responsibilities. A therapist will be accountable for offering great customer service, presenting a professional image, and contributing to the team's operational goals. In addition, most employers have policies and procedures specific to massage therapists that include client interaction, draping, standards of touch, code of ethics, and intake procedures.

There are numerous benefits to being an employee versus being self-employed. You will be working in a safe, controlled environment with supportive management staff. You will have the opportunity to meet and build lasting relationships with fellow team members. You will have a set schedule and a consistent flow of clients, which results in a reliable source of income. In addition, an employer typically takes the responsibility for marketing, client scheduling, supplies, and payroll so therapists are able to focus solely on what they love best—massage therapy. For many therapists, it doesn't get much better than that!

BOX 2-6	Personnel Policies for the Health and Wellness Massage Therapy Office

PROBATIONARY PERIOD

Your first 3 months are considered a probationary period, during which the owner can evaluate your progress with the new work. During this period, your employment may be terminated without notice. The massage therapist creates a Merit Rating Report at the termination of the probationary period and periodically thereafter. This report is used as the basis for salary increases and promotions.

PROMOTION

Your demonstrated ability to perform your job well, your attendance and punctuality record, and your relationships with employees have a bearing on your opportunities for promotion and advancement in salary. Any outside courses of study that result in skills in addition to those listed on your application are added to your record to ensure complete information when reviewing your record for advancement. All employees are reviewed every 6 months.

HOURS OF WORK

The office is open from 8:00 AM to 5:00 PM on Monday and Wednesday and from 8:00 AM to 9:00 PM on Tuesday and Thursday. On Fridays, the office is closed. Lunch hour is from 12:00 PM to 1:00 PM. The basic week of 35 working hours is assigned to each massage therapist.

OVERTIME

Overtime salary is paid for units of 30 minutes (0.5 hour). Fractions of less than 0.5 hour of overtime are not reported. If your salary is less than $2150 per month, compensation for work authorized by the massage therapist in excess of 35 hours is at the rate of time and one half beyond 35 hours in any week or for work on Saturdays, Sundays, and holidays.

HOLIDAYS

You are paid for the following legal holidays: New Year's Day, Memorial Day, Independence Day, Labor Day, Thanksgiving Day, and Christmas Day. When the office will be closed for a religious holiday or other holiday, an announcement is made in advance.

VACATIONS

Requests for vacation time in excess of 1 day must be made 30 days in advance. You will be entitled to 2 weeks of vacation after completing 12 months of continuous employment and 4 weeks of vacation after 10 years of employment. A legal holiday that falls within the vacation period adds 1 day to your vacation. When a vacation falls within a vacation period, your salary is paid in advance to the latest regular salary payment date falling within the vacation period.

ABSENCES AND LEAVES

Regular attendance and punctuality are necessary for smooth functioning of the massage office, and your record in this respect is considered in determining your advancement and salary adjustment. However, there are certain absences that are unavoidable and for which provision will be made. In each case, the massage therapists should be notified in advance when possible or before 7:30 AM on the day of your absence. If you fail to make proper notification, the unadvised absence will be counted as absence without salary.

When absence is for your own illness, salary is paid for up to 1 day for each month of employment, for a cumulative amount up to 30 days. If you need sick leave in addition to this amount, a request should be made to the owner for additional time without pay.

If you are required to serve as a juror or witness in court, your absence is considered as a leave with salary.

If there is a death in your immediate family, up to 3 days of leave may be granted with salary.

If you request a leave of absence for reasons other than those previously described or for a longer period than is provided with salary, several factors will be taken into consideration, including your previous work and attendance records, the length of leave you are requesting, the work needs of the office, and any other pertinent issues.

SALARIES

Your salary is paid by check on a weekly basis and covers the period through Wednesday of the current week. Salary checks are distributed each Friday. Salary increases are considered every 6 months. The quality of your work, the amount of responsibility you assume, your attendance and punctuality records, your attitude toward the staff and clients, and your length of service are factors that enter into the consideration. Deductions from salary regularly include federal and state withholding taxes and Social Security. Deductions for group insurance, hospital care, and other benefits are made only on written request.

INSURANCE

To help provide security in times of sickness and hospitalization, health insurance is available. Membership in a group health insurance plan is available to all those employed up to 1 year and is billed on a payroll deduction basis. Staff members may select this insurance at their own expense for the first 12 months of employment. Deductions for hospital care are made the first payday of each month. Coverage of your spouse and dependent children younger than 19 years may be included in your hospital care contract.

Social Security is provided through payments by you and the owner to the U.S. government. Your share of the cost is deducted from each salary payment.

ADDITIONAL BENEFITS

In addition to regular salary increases, the members of the staff are eligible for several additional benefits.

Uniform: The owner will provide uniforms. All massage therapists will wear blue scrubs with the business insignia and white gym shoes. The owner will provide the two uniforms but will not provide shoes.

Linens: All linens used for massage will be provided and laundered by a professional laundry service.

BOX 2-6	Personnel Policies for the Health and Wellness Massage Therapy Office—cont'd

INFECTION-CONTROL POLICY

An effective infection-control program has been implemented in the office for the protection of staff members, clients, and family members. It is recommended that you adhere to the provisions in the *Infection Control Policy Handbook* and that you are aware of all updates of this manual as they occur.

In the past, there have been three categorizations of tasks to differentiate exposure contact with blood, body fluids, and tissues. In reality, there are only two categories: A person has no contact with blood or has some or continuous exposure.

Category I: Tasks that involve exposure to blood, body fluids, or tissues

Category II: Tasks that involve no exposure to blood, body fluids, or tissues

Massage therapists are in category II.

TERMINATION OF EMPLOYMENT OR RESIGNATION

You are asked to give 2 weeks' written notice of resignation. If you have been employed for 6 months or more and you resign during the vacation period after giving 2 weeks' notice, you will be compensated for your vacation according to the vacation schedule.

PERSONAL TELEPHONE CALLS AND PERSONAL MAIL OR E-MAIL

Personal telephone calls affect the workload in two ways. They prohibit incoming calls from clients, and they take time from your job. Limit the number of personal calls, and receive incoming calls only in an emergency. Personal cell phones should be turned off or set on silent mode during office hours. Similarly, the volume of mail is heavy at the office; therefore, do not use the office address for personal mail or e-mail.

BOX 2-7	Business Responsibilities of the Massage Therapist

- Answering phones as necessary
- Client scheduling and appointment confirmation
- Conferring with clients about health histories
- SOAP (subjective, objective, assessment, and plan) notes or other types of documentation
- Daily maintenance of massage room, including emptying of garbage container
- Developing client treatment plans
- Filing records

- Greeting clients
- Maintaining treatment records
- Massage room preparation, including sanitation, preparing the draping material, and maintaining bolsters
- Preparing and blending massage oils
- Preparing clients for tests, therapy, or treatments
- Providing clients with rehabilitative exercises
- Upkeep of the restrooms and waiting area as needed

LEARNING ACTIVITY

In the space provided, develop a job description for your ideal job.

_____

_____

_____

_____

Legal Considerations in Hiring

Legal factors that must be considered when hiring an employee include application forms, citizenship status, and testing. An employer must ensure that application forms avoid any questions regarding race or ethnic background. Each applicant who completes an application form must be provided with the same type of form. Be certain that the application form used in the office does not violate any state requirements. For example, a state may consider it unlawful to use a lie detector test, and a question on an application asking the applicant to take a lie detector test would be in violation of the state law (Fig. 2-17).

It is in violation of federal law to hire an unauthorized (illegal) alien. An employer must require proof of an applicant's legal status, and the Immigration and Naturalization Service (INS) Form I-9 (Employment Eligibility Verification) must be filled out before employment. Documents accepted for verification include an original U.S. passport, a certificate of U.S. citizenship or naturalization, an alien registration card with a photograph, a state-issued driver's license, a Social Security card, or a birth certificate.

Pre-employment Testing

Employment testing may include standardized tests, polygraph tests, and drug and alcohol tests. Although a small massage therapy practice seldom uses all these tests, an institution such as a hospital or a large spa chain may use many tests.

Tests used to screen applicants can become discriminatory when they serve to disqualify members of a minority culture who are unfamiliar with the language or concepts but are fully qualified for the job. Many private-sector employers are considering drug and alcohol testing as a pre-employment requirement, which is likely to be part of a pre-employment physical examination.

An employer refusing to hire someone with acquired immunodeficiency syndrome (AIDS) violates federal and state disability discrimination laws. Protection under Title VII of the 1964 Civil Rights Act has been extended to disabled persons, including those infected with the human immunodeficiency virus (HIV) virus or who have tested positive for HIV.

Employment Interview

If you are seeking employment as a massage therapist, you will participate in an employment interview as the potential candidate (being interviewed). If you intend to be an employer, you will conduct employment interviews.

The employment interview is important for the person seeking a position and the employer. If you are interviewing for a position as a massage therapist, you are able to collect information during the interview about the employer and the business structure.

Before conducting an interview, the employer gathers information about each candidate (typically using the candidate's resume), develops an outline of questions, and determines the physical setting for the interview (Box 2-8).

As the interview begins, the employer should establish rapport with the candidate by introducing himself or herself, explain the purpose of the interview, and generate a relaxed atmosphere. This is not always the case because not all employers are effective interviewers. If you are the candidate being interviewed, you should establish rapport with the employer; introduce yourself; and maintain a relaxed, confident, and professional demeanor.

Application for Employment

Date _____

Name _____   Social Security # _____

Address _____   Zip _____   Telephone Number _____

If employed and you are under 18 can you furnish a work permit?   ☐Yes   ☐No

Are you legally eligible for employment in the U.S.A.?   ☐Yes   ☐No

Have you worked here before?   ☐Yes   ☐No   If Yes, when?_____

Are there any hours, shifts, or days you cannot or will not work?_____

Are you willing to work overtime if required?   ☐Yes   ☐No

List friends or relatives working here._____

Have you ever been convicted of a crime?   ☐Yes   ☐No   (A conviction record will not necessarily be a bar to employment)

EDUCATION

Circle Highest Grade Completed	Grade School 1 2 3 4 5 6 7 8	High School 9 10 11 12	College 1 2 3 4	Graduate 1 2 3 4	Degree Received	Course of Study
High School	*Name and Address*					
College(s)						
Graduate/Professional						
Specialized Training, Apprenticeship, Skills						
Honors and Awards and Accreditations						

MILITARY SERVICE RECORD   Have you served in the U.S. Armed Forces? _____   Dates of duty _____

POSITION(S) APPLIED FOR: 1) _____   2) _____

You must indicate a specific position. Applications stating "ANY POSITION" will not be considered.

Wage or salary requirements $ _____   When can you start? _____

FIGURE 2-17. Employment application. (*Modified from Gerdin J: Health Careers Today, ed 4, St. Louis, 2007, Mosby.*)

The main part of the interview consists of asking questions, listening to responses, answering questions, and providing a transition from one discussion topic to another. Typical inquiries include the following: "Tell me about your previous job experiences." "What is your attitude toward your previous working experience?" "What do you feel your strengths and weaknesses are for the position available?"

Common types of questions asked during an interview include direct, indirect, and hypothetical. The direct question usually elicits an expected response. An indirect question does not seek a "yes" or "no" response. The following examples illustrate the differences in these types of questions:

Direct: Would you be opposed to traveling to a satellite office?

Indirect: How would you feel about traveling to a satellite office?

Hypothetical: If one of our clients told you he did not like the way he was treated by a different massage therapist in the company, how would you respond?

A hypothetical question describes a situation and elicits a response from the candidate. This type of question is valuable because it is the closest the interviewer will get to observing the candidate's behavior.

During the interview, the interviewer intends to gather information about the candidate's qualifications for the job in a nondiscriminatory manner and to convey information to the candidate about the business and specific job responsibilities (see Box 2-7). There are certain legal considerations

---

Application for Employment—cont'd

WORK HISTORY

If presently employed, may we contact your employer?   ❑ Yes   ❑ No

(1) **Present or Most Recent Employer**		Address	Phone
Date Started	Starting Salary		Starting Position
Date Left	Salary on Leaving		Position on Leaving
Name and Title of Supervisor			
Description of Duties			Reason for Leaving

(2) **Previous Employer**		Address	Phone
Date Started	Starting Salary		Starting Position
Date Left	Salary on Leaving		Position on Leaving
Name and Title of Supervisor			
Description of Duties			Reason for Leaving

(3) **Previous Employer**		Address	Phone
Date Started	Starting Salary		Starting Position
Date Left	Salary on Leaving		Position on Leaving
Name and Title of Supervisor			
Description of Duties			Reason for Leaving

FIGURE 2-17, cont'd

(Continued)

related to interviewing. Rules of thumb for appropriate interview questions are shown in Box 2-9. Guidelines by the U.S. Department of Labor and the EEOC prohibit discriminatory hiring based on race, creed, color, sex, national origin, handicap, or age. Questions related to any of these topics or to marital status, children, ownership of a house or car, credit rating, or type of military discharge can also be considered discriminatory. Questions that should and should not be asked during an interview include many of those shown in Box 2-10, and topics that should be avoided are listed in Box 2-11.

The interview should include information for the prospective candidate from all of the following areas:

- Specific job responsibilities
- Orientation procedures

- Opportunities for advancement
- Management procedures
- Professional responsibilities
- Work hours, salary, and fringe benefits

After all candidates have been interviewed and the decision made about each, the person to be hired should be contacted promptly. A letter of confirmation should be sent to the new employee stating the conditions of employment (e.g., wages, hours, promotions, starting date) and other conditions agreed on during previous discussions. The letter should identify probationary periods, which allow either party to terminate employment within an established period without fear of penalty. It is wise to have the new employee sign the letter. A copy is then

---

ADDITIONAL INFORMATION

OTHER QUALIFICATIONS
Summarize special job-related skills and qualifications acquired from employment or other experience.

_____
_____
_____

SPECIALIZED SKILLS   (CHECK SKILLS/EQUIPMENT OPERATED)

_____ CRT	_____ Fax	Other (list):
_____ PC	_____ Lotus 1-2-3	_____
_____ Calculator	_____ PBX System	_____
_____ Typewriter	_____ WordPerfect	_____

State any additional information you feel may be helpful to us in considering your application.

_____
_____
_____
_____

Note to Applicants: DO NOT ANSWER THIS QUESTION UNLESS YOU HAVE BEEN INFORMED ABOUT THE REQUIREMENTS OF THE JOB FOR WHICH YOU ARE APPLYING.
Are you capable of performing in a reasonable manner—with or without a reasonable accommodation—the activities involved in the job or occupation for which you have applied? A description of the activities involved in such a job or occupation is attached.   ❏ Yes   ❏ No

REFERENCES

1. _____
                        (Name)   Phone #
   _____
                        (Address)

2. _____
                        (Name)   Phone #
   _____
                        (Address)

3. _____
                        (Name)   Phone #
   _____
                        (Address)

UNDER MARYLAND LAW, AN EMPLOYER MAY NOT REQUIRE OR DEMAND, AS A CONDITION OF EMPLOYMENT, PROSPECTIVE EMPLOYMENT, OR CONTINUED EMPLOYMENT, THAT AN INDIVIDUAL SUBMIT TO OR TAKE A LIE DETECTOR OR SIMILAR TEST. AN EMPLOYER WHO VIOLATES THIS LAW IS GUILTY OF A MISDEMEANOR AND SUBJECT TO A FINE NOT EXCEEDING $100.00.
By my signature below, I certify that I have read the above and understand it completely.

_____   _____
            Signature   Date

FIGURE 2-17, cont'd

BOX 2-8	Suggestions for Job Interview Preparation

- Perform a task analysis of the proposed job.
- Determine the competencies needed to fulfill the job requirements.
- Prepare a well-defined job description.
- Have the applicant complete a job application.
- Determine how to measure an applicant's ability. Tests may be used to measure certain abilities, such as performing a demonstration massage.
- Explain the requirements of the job completely.
- Determine key questions to ask in the interview.
- Review reactions toward the applicant. Were you comfortable? Was the applicant an active participant in the conversation? Was the individual shy or domineering?
- Make accurate observations about the applicant's answers, grammar, and nonverbal cues during the interview. Use a check-off form to ensure that each candidate is evaluated on the same basis.
- Record evaluations as soon as the interview is completed to ensure that you do not forget the responses.
- Investigate the references provided by the applicant. This confirms the accuracy of the applicant's statements.

BOX 2-9	Three Rules of Thumb for Interviewing

1. Ask only for information that you intend to use to make hiring decisions.
2. Know how you will use the information to make a decision.
3. Recognize that it is difficult to defend the practice of seeking information that you do not use.

retained by the employee, and a copy is placed in the employee's file.

A letter should be sent to candidates not being hired, and their applications may remain on file if desired. Understanding how an interview is conducted and what factors influence the decision to hire an individual can help the person seeking employment respond effectively during the employment interview.

LEARNING ACTIVITY

Pairing with a partner and using your ideal job description, practice interviewing each other for that job. Play the roles of interviewer and interviewee. Pair with a different partner, and repeat the process. Complete the process at least three times. More is better. Make sure to follow the criteria for conducting a thorough and legal interview. Information available on the Small Business Association Web site is helpful.

BOX 2-10	Appropriate Questions to Ask and Inappropriate Questions Not to Ask During an Interview

APPROPRIATE QUESTIONS

1. What was your absentee record at your prior place of employment?
2. Do you know of any reason (e.g., transportation) why you would be unable to get to work on time and on a regular basis?
3. Are you available to work overtime?
4. We are looking for employees with a commitment to this position. Are there any reasons why you may not stay with us?
5. What are your career objectives?
6. Do you foresee any reasons why you could not be assigned to a branch or satellite office?
7. Where do you see yourself in 5 years?

INAPPROPRIATE QUESTIONS

1. Where were you born?
2. Where and when did you graduate from high school?
3. Do you have any handicaps?
4. What religious holidays do you practice?
5. Are you married?
6. Do you plan to have children? How many?
7. Do you own a home?
8. Do you own a car?
9. Do you have any debts?
10. Can you provide three credit references?
11. Is your spouse likely to be transferred?
12. Is your spouse from this area?
13. How old are you?
14. How do you feel about working with members of a different race?
15. What languages do your parents speak?

BOX 2-11	Topics to Avoid During the Interview Process

- Arrest records
- Marital status
- Maiden name
- Spouse's name
- Spouse's education
- Spouse's income
- Form of birth control
- Child care arrangements
- Lawsuits or legal complaints
- Ownership of car or residence
- Loans
- Insurance claims
- National origin
- Mother's maiden name
- Place of birth
- Disabilities
- Weight
- Age
- Date of high school graduation
- Religion
- Social organizations

New Employee Training

After you are hired, it is important to participate in an orientation and training procedure. An employee handbook provides guidelines along with responsibilities and policies that assist in the new position (Box 2-12). A well-organized business can provide a smooth transition for the new employee into the practice. Time for the new employee to become well established in the office varies according to the individual business. New employee training includes the following:

- Describe how the practice is run and what standards are required of the staff.

- Explain the organizational chart and job descriptions.
- Complete employee documents, including federal and state tax forms.
- Review procedural techniques.
- Allow time for observation, but let the skills and responsibilities of the new employee be used as soon as possible.
- Evaluate the performance of the new employee regularly. This allows changes to be made in performance and provides the employee with knowledge of his or her status.
- Review progress with adequate promotion by means of benefits or a pay increase.

BOX 2-12 Sections for Employee Handbooks

- Company Logo and Company Name
- Title Page
- Welcome to XYZ Massage Therapy Business
- Disclaimer
- Introduction
- XYZ Massage Therapy Business Mission Statement
- Career Opportunities
- Code of Conduct
- Employment
- Equal Opportunity Employment
- Eligibility for Employment
- Part-Time Employment
- Minimum Wage
- Criminal Convictions
- Violence
- Weapons
- Alcohol, Drugs, and Illegal Substance Abuse
- Sexual and Other Unlawful Harassment
- Domestic Violence Statement
- Job Posting
- Seniority
- Employment Evaluation
- Personnel File
- Policies and Procedures
- Attendance
- Parking
- Schedule
- Staff Meetings
- Bulletin Boards
- Suggestion Box
- Time Cards
- Lunch Break
- Breaks

- Dress Code
- Medical Attention
- Compensation
- Overtime
- Commissioned Sale
- Wage and Salary Disclosure
- Payroll Schedules
- Your Paycheck
- Payroll Deductions for Taxes, FICA, and Medicare
- Individual Retirement Accounts (IRAs)
- Working Away from the Office
- Performance and Evaluation Reviews
- Reimbursement of Expenses
- Reporting Personal Information Changes
- Gifts, Entertainment, and Meals
- Visitors
- Personal Property
- Personal Safety
- Food and Beverage
- Smoking
- Office Parties
- Solicitation
- Moonlighting
- Company Property
- Facilities Security
- Office Supplies, Postage, and Company Accounts
- Company Equipment
- Phone Systems, Voicemail, and Personal Calls
- Conservation and Recycling
- Computers and Related Equipment
- Internet, E-Mail, and Electronic Communication

- Policies for Leave of Absence
- Eligibility
- Personal Leave of Absence
- Sick Leave
- Personal Time
- Short-Term Disability Leave
- Unpaid Family and Medical Leave
- Funeral Leave
- Jury Duty
- Military Duty
- Severe Weather Closings
- Benefits
- Eligibility
- Group Medical Insurance
- Retirement
- Worker's Compensation
- Holidays
- Vacations
- Vacation Schedules
- Education and Tuition Reimbursement
- Employee Discounts
- Discipline Policies
- Problem Resolutions
- Violation of Company Policy
- Termination of Employment
- Termination
- Severance
- Acknowledgement
- Notice
- Drug Testing Policy and Consent Form
- Noncompete and Nondisclosure Agreement

Examples are posted on Evolve at http://evolve.elsevier.com/Fritz/business.

Data from http://www.dtcc.edu/stanton-wilmington/documents/faculty_hand-book.pdf *and* http://www.grants.nmsu.edu/pub/documents/safety.pdf

Good Stuff from the Government

SMALL BUSINESS TRAINING NETWORK ONLINE TRAINING

All web links mentioned below are annotated on the Evolve site at http://evolve.elsevier.com/Fritz/business.

The Small Business Training Network (SBTN) is a virtual campus providing quality and targeted online training to meet the information needs of prospective and existing small business owners. It is an electronic government initiative, powering a comprehensive menu of business courses that are designed to serve more customers more efficiently. The SBTN operates like an electronic umbrella, under which many SBA and agency resource training programs are captured, aggregated, sorted by content, and made available in multiple formats.

The SBTN is a customer-focused SBA strategy designed to enrich, educate, and empower small businesses. It is an Internet-based learning environment that operates like a virtual campus by offering online courses, workshops, publications, information resources, learning tools, and direct access to electronic counseling and other forms of technical assistance that support professionals. Not all training can be effectively achieved or is best suited for an online environment. In addition to a robust selection of online offerings, the SBTN serves as a window to all of the traditional, face-to-face technical assistance programs offered by the agency. Traditional training opportunities offered by SBA and its resource partners around the country can be easily identified by clicking on the National Training Events site (http://www.sba.gov/news/calendar/).

When you log on, check out the course on strategic planning and execution. This course presents the fundamental devices used in crafting a strategy for a business venture. The course presents the innovative mechanisms of internal and external strategies. These innovations are based on the findings of a new body of research into the strategy-making processes of successful growing ventures. The course shows how to craft missions, visions, goals, and strategies for your business. It shows you how to best present and execute your strategy through strategic stories, the act of organizing genius, and tipping point leadership tactics (http://www.sba.gov/training/index.html).

The SBA also offers information on management of employees. Log on to find out more about the following topics (http://www.sba.gov/smallbusinessplanner/manage/manageemployees/):

Writing effective job descriptions
Employees versus contractors: what's the difference?
The interview process: how to select the "right" person
When potential employees lie
Immigration FAQs
Hiring employees FAQs
The U.S. Department of Labor's employment law guide
Verify a Social Security Number
Plain English guide to employee handbooks
Planning for the future
Another great resource is the find a mentor feature.

Never think you can do it alone! One of the best ways to insulate yourself against business failure is to find and work with a mentor, someone with business experience who can guide and assist you.

Another great government site is www.business.gov. It is the official link to the U.S. government business portal to many different helpful sites. Log on and explore employment and labor laws and workplace safety and health.

The Department of Labor site also has useful information. The Department of Labor Occupational Safety and Health Administration (OSHA) offers a small business handbook that can be downloaded. It can provide content for office procedural manuals.

Employers are responsible for providing a safe and healthful workplace for their employees. OSHA's role is to ensure the safety and health of America's workers by setting and enforcing standards; providing training, outreach, and education; establishing partnerships; and encouraging continual improvement in workplace safety and health. The entire text of the *Small Business Handbook* is available on OSHA's Web site.

SUMMARY

Professionalism emphasizes the importance of learning to identify and trust your inspiration, intention, and intuition, which provide a pathway for developing massage practice goals and objectives. Business office etiquette includes respect for diversity and demands self-assessment to identify areas that need improvement. Effective management is related to communication skills, conflict management, time management, and thoughtful hiring practices. Employees benefit from a procedure manual, which consolidates the policies and procedures of the office for smooth and successful business operations.

Using professional associations and governmental resources can help professional message therapists investigate areas of interest and expand learning beyond the pages of this textbook.

Bibliography

Adams B, Arquette L, Deutscher N et al: *Streetwise Managing People: Lead Your Staff to Peak Performance*, Holbrook, MA, 1998, Adams Media Corporation.

Bruce V, Green PR, Georgeson MA: *Visual Perception: Physiology, Psychology and Ecology*, ed 3, London, 1996, Taylor & Francis.

Freeman WJ: The physiology of perception, *Sci Am* 264:78-85, 1991.

Fulton-Calkins PJ: *General Office Procedures for Colleges*, ed 12, Cincinnati, OH, 2003, South-Western.

Hastings W, Potter R: *Trust Me*, Colorado Springs, CO, 2004, WaterBrook Press.

Thill JV, Bovée CL: *Excellence in Business Communication*, ed 5, Upper Saddle River, NJ, 2002, Prentice-Hall.

⊖ Evolve Annotated Web Links

http://evolve.elsevier.com/Fritz/business

Bureau of Labor Statistics, U.S. Department of Labor, Occupational Outlook Handbook, 2008-2009 edition: www.bls.gov/oco/ocos295.htm

United States Equal Employment Opportunity Commission: http://www.eeoc.gov/

Employment and labor laws and workplace safety and health: http://www.business.gov/

Delaware Technical and Community College employee handbook: http://www.dtcc.edu/stanton-wilmington/documents/faculty_handbook.pdf

New Mexico State University: http://www.grants.nmsu.edu/pub/documents/safety.pdf

U.S. Small Business Administration online courses: http://www.sba.gov/training/index.html

U.S. Small Business Administration small business planner, managing employees: http://www.sba.gov/smallbusinessplanner/manage/manageemployees/index.html

---

Workbook

1. Write job descriptions for a massage therapist in a spa-setting job and a chiropractic office, and for a part-time massage therapist sharing a massage office with a sole massage practitioner.

    _____
    _____
    _____
    _____
    _____

2. Create an interview outline that lists the sequence of events of an interview. Develop a series of questions that can determine a candidate's skills for a job. Interview fellow classmates to practice being the interviewer and the candidate.

    _____
    _____
    _____
    _____
    _____

3. Describe how you would handle the following conflict situations:

A massage therapist reprimands a coworker for wearing facial piercings, which is a violation of the office procedural manual for clinical assistants. What is your response?

    _____
    _____
    _____
    _____
    _____

Office hours for the staff are 8:15 AM to 5:00 PM. The receptionist is chronically late, arriving 15 to 20 minutes after the assigned time each day. This person always leaves by 5:00 PM and seldom is late leaving for lunch. Friction is occurring among the staff. Is this really a problem? What are the issues involved? Can there be a resolution? What action should be taken, and who should take action?

    _____
    _____
    _____
    _____
    _____

FOCUS ON THE CLIENT

KEY TERMS

Client-centered therapy

Clients' rights

Defense mechanisms

Hierarchy of needs

Implied outcomes

Nonverbal cues

Office policy

Stated outcomes

Open-ended questions

LEARNING OUTCOMES

Mastery of the content in this chapter will enable the reader to:

- Define glossary terms
- Understand clients' needs
- Explain the special needs of clients
- Identify barriers to communication

- Recognize nonverbal cues
- Manage interpersonal communication in the reception area
- Design an office policy statement
- Understand client rights

ℯ Guidelines for the Learning Activities and answers to the Workbook questions are located on Evolve at http://evolve.elsevier.com/Fritz/business.

So, chapter 3 begins looking how to assess the needs of our clients

First & foremost, massage is a "service" profession

People are an essential part of the massage practice. It may be a cliché, but the most important person in a massage practice is the client. This is a service profession based on a professional relationship. The key words are *service, professional,* and *relationship.* You must never overlook the fact that each client has a different background and different needs. While communicating with clients, it is important that you recognize each as an individual with specific needs and that you determine how to be sensitive to those needs.

Therapeutic massage is a helping profession, and every effort needs to be made to achieve appropriate outcomes for the client. *Stated outcomes* are determined during the development of the massage care plan. *Implied outcomes* are more ambiguous. The reasons for and results of massage often go unstated, but they may be the motivation for the massage sessions. For example, a stated outcome is that the client wants to be able to run a marathon, but the implied outcome is different: help me believe in myself. In another example, the stated outcome is pain management, but the implied outcome is something else: Help me be more in control of my life. The implied outcomes typically emerge over time and through ongoing communication. The topic of communication continues to appear because it is important. In Chapter 1, communication content included listening described in the context of a service profession and the importance of focused listening to understand the client. Chapter 2 dealt with communication skills, especially in terms of conflict resolution. In this chapter, we discuss communication in more depth and review interpersonal relationships.

Clear, concise, and friendly communication is essential. Communication is difficult if a person is behaving in a defensive way. Defense mechanisms are psychological methods of dealing with stressful situations, and they include sarcasm, denial, making excuses, blaming, and other forms of ineffective communication. Listening is one of the most important skills in communication. Listening involves silence and active feedback. Open-ended questions help to restate what the client, coworker, or supervisor is saying to be sure that the message is understood clearly.

UNDERSTANDING CLIENT NEEDS

Each person who comes in contact with the massage clients should have an understanding of the basic drives involved in motivating clients. Unless the massage therapist and others in the work environment understand these drives, they will become discouraged after many attempts fail to motivate clients to maintain a regular appointment schedule and participate in self-help activities.

Massage embraces the concepts of wholeness, and appreciation of the human experience supports business success. It therefore seems appropriate for massage therapists to be aware of the contributions of two humanistic psychologists, Abraham Maslow and Carl Rogers.

Maslow's Hierarchy of Needs

Maslow described a hierarchy of needs (Fig. 3-1) to assist in understanding how a person's needs motivate his or her behavior. Maslow identified five levels of needs, ranging from basic biologic needs to complex social or psychological drives.

1. *Physiologic or biologic needs:* Bodily needs are the first to be satisfied. Physical needs must be satisfied to sustain life. If you are healthy, eat regularly, and are housed adequately, you can advance to the next level of the hierarchy with a sense of well-being.
2. *Safety or security needs:* After the basic biologic needs are met, you are ready to explore your environment. Just as small children begin to explore their environment after their food and comfort needs have been met, adults begin to explore issues concerning safety and freedom from danger, threats, or other deprivation. If you have a job that is nonthreatening and live in a safe environment, you will feel secure and will be able to advance to the next level.

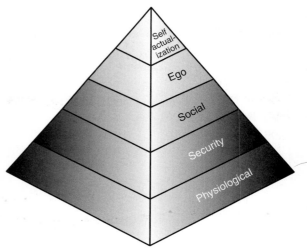

FIGURE 3-1. Maslow's hierarchy of needs. (*Modified from Finkbeiner BL, Finkbeiner CA:* Practice Management for the Dental Team, *ed 6, St. Louis, 2006, Mosby.*)

SELF-REFLECTION

What are the defensive mechanisms I use when stressed? Defense mechanisms include sarcasm, denial, making excuses, blaming, crying, stomping off, refusing to talk, bringing up the past, being a victim ("poor me"), lying, exaggerating, and pouting. Which of these behaviors bother me when others act out? How do I respond to others' defensive behavior? How do others respond to my defensive behavior? How may these behaviors interfere with my massage career?

3. *Social or love needs*: After you are secure in your environment, you can advance to the level of social interaction. The poet John Donne wrote, "No man is an island, complete to itself." Donne realized that to be human means to interact with others. Maslow realized that you need to interact with others who share similar beliefs and who provide you with reinforcement to continue your social relationships. Love or social interaction gives you confidence to advance to the next level on the hierarchy.

4. *Ego or esteem needs*: From interaction with others, you will generate goals for yourself. These ego needs relate to your self-esteem, reputation, and recognition. You look forward to achieving your goals, and from accomplishment, you derive self-esteem. Typically, the self-satisfaction achieved from accomplishing these goals provides an impetus to establish new goals and begin the cycle again.

5. *Self-actualization needs*: Self-actualized people are motivated by the need to grow. They must have achieved self-esteem and self-confidence. Maslow explained that to achieve this level of self-actualization, people must be relatively free of illness, sufficiently satisfied in their basic needs, positively using their capacities, and motivated by some existing or sought-after personal values. A person at this level often wants to help others achieve their goals by sharing what he or she learned in the earlier stages of development. Some people never reach this level because they have not aspired to its recognition.

Relating this hierarchy to massage therapy allows massage therapists to better understand clients and coworkers. Before a massage therapist can motivate a client to embrace massage as an important aspect of self-care, it must be understood where the client is on the hierarchy of needs. For example, one of your clients is a bank president who is respected for his civic activities and has a warm, loving family and a fine home. The client develops low back pain. The pain has moved from the acute stage to the chronic stage. It is difficult for him to sit for extended periods, sleep is interrupted, and he is irritable. This person has dropped from a self-esteem level to the physiologic level, and you must satisfy the physiologic needs for pain management, sleep restoration, and daily function before attempting to suggest further intervention. This amounts to helping the client return to the previous level on the hierarchy of needs.

Setting fees for massage services and payment plans for a client often exposes a conflict of needs. A client must ensure that basic needs of food, housing, and clothing are met, but there may be a desire to meet social and touch needs because the person is going through relationship transitions. A conflict arises in the decision-making process when the client is confronted with conflict over how to satisfy all of these needs within a specified income. A primary business goal is to support a satisfied, retained client. The massage therapist needs to make an effort to determine the client's needs, realize the client's potential conflict areas, and present an alternative treatment plan that provides some options. For example, a single mother who is cashier at a grocery store is in pain from standing in one spot for extended periods. She is barely making ends meet. You (a practicing massage therapist charging $50 per session) and she know massage can help, but she cannot justify the cost. An alternative is to refer her to the local massage school clinic where massage is offered by students at a reduced fee. Although the student at the school clinic has limited skills, the availability of massage at a fee that is affordable is a viable option.

The hierarchy of needs also can be applied to interactions between coworkers. Typically, all have the same needs, and each is concerned, like a client, about security today and in the future. When there are enough clients and resources to meet the needs of all concerned, conflict is reduced, but if there is competition for clients or limited resources, the need for security can fuel conflict. Consider the referral in the previous example. If the massage therapist was struggling financially as much as the potential client, the massage therapist may consider reducing fees to retain the individual, rather than referring her. Where you are on the hierarchy of needs influences the decision you make.

SELF-REFLECTION

Where am I on Maslow's hierarchy of needs in my professional world? What about my personal world? What could occur to move me down the hierarchy? What is my plan if that happens? What do I need to do to move up to the next level? What resources are available to support personal and professional growth?

Conflict often arises when a person becomes fixed at one level on the hierarchy of needs. There may appear to be no change in motivation, and the person's perspective remains unchanged. This pattern becomes evident when a person has an interest in making money or increasing a social status without regard for other people's levels of motivation.

One of the best lessons you can learn from Maslow's theory is that an individual has a choice in determining his or her behavior. Although basic physiologic and environmental needs have a strong influence, an individual makes choices voluntarily. A similar thought process affects people experiencing pain and suffering. Pain occurs in our lives. How we deal with pain determines how we live our lives. Suffering is a choice. We can choose to not suffer by countering the pain with a focus on life's purpose and by regaining an internal sense of control in our lives.

Rogers' Client-Centered Therapy: Reflective Listening

Carl Rogers, another humanistic psychologist, believed that it is "the client who knows what hurts, what direction to go, what problems are crucial, what experiences have been deeply buried." Rogers also suggests that you must accept the client or other person as a genuine person with his or her own set of values and goals and that these people must be treated with "unconditional positive regard."

Client-centered therapy assumes that clients know how they feel, what they want, and what their priorities are. Applied to therapeutic massage, this philosophy encourages you to listen to the client. This means that they talk more than you do. This concept suggests that you must respect clients as human beings, not just numbers, case studies, or research projects. The combined concepts of Maslow and Rogers provide the groundwork for a humanistic, caring attitude, which should be a requisite for all health care providers, including massage therapists.

WHAT DO YOU SEE AS A BARRIER TO

Barriers to Communication with Clients COMMUNICATION

We often are unable to communicate with clients because barriers have been established, and one of the first may create be prejudging a person. A massage therapist may hesitate to set an appointment because of the way the individual dresses or the type of car he or she drives. As a result, the person is not considered a possible retention client because his or her economic status has been prejudged. People with disabilities often are prejudged. When an individual who has an artificial limb, is in a wheelchair, or has a visible birthmark on the face comes in for a massage session, the first noticeable feature frequently is the disability. If this individual is with a spouse or another person, the potential client may go unnoticed while questions are directed to the accompanying person. Massage professionals must treat people with disabilities as they would treat any other clients and direct all communication to them.

Another barrier occurs when the massage therapist hears but does not *listen*. A massage professional should never be too busy to listen with understanding to a client. You must listen to the *meaning* of the words and recognize the feeling behind the meaning. Before presenting your point of view, you must be able to restate what has been said to the client's satisfaction (i.e., reflective listening). This is not as easy as it sounds. You may be too eager to present your own point of view and fail to understand the real meaning of what the client is attempting to say. When the client says, "I think I'll just call later when I think I need another massage," what is she really saying? If you respond, "Oh, that's okay, Mrs. Gates, I understand," you will not discover the true intentions of the client. You may cut off communication. The client may really be saying, "I can't afford it," or "I don't like the way you treat me." The best way to arrive at the real meaning is to continue the dialog until you discern the client's true feelings, as in the following example:

Massage therapist: Mrs. Romano, do you feel that you want to call later for the next appointment?
Client: Yes.

Massage therapist: Do you want to wait because you are too busy now? (The client may say "yes" and terminate the conversation at this point, or the conversation may continue.)
Client: No, it's just that I don't know if I should spend the money right now.
Massage therapist: Do you feel that weekly massage sessions are more than you can afford just now?
Client: Well, it's not that I can't afford it. I guess what it boils down to is being comfortable with spending money on me when my daughter is ready to go to college.
Massage therapist: In other words, there is a concern about the need to support your daughter and importance of caring for you?
Client: Yes, I guess that's it. I have always taken care of the kids first.

The hidden meaning becomes evident in the last response. Notice in this dialog that the massage therapist never offered a solution to the problem, such as an alternative payment plan or a later appointment date. Instead, the dialog with the client is encouraged, and content is rephrased to arrive at the real meaning.

A third barrier is preoccupation. During daily routines, many demands are placed on your time, and you may begin to think about other activities while trying to communicate with a client. Everyone has been in that position at one time or another. A client is trying to explain how his leg became bruised, and you suddenly realize you have not heard a word that was said because you were concentrating on another problem. Unfortunately, clients are quick to recognize such preoccupation and may suddenly stop talking or may even stop coming for massage. This type of situation emphasizes the service model illustrated in Chapter 1. The client is the most important person in the massage practice and should be given your complete attention. When you do lose focus on the client, admit it, and apologize. For example, "I apologize for not concentrating on what you just told me. Please tell me again."

Unawareness of importance, impatience, and even hearing loss are barriers to communication. You may not realize how important the problem is to a client and ignore it as a whim. You may inadvertently find yourself becoming impatient with a chatty young child or an older person who is slow. You may not be hearing everything a person says because of an unrecognized hearing loss.

To prevent or correct these barriers, you must be willing to evaluate yourself. Before each contact with a client, decide to ignore extraneous activities and be willing to listen and understand a client's problem before you offer a solution. Following Rogers' concept of listening to the client long enough can provide the solution. Practice asking good questions to elicit responses:

- If you could massage yourself, what would you do?
- Show me what you think needs to be done.
- What do you think the underlying cause is?

This part should be easy. This is what we do!

Recognizing Nonverbal Cues

Many books have defined and guided the reader to recognize nonverbal communication cues. *Nonverbal cues* refer to the gestures and body movements a person makes in a given situation. Just as a picture is worth a thousand words, a gesture can give meaning to a person's inner feelings. Nonverbal communication provides feedback on the client's reactions.

The alert massage therapist is able to pick up these cues and interpret them while communicating with a client. Care should be taken not to be misled by one gesture. A series of gestures usually gives a more realistic indication of a person's attitude. Therapeutic massage presents many opportunities

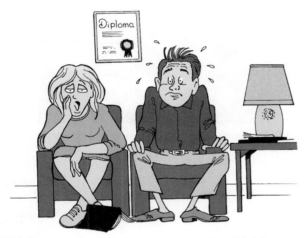

FIGURE 3-2. A client displays nervousness. *(Modified from Finkbeiner BL, Finkbeiner CA: Practice Management for the Dental Team, ed 6, St. Louis, 2006, Mosby.)*

to use and to receive nonverbal cues because the practice is body oriented, but you must be careful to avoid prejudging, assuming, and stereotyping. Although crossing an arm over the chest may mean closing off communication, it can also be a way of supporting the low back when it is aching. Do not jump to conclusions, and keep an open mind.

Nonverbal cues include the following:

Nervousness: A client who enters the reception room and sits down, locking the ankles together and clenching the hands, may be expressing fear by holding back emotions (Fig. 3-2). When the client relaxes, he or she will automatically unlock the ankles.

Defensiveness: A client or coworker may use a gesture of crossed arms and clenched fists as signals to indicate disagreement or defensiveness. This gesture may even indicate the person has withdrawn from the conversation (Fig. 3-3).

Touching: The massage therapist has many opportunities to use this gesture, which indicates compassion and support (Fig. 3-4). A hand on a small child's shoulder may show concern, or an arm around the shoulder of a senior citizen may give reassurance (Fig. 3-5).

Openness: During intake and assessment, the massage therapist should express openness rather than assume an authoritative posture behind a desk. Having the client seated beside the desk removes this barrier and allows the massage therapist an opportunity for more open gestures (Fig. 3-6).

Embarrassment: Clients may pull on clothing because they are attempting to cover some area of the body they are embarrassed for the massage therapist to see or touch (Fig. 3-7).

It is important that you become aware of the meaning and the potential of nonverbal communication. Although

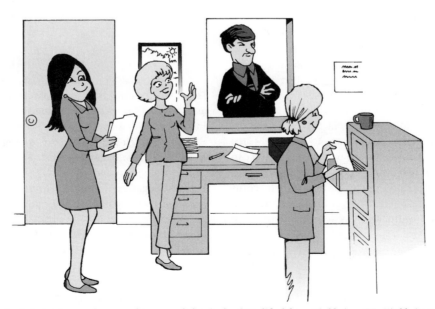

FIGURE 3-3. A client who is being ignored crosses his arms defensively. *(Modified from Finkbeiner BL, Finkbeiner CA: Practice Management for the Dental Team, ed 6, St. Louis, 2006, Mosby.)*

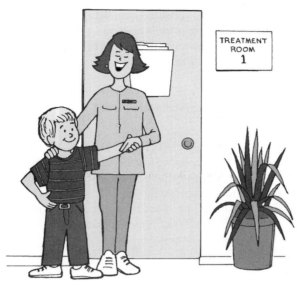

FIGURE 3-4. A massage therapist displays caring by touching a child. *(Modified from Finkbeiner BL, Finkbeiner CA:* Practice Management for the Dental Team, *ed 6, St. Louis, 2006, Mosby.)*

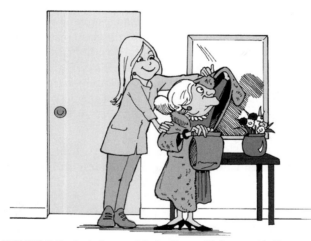

FIGURE 3-5. Assisting an elderly client with her coat indicates caring. *(Modified from Finkbeiner BL, Finkbeiner CA:* Practice Management for the Dental Team, *ed 6. St. Louis, 2006, Mosby.)*

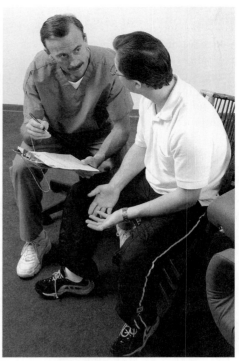

FIGURE 3-6. A massage therapist consults with a client. *(Modified from Finkbeiner BL, Finkbeiner CA:* Practice Management for the Dental Team, *ed 6, St. Louis, 2006, Mosby.)*

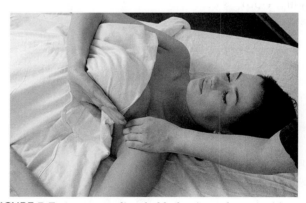

FIGURE 3-7. A massage client holds draping to keep sensitive areas covered. *(From Salvo S:* Massage Therapy: Principles and Practice, *ed 3, St. Louis, 2008, WB Saunders.)*

the previous suggestions can provide a place to begin understanding nonverbal communication, learn to use your intuition to read between the lines. No one tool or technique can ensure successful communication, and becoming an effective communicator is a lifelong pursuit. These efforts, combined with a sincere interest in satisfying a client's needs, will provide a successful communication system in the massage office.

Improving Verbal Images

A massage professional has an obligation to allay fears and hesitancy about getting a massage and to comfort clients. The best way of accomplishing these tasks is to create a good image about massage in the client's mind. In a massage practice, you need to eliminate the use of words or phrases that conjure negative thoughts. For instance, when you say, "I don't care what you look like," you have told the client there is a possibility that you do notice. If you had said, "Draping is used to maintain warmth and modesty," you would have let the client know you were there to help him or her be comfortable. In Chapter 10, terms and phrases frequently used to support clients are discussed in greater detail. Try replacing discomforting terms with words that create a more positive environment. When discussing treatment, use language the client can understand. You had to learn the scientific and medical terminology in school, but it does not impress clients who have no clue what you are talking about.

[handwritten: TIED INTO ALL THIS — IT IS IMPORTANT TO]

THE CLIENT *[handwritten: REMEMBER THAT THE CLIENT HAS SOME RESPONSIBILITY, TOO]*

The most important person in the massage practice is the client. Although massage is a business, it should never be forgotten that it is first a health care service profession. Much is expected of a client: following directions, keeping appointments, and paying fees promptly. In return, we must take time to recognize the client as a person and realize that the client has some special needs and inherent rights.

Clients' Rights *[handwritten: AND WHAT ABOUT THOSE CLIENT RIGHTS?]*

[handwritten vertical margin: AMTA Code of Ethics]

The phrase *patients' rights* is used often and is the result of most health care professions' decisions to design a patient's bill of rights. In some health care agencies, the care unfortunately has become so impersonal that it is necessary for a professional association or agency to formally document the things that are naturally considered to be patients' rights. Some health care workers see this action as confirmation of an individual's inherent rights, not the result of a lack of consideration. The massage profession has yet to develop a client's bill of rights, but the various codes of ethics in the profession imply a foundation of respect for the individual.

As our society becomes increasingly concerned with individual rights, members of the massage health care team cannot afford to neglect clients' rights. Take time to recognize the client as a person, and consider the list of rights in Box 3-1 as rights of the client and not as threats to the profession of massage. The content in the box is adapted from client rights used in health care. *[handwritten: PT. BILL OF RIGHTS]*

Managing the Client's Special Needs

Many individuals with special needs seek massage therapy services. The Americans with Disabilities Act (ADA) of 1990 sets specific guidelines for businesses. This topic was introduced in Chapter 2. Several issues regarding the structural design of a building for access are discussed in Chapter 6. Other factors in the ADA require the massage therapist not to discriminate against a person who requests massage services. If they can get into a treatment room, most disabled persons can receive treatment. Perhaps the biggest challenge a massage therapist faces is attempting to give a massage to a client who struggles to mentally or physically cooperate, such as when a client has cerebral palsy or is a quadriplegic whose high-level neck injuries make moving from a wheelchair to a massage table dangerous. An individual with early-stage dementia may forget to tell you about some medication that he or she is taking. It is necessary to be creative in how you solve these problems.

BOX 3-1   Client Rights

Clients in a massage practice are entitled to
- Be treated with adequate, appropriate, compassionate care at all times and under all circumstances.
- Be treated without discrimination based on race, religion, color, national origin, sex, age, handicap, marital status, sexual preference, or source of payment.
- Be informed of all aspects of treatment.
- Be informed of appointment and fee schedules.
- Review their financial and clinical records.
- Obtain a thorough evaluation of their needs.
- Be treated as a partner in care and decision making related to treatment planning.
- Receive current information and be assured of quality treatment.
- Be able to refuse treatment to the extent provided by law and to be informed of the medical/massage consequences of that refusal.
- Expect confidentiality of all records pertinent to their massage care.
- Be informed if the massage therapist participates in different third-party payment plans.
- Request and expect appropriate referrals for consultation.
- Expect continuity of treatment.
- Be charged a fair and equitable fee.
- Have appointment schedules and times maintained.
- Be treated by a staff of professionals who maintain good health and hygiene.
- Be respected for requesting a second opinion.
- Be respected as human beings who have feelings and needs.

It may be necessary for you to make a special effort in communication with some clients. For instance, if the disabilities include vision or hearing impairments or the client uses a wheelchair or walker, you may find it necessary to take special care when communicating. For clients who have difficulty hearing, you may need to stand in front of them when talking to ensure that they are able to read your lips. For clients with poor vision, you may need to read the questions on the history form and fill in the information. For people using wheelchairs, walkers, or crutches, it may be necessary to take extra time when asking them to move about or lie on the massage table. *[handwritten: You may need to accomodate by working on them in their wheel chair]*

LEARNING ACTIVITY

In the space provided, write a massage client's bill of rights for your future professional practice.

_____

_____

_____

Recognizing Abuse

In our society, abuse is evident in many forms but is most commonly noticed in children, adult women, and the elderly. Each year, more than 2.7 million children are abused or neglected by caregivers, relatives, or strangers. More than 1000 children die annually as a result of this abuse. Child abuse may be classified as physical, sexual, emotional, or neglectful. Those who are elderly and dependent on others for care and adults in volatile relationships may also be victims of abuse. *You are most likely to see*

Although uncommon, massage therapists may be faced with reporting an abuse situation. Abused children or adults may show overall signs of neglect, abnormal fears or neuroses, or evidence of scarring or bruises of various colors on exposed areas of the body. Reports of suspected abuse should be made to the state or county social services office. Individual states vary in their requirements for reporting, and it is necessary to contact the appropriate state agency to find out the specifics for your area.

ALWAYS REPORT SUSPECTED ABUSE.

SEXUAL APPROPRIATENESS

Sexual behavior by the therapist toward the client or by the client toward the therapist is always unethical and inappropriate. It is always the responsibility of the therapist or health professional to ensure that sexual misconduct does not occur. If inappropriate sexual behavior occurs by the client or the massage therapist, the incident should be reported immediately to supervisory personnel. If a supervisor or manager is unavailable, the incident should be written up with documentation and the session ended. If the massage therapist is at fault than the charge for the massage is to be refunded. If the incident could be considered solicitation for prostitution, the client should report to the police. If the client acts inappropriately, he or she should be refused massage services based on sexually inappropriate behavior. If there is concern about appropriate behavior, it should be addressed with a statement in the policy and procedures brochure. The statement could read as follows: Massage therapy is a professional health service and a nonsexual environment. Sexual impropriety is not tolerated.

Sexual impropriety includes the following behaviors:

WHAT CONSTITUTES SEXUAL IMPROPRIETY?

- Engaging in any conduct that is sexual or reasonably may be interpreted as sexual
- Any behavior, gestures, or expressions that are seductive or sexually demeaning to a client or by a client toward the massage therapist
- Disrobing or draping practices that reflect a lack of respect for the client's or massage therapist's privacy
- Inappropriate comments about or to the client or by the client about the massage therapist, such as
  Sexualized or sexually demeaning comments

Comments concerning sexual orientation
  Discussion of potential sexual performance
  Conversations about sexual preferences or fantasies
- Therapist–client sex, whether initiated by the client or massage professional

---

THE RECEPTION ROOM

The reception room creates an impression of the massage environment and the massage therapist. Business success is influenced by how you set up and maintain the reception area. If you have your own business, the design of the reception area is your responsibility. You must also take on the role of receptionist. If you are employed, the employer is responsible for the business environment, including the reception room and designating someone who takes care of the receptionist duties. You may be able to have productive input about improving and maintaining a reception process.

Role of the Receptionist

In the small, single-person massage practice, you assume many roles, including receptionist. If you are working in a larger setting, a receptionist may be hired to handle the responsibilities of the reception room. *LIKE ANY OTHER BUSINE[SS]*

The receptionist usually is the first person to greet clients as they enter the office, and he or she should appear neat and professional. In health care business offices, the receptionist can wear appropriate business dress or a uniform. The receptionist's clothing or uniform should be clean, shoes should be well polished and clean, and hair should be neatly styled. The positive image of the receptionist indicates a clean and well-organized office (Box 3-2). Because the image portrayed in this role must remain with the client, this is no place to try out new clothing styles, experiment with garish jewelry, or wear facial and oral piercings.

As the client enters the office, the receptionist acknowledges the client immediately with a pleasant smile and a cheerful "hello" and calls him or her by name. Everyone likes the feeling of being recognized. Even if the receptionist is busy with a telephone call, she or he should look up and smile to acknowledge the client.

Reception Room Appeal

A bright, cheerful, and pleasantly decorated office usually makes a favorable impression on the client. If the room appears to have a warm and friendly atmosphere, the client will relax. Design of the reception room for the client's comfort is discussed in Chapter 6.

The reception room should have a good selection of reading material that is current and appeals to a wide variety of interests. Health-related magazines, cookbooks, and recipe

BOX 3-2	Tips for Professional Etiquette in the Massage Office

- Use correct grammar; pronounce words correctly; expand your vocabulary.
- Explain technical terms in understandable language without being demeaning.
- Make clients feel important; discuss issues of interest to them.
- Perform proper introductions of the client and staff members.
- Introduce yourself to a new client; shake hands heartily to extend a warm welcome.
- If a client is engaged in a conversation with another person, avoid standing within hearing range. If you wish to talk to one of them, leave the area and return later.
- Don't eat or drink in front of clients.
- Say "Thank you" when a client is helpful, has cooperated during treatment, or has complimented you.
- Send thank-you notes for referrals or other thoughtful acts.
- Respect the client's privacy.
- If the telephone rings while you are talking to a client, excuse yourself to answer it. If a lengthy conversation is expected, ask the caller if you can return the call, then complete the business with the client.

The answer to...

What's for dinner?

COMPLIMENTS OF

RECIPE   Luke Fritz, MT, NCTMB   SERVES
                123-456-7890

FIGURE 3-8. A recipe card is available in the reception room for copying information from magazines. *(Modified from Finkbeiner BL, Finkbeiner CA:* Practice Management for the Dental Team, *ed 6, St. Louis, 2006, Mosby.)*

or magazine related to massage therapy to read so that your wait time is productive.

cards for jotting down information that clients find interesting are helpful (Fig. 3-8).

Avoid dirty carpets, frayed furniture, and unsightly plants. Children's books and quiet games and toys should be available if children are part of the massage practice. An area designated as a children's play area is helpful. If background music is played in the office, be sure to select music that has a soothing effect rather than loud rock or heavy concert music. A drinking fountain or water cooler with paper cups should be available for clients while they wait and after their appointments.

One of the responsibilities of the receptionist is to keep clients informed about delays or to indicate what the waiting time will be. Unexpected delays or emergencies should be explained honestly, and the client should be contacted if possible about the length of wait time.

The Greeting Process for On-Site Massage

If your massage business is based on going to a client's home or business location, you still need to attend to the concept of the reception room. You need to announce your presence by knocking, ringing a doorbell, or talking with the client's business receptionist. You then enter the area in an unobtrusive manner. The area you set up for massage needs to be pleasant. When the client is ready for massage, the initial greeting needs to be professional. This is more difficult in the relaxed atmosphere of a client's home. You may be the one waiting because the client is more likely to be delayed by a family or business concern. Always carry with you a book

CLIENT POLICY AND PROCEDURES BROCHURE

Purpose

The client policy and procedures brochure is the key to establishing an understanding between the client and the massage therapist and staff. The brochure should be a written statement of the philosophy and policies, defining the responsibilities of the client and those of the massage staff. It is given to a new client at the first visit and serves as an informational device and a good public relations tool.

A new practitioner often neglects to establish a client policy and procedures document, only to be confronted with misunderstandings with clients at a later date. The client policy and procedures brochure should be implemented when the business is first opened and should be revised as the practice grows and changes. However, the policy can be integrated into an established practice with minimal effort. If you are considering employment as a massage therapist, make sure that the business you are considering working with has reasonable policies and procedures written down and that you are willing and able to be in compliance with them.

Brochure Contents

Each practice has specific needs, but all brochures should include the following elements (Box 3-3):

Philosophy: This is a statement of the massage therapist's attitude toward the practice of massage and, more

BOX 3-3	Developing a Client Brochure and Policy Statement

A massage professional should cover the following important points in developing a client brochure and policy statement.

TYPE OF SERVICE
- Explain the type of work you provide.
- Explain the benefits and limitations of this particular style of massage.
- Specify whether you specialize in working with a particular group, such as elderly people, athletes, or people with specific problems such as headaches or back pain.
- Indicate any situations or conditions with which you do not care to work, such as pregnancy or certain medical conditions.

TRAINING AND EXPERIENCE
- If your state requires licensing or if you are nationally certified, provide documentation.
- State how long you have been in practice, what school you attended, whether the school was approved by any state or accrediting body, and how many classroom hours were required for graduation.
- Provide information about continuing education you have pursued.
- Provide information about any additional education; for example, that you are also an athletic trainer.
- Provide the names of any professional organizations of which you are an active member.

APPOINTMENT POLICIES
- Specify the length of an average session.
- Inform the client of the days you work, your hours, and whether you do on-site residential or business work.
- Inform the client that the first appointment for intake will be longer than subsequent appointments; also state whether you take emergency appointments and how often you suggest that clients come for massage sessions.
- Be clear about the cancellation policy and your policy for late appointments.
- Explain to the client any change in or restriction on physical activity before or after the session.

EXPECTATIONS OF CLIENTS AND PRACTITIONERS
- Explain in detail what happens at the first massage session (i.e., paperwork, medical history, other preliminaries).
- Make sure that clients know they can partly undress or undress down to their underclothes and that they are always covered and draped during the session.
- Explain the order in which you massage (face up or face down to begin), the parts of the body on which you work and in what order, whether you use oils or creams, if a shower is available before or after the massage, and if bathing at home before the massage appointment is expected.
- Make sure the client understands whether talking is appropriate during the session and that you should be informed if anything feels uncomfortable.
- If you have low lighting and music during the session, be sure the client is comfortable with that atmosphere.
- Make sure the client understands when a reaction might be expected, such as tenderness over a trigger point when direct pressure methods are used.
- Tell clients that before the session you will discuss with them the goals for the massage, as well as the proposed styles and methods of massage, and that consent must be given for all massage procedures.
- Inform the client that your profession has a code of ethics and explain your policy on confidentiality.
- Let clients know that if they are uncomfortable in any way, a friend or relative may accompany them.

FEES
Make sure your fee structure is clearly defined regarding the following:
- How often you raise your fees
- Whether you have a sliding fee scale
- Whether you take only cash or will accept money orders, checks, or credit cards
- Whether you bill
- Whether you accept insurance
- How often insurance covers your services
- Different fees for variations in the length of a session
- Whether a series of sessions can be bought at a discount

Let's take 15 minutes to write an outline (two sentences for each heading) for your business's client brochure + policy statement.
Learning Activity Pg. 59

specifically, the moral and ethical obligation to the client. In this section, the massage therapist can make a statement about how the practice is unique and what special features are likely to attract and retain clients.

Office hours: Although business hours may occasionally vary, specific hours should be listed for the client's benefit.

Appointment control: A statement should be included designating the person who makes appointments. A broken appointment policy should be included in the office policy and should be adhered to consistently.

Payment policy: The massage therapist should outline acceptable payment options, and they should be described in detail. The person responsible for implementing the payment options should be identified.

Hygiene: The value of hygiene before receiving a massage can be emphasized by statements such as, "Please bathe before the massage appointment."

Attitude toward children: The treatment of children must be explained. A parent or guardian must be present during the massage.

Infection-control policies: These policies should be explained to assure clients that the latest barrier techniques and preventive concepts are being used for their protection.

Quality assurance: This is an explanation of efforts taken to ensure that procedures and techniques used in the office are routinely evaluated to maintain good quality.

Continuing education: Clients appreciate knowing that the massage therapist makes efforts to update his or her skills.

Office data: The massage therapist's name, address, phone number, fax, and e-mail address should appear on the cover or be easy to find within the policy for the client's convenience.

The style of the brochure should be attractive, well organized, brief, and sized to be easily handled by clients (Fig. 3-9). Many businesses prefer to use a printing service to achieve a professional-looking pamphlet. In Figure 3-10, the policy has been printed on both sides of heavy, 8.5 by 11 inch bond paper that is folded in half. A simpler, less expensive statement printed on business letterhead is shown in Figure 3-11. The business policy and procedures pamphlet

has two primary purposes: it is a practice builder, and it informs the client about office procedures and the massage therapist's philosophy. When it achieves both purposes, the office policy becomes a valuable public relations device.

LEARNING ACTIVITY

Using the components listed in this chapter, develop a client policy and procedures brochure. Each practice has its own specific needs, but the brochure should include the following elements:

- Philosophy
- Office hours
- Appointment control
- Payment policy
- Hygiene
- Attitude toward children
- Infection-control policies
- Quality assurance
- Continuing education
- Office data

RECOURSE POLICY

If a client is unhappy or dissatisfied, how do you plan to deal with the situation? Do you offer a refund or a free session, do nothing, or discuss it with the client? You do need to let the client know that if the matter is not handled satisfactorily, complaints can be registered at a professional organization or licensing board.

Some professionals send out client policy and procedures booklets before the scheduled appointment. If this is done, include a personalized cover letter asking the client to read the booklet carefully and stating that you will discuss it with him or her at the first appointment.

The policies you set for your business practice demand serious thought. If you are self-employed, you have discretion about what polices you set and how to enforce them. If you are employed, the employer is responsible for this task.

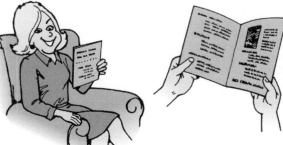
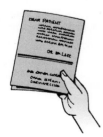
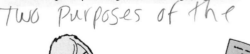

FIGURE 3-9. A client reads the office policy. *(Modified from Finkbeiner BL, Finkbeiner CA: Practice Management for the Dental Team, ed 6, St. Louis, 2006, Mosby.)*

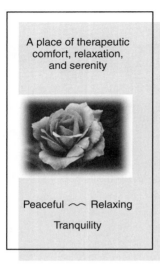

A place of therapeutic comfort, relaxation, and serenity

Peaceful ～～ Relaxing

Tranquility

1. *Appointment cancellation.* A broken appointment that is not caused by an emergency 24 hours before the appointment may result in a cancellation fee of $25.00.

2. *Hygiene.* Please bathe before the massage appointment.

3. *Children.* A parent or guardian must be present during the massage.

4. *Infection control.* The latest barrier techniques and current preventative concepts are being used for everyone's protection.

5. *Quality assurance.* The office policies and procedures are routinely evaluated to maintain good quality.

6. *Training.* Every year, the minimum of 3 credit hours of education is obtained to stay current on research, trends, and treatment.

YOUR MASSAGE SESSION

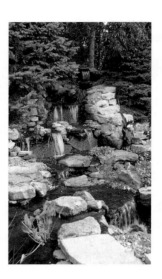

Luke Fritz
204 W Nepessing St
Lapeer, MI 48446
Phone 123-456-7890
E-mail hec@sbcglobal.net

All Services Are by Appointment Only

Available Hours
Monday–Friday: 10 AM–8:45 PM
Last massage starts at 7:30 PM
Saturday: 9 AM–5:30 PM
Last massage starts at 4 PM
Sunday: 10 AM–5 PM
Last massage starts at 3:30 PM

Forms of Payment Accepted
Cash, checks, and money orders are accepted. Credit cards are not.

Travel to Client
An additional charge for travel to the client depends on the time and distance involved. The minimum additional charge is $30.00.

Contraindications to Massage
Massage or bodywork may not be advised for certain medical conditions, such as a fever, which indicates an infection. If a massage is potentially harmful to a client's condition, the massage therapist has the right to decline to perform the massage.

Insurance Claims
I do not handle insurance forms but will provide a receipt for you to submit to your insurance company for possible reimbursement.

What to Expect during Your Bodywork or Massage Session

Your massage or bodywork session takes place in a warm, comfortable, quiet room. Soft music usually is played, and you may request a particular style of music, including classical, nature sounds, new age, or jazz.

No two massages are exactly alike. Because the body is always in a state of flux and what you may want to address in one session may not be relevant in another, you may request the massage therapist use a certain technique or modality. Most massage and bodywork sessions are traditionally performed with the client unclothed, with underwear left on. However, you may decide what amount of clothing you prefer to wear for your own comfort. The massage practitioner leaves the room so you can undress in privacy and then lie underneath the top draping material. You will remain properly draped during the massage session, which is performed with you underneath a set of sheets and perhaps a blanket for extra warmth. A typical full-body session includes work on your back, arms, legs, head, neck, and shoulders. The buttock area is massaged in relation to the back and legs unless you request differently. You are not touched

inappropriately—on or near your genitals (male or female) or breasts (female). A light oil or massage cream (with or without aroma therapy essential oils) may be used to permit muscles to be worked on without causing excessive friction on the skin. In a general full-body massage, the session may start with broad, flowing strokes that help to calm the nervous system and relax exterior muscle tension. As your body becomes relaxed, pressure may gradually be increased to relax specific areas and to relieve muscular tension. You should communicate with the therapist immediately if you feel any discomfort or pain.

Therapy sessions are 35, 70, or 90 minutes long. Many people prefer the longer sessions for optimal relaxation. Always allow relaxation time before and after the massage session. After a massage, most people feel very relaxed, and some experience freedom from long-term aches and pains caused by tension or repetitive activity. An initial period of feeling slowed down is often replaced by an experience of increased energy, heightened awareness, and greater productivity, which can last for days.

FIGURE 3-10. Example of a brochure explaining the massage therapy office policy. *(Modified from Associated Bodywork and Massage Professionals.)* ⊜ Brochure templates for your use are located on the Evolve Web site at http://evolve.elsevier.com/Fritz/business.

Luke Fritz, MT, NCTMB
2050 Leisure Lane, Lapeer, MI 48446
(123) 456-7890 / leisurelymassage@hec.com

All Services Are by Appointment Only

Available Hours
Monday–Friday: 10 AM–8:45 PM   Last massage starts at 7:30 PM
Saturday: 9 AM–5:30 PM   Last massage starts at 4 PM
Sunday: 10 AM–5 PM   Last massage starts at 3:30 PM

Forms of Payment Accepted
Cash, checks, and money orders are accepted. Credit cards are not.

Travel to Client
An additional charge for travel to the client depends on the time and distance involved. The minimum additional charge is $30.00.

Contraindications to Massage
Massage or bodywork may not be advised for certain medical conditions, such as a fever, which indicates an infection. If a massage is potentially harmful to a client's condition, the massage therapist has the right to decline to perform the massage.

Insurance Claims
I do not handle insurance forms but will provide a receipt for you to submit to your insurance company for possible reimbursement.

What to Expect during Your Bodywork or Massage Session
Your massage or bodywork session takes place in a warm, comfortable, quiet room. Soft music usually is played, and you may request a particular style of music, including classical, nature sounds, new age, or jazz.

No two massages are exactly alike. Because the body is always in a state of flux and what you may want to address in one session may not be relevant in another, you may request the massage therapist use a certain technique or modality.

Most massage and bodywork sessions are traditionally performed with the client unclothed, with underwear left on. However, you may decide what amount of clothing you prefer to wear for your own comfort. The massage practitioner leaves the room so you can undress in privacy and then lie underneath the top draping material. You will remain properly draped during the massage session, which is performed with you underneath a set of sheets and perhaps a blanket for extra warmth.

A typical full-body session includes work on your back, arms, legs, head, neck, and shoulders. The buttock area is massaged in relation to the back and legs unless you request differently. You are not touched inappropriately—on or near your genitals (male or female) or breasts (female). A light oil or massage cream (with or without aroma therapy essential oils) may be used to permit muscles to be worked on without causing excessive friction on the skin.

In a general full-body massage, the session may start with broad, flowing strokes that help to calm the nervous system and relax exterior muscle tension. As your body becomes relaxed, pressure may gradually be increased to relax specific areas and to relieve muscular tension. You should communicate with the therapist immediately if you feel any discomfort or pain.

Therapy sessions are 35, 70, or 90 minutes long. Many people prefer the longer sessions for optimal relaxation. Always allow relaxation time before and after the massage session. After a massage, most people feel very relaxed, and some experience freedom from long-term aches and pains caused by tension or repetitive activity. An initial period of feeling slowed down is often replaced by an experience of increased energy, heightened awareness, and greater productivity, which can last for days.

FIGURE 3-11.   Massage therapy office policy example: simple piece of paper. *(Modified from Associated Bodywork and Massage Professionals.)* ⊖ Templates for brochures are located on the Evolve Web site at http://evolve.elsevier.com/Fritz/business.

You need to be informed about the policies and procedures of the employer to be able to explain them to clients. One criterion for a good employment fit is whether you agree with the office's policies and procedures and are willing to support their enforcement. If the policies are similar to those that you would set for yourself, it is an indication that you will be comfortable in the environment. However, if you have a disagreement about how clients are cared for, it will be difficult for you to be comfortable and, therefore, to be a productive employee.

SUMMARY

The importance of meeting clients' needs can be understood in terms of Maslow's hierarchy of needs and Rogers' client-centered therapy. Not all communication is verbal. Nonverbal communication is often a more accurate projection of feelings, but it is important to not assume the meaning of body language. The rights of clients permeate many aspects of professional behavior, such as respect, confidentiality, quality care, and accommodation for those with special needs.

 ## Good Stuff from the Government

SMALL BUSINESS ASSOCIATION: CUSTOMER SERVICE IS AN IMPERATIVE

The Golden Rule—do unto others as you would have them do unto you—may seem self-evident in the way we try to conduct our personal lives. However, this axiom is assuming new importance as a guiding principle in the world of business. The climate of the recession-ridden early 1980s, when customers blithely traded away high-quality service in exchange for price reductions or convenience, no longer exists. Customers are again demanding service. Companies of all sizes realize that their strongest selling point can boil down to treating customers as they would like to be treated or better. "Consumers are beginning to feel that their needs haven't been met," explains Bonnie Jansen of the U.S. Office of Consumer Affairs. "They're sick of getting poor service all the time."

The message is getting through. According to John Goodman, president of the Technical Assistance Research Programs Institute (TARP), "In the past few years, companies began to realize that service was really a competitive factor, and they began to view it as an integral part of their product."

The growing significance of meeting or exceeding customer demands for quality service has special implications for small businesses. In this arena, small companies can in the least expensive way set themselves apart from the competition.

A 3-year study by the National Federation of Independent Businesses (NFIB) in Washington, DC, showed that small businesses that strongly emphasized customer service were more likely to survive and succeed than competitors who emphasized advantages such as lower prices or type of product.

GOLDEN RULE 1: PUT THE CUSTOMER FIRST

"A strong customer ethic must guide your business from the inception," writes author and business owner Paul Hawken in his book *Growing a Business*. "No matter whether you manufacture, grow, produce, distribute, or sell, you are 'in service.'"

Quality customer service begins with your employees. An owner of a successful chain of hair salons advises that the first step is to set standards and then ensure that everyone in the company understands them. He recommends rewarding employees for achieving your service goals. Be sure to seek and solve any annoyances employees have that may lead to poor

morale. An employee with a complaint cannot be completely effective in dealing with customers. Hawken says, "If you take care of your employees, they will take care of your customers." However, he also warns that if your employees are not customer oriented, no standards or goals can change the situation: "We concentrate on hiring people who embody the quality of service for which we strive. It is difficult to teach someone to be helpful and serve others if he or she is misanthropic to begin with."

Hiring the best people means trusting them. Your employees should be able to do what is necessary to make the customer happy without fear of reprisal. Hawken says, "Policies and procedures are helpful only as guides toward an end result. When employees run out of possibilities to make the customer happy, they must have the latitude to improvise to make it right. Most employees operate in a state of fear that their own generosity with a customer will be viewed as foolishness by their boss. This situation will stifle flexible customer service."

GOLDEN RULE 2: STAY CLOSE TO YOUR CUSTOMERS

In the smartest companies, asking questions and listening carefully to the answers is an important part of customer service. These firms train their employees to focus on what the customer is saying and then tailor products or services to meet customers' needs. Says one corporate executive whose words also hold true for smaller firms, "Knowing what's on the customer's mind is the smartest thing we can do."

It is also cheaper than attracting new customers. According to the Customer Service Institute, 65% of a company's business comes from existing customers, and it costs five times as much to attract a new customer than to keep an existing one satisfied.

Losing a customer is even more expensive. According to studies by the TARP, 91% of unhappy customers will never again buy from a company that has displeased them; they will also voice their dissatisfaction to at least seven other people.

The responsibility to be receptive does not lie solely with your employees. If you want your business to be successful, you must listen to and talk with customers. There is no substitute for getting out and learning from the customers themselves how you may serve them better. The best business owners are committed to staying close to their clientele, and they identify with them. Owners give their customers the

Good Stuff from the Government—cont'd

level of service the owners would expect to receive. A good relationship with customers necessitates paying attention to every link in the distribution chain; this means listening to everyone who helps get your products to market and asking them for suggestions on improving your service. Be sure to take advantage of feedback from employees, especially those whose everyday job is dealing with customers. They can serve as tremendous reservoirs of information.

"Our goal as a company is to create customer service that is not just the best, but legendary," Paul Hawken asserts. "'Legendary' gives everyone who deals with customers a rich sense of the possibilities."

GOLDEN RULE 3: PAY ATTENTION TO DETAILS

Many owners search for a special touch that will make them stand out from the crowd. Discount coupons, longer hours, home delivery, or free coffee, for example, show customers you want to take that extra step to please them.

Some of the most effective extras are really basic adages of conducting good business, although customers are often surprised when they take place. These actions include answering the phone by the third ring, treating customers respectfully and courteously at all times, greeting them by name, promptly answering their questions (and if you cannot, getting back to them with an answer as quickly as possible), and manufacturing high-quality goods that work the first time and keep working.

FIVE RULES OF CUSTOMER CARE

Essential to keeping customers happy is understanding the way they think. For example, customers do business on the basis of emotional desire—they want what they want when they want it. Customers also tend to gravitate toward a company or group of people they like. Most customers have a strong tendency to stick with businesses with which they are familiar, and they are slow to change buying habits unless given a good reason. However, when they are displeased, even by a small disappointment

or discourteous word, various surveys have revealed that customers tell 7 to 11 people about their dissatisfaction.

An important key to serving customers well is this: do not try to change them. Here are five specific steps to help you take full advantage of the critical element of customer care:

1. Conduct your own survey. Profit from the ideas, suggestions, and complaints of your present and former customers. Meet and talk with your customers. Ask questions. Learn their attitudes, what they want, and what they dislike.
2. Check employees' telephone manners periodically. This is particularly important for small businesses, because bad telephone handling can undermine other constructive efforts to build a profitable enterprise.
3. Rules such as prompt answering and a cheerful attitude of helpfulness are essential. Have someone whose voice is unfamiliar play the role of a customer or prospective customer, preferably a difficult one.
4. Make customer service a team effort. Use group meetings, memos, posters, and in-house publications to build customer consciousness throughout the organization. Continually drive home the crucial rule that getting and holding customers requires team play, and invite employees' ideas.
5. Extend your efforts after hours. It is the friendly feelings people have that drew them to you and your business. Take advantage of the relaxed atmosphere of social occasions or a neighborly chat over the back fence to turn friends into customers or to reinforce the loyalty of existing ones.

Customer service is enjoying a resurgence, and no business can afford to take customers for granted. To succeed, you must give your customers what they want, not what you think they want. That means providing courteous, friendly service to your customers, your suppliers, and others with whom you come in contact. If you want to keep customers coming back for more, practicing the Golden Rule in all domains of business makes sense.

From The U.S. Small Business Administration, available at http://www.sba.gov/smallbusinessplanner/manage/marketandprice/.

The client's perception of the business may be based on the appearance of the massage facility and the demeanor of the welcoming staff. Clients also have obligations, which should be carefully outlined in the policy and procedures brochure provided to the client. Clients are the most important persons in the massage business operation, and when satisfied, they are your best form of marketing. The good stuff from the government allows you to view interviews with successful business people to learn how to develop your massage therapy business.

Bibliography

Bernstein DA, Nash PW: *Essentials of Psychology*, ed 2, Boston, 2002, Houghton Mifflin.

Frazier GL: *Connecting with Customers*, ed 2, Upper Saddle River, NJ, 2004, Prentice-Hall.

Locker KO, Kyo Kaczmarek S: *Business Communication: Building Critical Skills*, ed 2, New York, 2003, Irwin/McGraw-Hill.

Mosley DC, Meggisson LC, Pietri PH: *Supervisory Management*, ed 4, Cincinnati, OH, 2001, South-Western.

Rathfus SA: *Psychology in the New Millennium*, ed 7, Orlando, FL, 1999, Harcourt Brace.

Evolve Annotated Web Links

http://evolve.elsevier.com/Fritz/business

Small Business Association: http://www.sba.gov/tools/audiovideo/deliveringsuccess/index.html

American Massage Therapy Association: www.amtamassage.org

Associated Bodywork and Massage Professionals: www.abmp.org

1. Identify and give examples of barriers in communication.

_____

_____

_____

_____

_____

_____

_____

2. Describe the duties of a receptionist in communicating with clients and putting them at ease.

_____

_____

_____

_____

_____

_____

3. Explain Maslow's hierarchy of needs and Carl Rogers' client-centered therapy as they relate to therapeutic massage.

_____

4. List five rights of the client that should be considered during a treatment procedure.

_____

_____

_____

_____

_____

_____

_____

5. Observe nonverbal behavior. During your daily activities, become aware of nonverbal cues given to you. What types of facial expressions, hand movements, and torso movements do you notice? Do they affect your behavior?

_____

_____

_____

_____

_____

_____

6. List the preconceptions that a client may have about a massage practice and any associated staff.

_____

_____

_____

_____

_____

_____

7. List attitudes that a massage therapist may have about a client. Are there similarities or differences in the perceptions of each of these people?

_____

_____

_____

_____

_____

_____

_____

4

LEGAL AND ETHICAL ISSUES IN THE MASSAGE PROFESSIONAL PRACTICE

OUTLINE

Professional Practice
Definition of Law
Classifications of Law
  Crimes and Torts
  Good Samaritan Law
  Americans with Disabilities Act
  Contracts
  Legal and Ethical Monetary Responsibilities
  Managed Care Legalities
Records Management
Litigation
Massage Practice Acts and Credentialing
  Federation of State Massage Therapy Boards and the
    Massage and Bodywork Licensing Examination

Voluntary Credentialing: Validation of Excellence
Value of Credentialing beyond Licensure
Educational Standards for Legal and Ethical Massage
  Therapy Practice
Ethics
  Ethics in Massage Therapy
  Maintaining Quality Service
  Consent
  Making Ethical Decisions
Summary

KEY TERMS

Accreditation
Americans with Disabilities Act
Beneficence
Certification
Civil law
Computer security
Consent
Contract
Credentialing
Crime
Criminal law
Defamation of character
Defendant

Ethics
Expert witness
Fact witness
Felony
Fraud
Informed consent
Invasion of privacy
Justice
Laws
Lawsuit
Litigation
Malpractice
Managed care

Misdemeanor
Massage Practice Act
Morals
Nonmalfeasance
Negligence
Piracy
Plaintiff
Standard of care
Supervision
Tort
Values

e Guidelines for the Learning Activities and answers to the Workbook questions are located on Evolve at http://evolve.elsevier.com/Fritz/business.

LEARNING OUTCOMES

Mastery of the content in this chapter will enable the reader to

- Define glossary terms
- Explain the impact of ethics and law on the massage professional practice
- Differentiate between the various types of law that affect the practice of massage therapy
- Explain various types of consent

- Describe situations in the massage business office that can lead to potential litigation
- Describe the code of ethics of professional massage organizations
- Identify nine steps in making ethical decisions

Each day, massage professionals are faced with issues involving the legal requirements and standards of care in the delivery of massage treatment. The Massage Practice Act (i.e., licensing) of each state defines the requirements necessary to practice therapeutic massage and the scope of massage practice for that particular state. Standards for massage care may arise from professional organizations and statutory law (enacted by a legislative body). Although most states have licensing laws for massage practice, not all regulate massage. The massage professional also is governed by voluntary standards, such as the principles of *ethics*, developed and implemented by the massage profession itself. The ⊝ Evolve Web site provides links to the various state regulations.

PROFESSIONAL PRACTICE

Legal and voluntary requirements and standards are implemented for the protection of society and, ultimately, the client. This process of regulation is illustrated in Figure 4-1. The massage therapist needs to have an understanding of the effect of law on the massage practice and an awareness of its importance on his or her performance of daily duties. Each member of a professional organization should be familiar with the code of ethics for its professional group.

Membership in a professional organization is voluntary, and the standards of these organizations are considered voluntary. However, the standards are used as guidelines in peer review. Professional organizations continually reassess the functions of their standards and the qualifications of their members. Examples of voluntary standards are illustrated in the profession's code of ethics, professional standards for *accreditation* of educational programs, and standards for *credentialing*.

Legal standards for massage result in standards such as the informed consent doctrine (discussed later). Legislative action through various Massage Practice Acts establishes the legal requirements and scope of the practice within a state, province, and, in some instances, country. This action establishes education, credentialing, and licensure requirements for the massage therapist.

Copies of the principles of ethics for any of the massage professional organizations may be obtained from their national offices or official Web sites. To obtain a copy of a state Massage Practice Act, contact the Board of Massage in your state (province in Canada) or the Federation of State Massage Therapy Boards (FSMTB), or obtain information on the Massage and Bodywork Licensing Examination (MBLEx).

DEFINITION OF LAW

Law consists of enforceable rules governing relationships among individuals and between individuals and their society. A broad definition of the law implies that there must be established rules, such as constitutions, statutes, administrative agency rules, and judicial decisions. Rules of law must be enforceable and establish limits of conduct for governments and individuals in society.

In many states, the Board of Massage is an administrative agency at the state level. The executive officers of an administrative agency perform specific functions, including enforcing laws within their agency. The state boards have the power to make rules and regulations that conform to enacted laws that govern therapeutic massage. The FSMTB (http://www.fsmtb.org/) is an organization made up of the various massage therapy boards in the United States.

Rules and regulations adopted by each state massage board are components of the body of law, referred to as administrative laws. State statutes must conform to the state's constitution and the federal constitution.

CLASSIFICATIONS OF LAW

Because it is common for massage to be regulated by legislation, it becomes necessary for you to understand what laws are. Laws can be divided into two classifications: civil and criminal. *Civil law* relates to duties between persons or between citizens and their government. *Criminal law* deals with wrongs committed against the public as a whole.

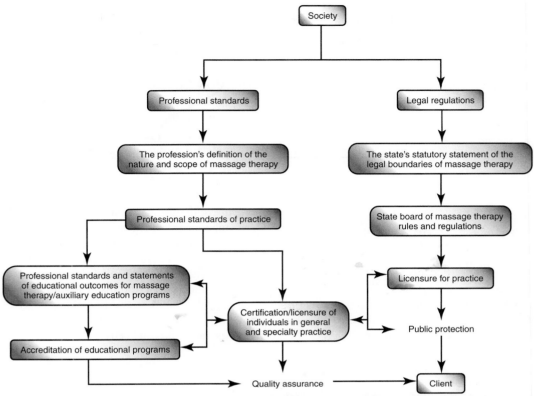

FIGURE 4-1. Diagram of professional and legal regulations of massage therapy. (*Adapted from Finkbeiner BL, Finkbeiner CA: Practice Management for the Dental Team, ed 6, St. Louis, 2006, Mosby.*)

In a civil case, one party tries to correct interference with his or her interest by another party. The other party might have failed to comply with a duty or otherwise breached an acceptable standard of conduct. The other party may be required to pay for the damages caused by failure to comply with that duty. In criminal law, the interests of society are at stake, and the government may seek to impose a penalty, such as a fine or imprisonment, on the guilty person.

Crimes and Torts

A *crime* is a wrongdoing against the public at large, and it is prosecuted by a public official. In most cases when a crime is committed, there is intent to do wrong. However, a person or entity that breaks certain laws may be guilty of a crime whether there was intent or not. Criminal liability typically involves the performance of a prohibited act and a specified state of mind or intent on the part of the person or entity committing the crime. In some cases, the omission of an act can be a crime if the person or entity has a legal duty to perform the act, such as failure to file a federal income tax return.

A crime can be classified as a *misdemeanor* or a *felony*. A misdemeanor is less serious than a felony and is punishable by a fine or imprisonment up to 1 year. A felony is a more serious crime and usually is punishable by imprisonment for a longer period.

A *tort* is a civil wrongdoing. It is an interference with a recognized interest or a breach of a legal duty owed by a *defendant* to a *plaintiff*. The plaintiff in most instances must show that the defendant's action or omission was a cause of loss or harm to the plaintiff. A tort usually is resolved through a civil trial with a monetary settlement for damages. Included in torts are the areas of negligence, assault and battery, infliction of mental distress, defamation, and fraud.

Torts may be intentional or unintentional acts of wrongdoing. If intentional, the person committing the tort intended to commit the wrongful act. Intentional torts for which a massage therapist can be held liable include assault and battery, defamation of character, invasion of privacy, immoral conduct, and fraud.

Unintentional torts do not require a particular mental state. Failure to exercise a *standard of care*, such as performing a treatment that a reasonably prudent professional would perform in similar circumstances, is an example of an unintentional tort. Even if a massage professional neither wishes to bring about the consequences of the act nor believes that they will occur, negligence may be alleged whereby someone suffers injury because another failed to live up to a particular standard of care. Questions relating to the failure to exercise

---

BOX 4-1	Common Negligent Acts in a Massage Office

- Failure to protect clients from allergic reactions
- Use of defective equipment
- Failure to observe client reactions to massage and take appropriate action
- Failure to exercise good judgment
- Failure to communicate
- Loss of or damage to client's personal property
- Disease transmission

---

a standard of care need to be answered. The following four elements make up the unintentional tort of negligence:

1. Was there a duty to follow a standard of care?
2. Was this duty breached?
3. Did the plaintiff suffer injury?
4. Was the injury a direct result of that breach of duty?

Strict liability is an unintentional tort. It relates to a person being liable for actions regardless of the care exercised and for damages or injuries caused by the act.

NEGLIGENCE

Negligence is the performance of an act that a reasonably careful person under similar circumstances would not do or the failure to perform an act that a reasonably careful person would do under similar circumstances.

Negligence is an act of omission (i.e., neglecting to do something that a reasonably prudent person would do) or commission (i.e., doing something that a reasonably prudent person would not do). To prove negligence, it is necessary to prove that there has been a breach of duty owed, including deviation from the standard of care. In a massage negligence case, it is often necessary to provide expert testimony. To prove negligence, the plaintiff must show that there is an obligation to provide care according to a specified standard; that there was failure to meet that standard; that the failure to meet the standard led to injury; and that there was actual injury to the client.

MALPRACTICE

Professionals usually consider *malpractice* a form of negligence, but in a broader sense, it can mean any wrongdoing by a professional. Malpractice can refer to any professional misconduct, evil practice, or illegal or immoral conduct, not just negligence. Malpractice can be unintentional or intentional. Box 4-1 contains a list of negligent acts that may occur in a massage office.

DEFAMATION OF CHARACTER

Defamation of character is the communication of false information to a third party about a person that results in injury to that person's reputation. The communication can be verbal (slander) or written (libel). The false statement may be about a person's product, business, profession, or title to

property. A massage professional should make statements about a client or other professional only as it relates to the rendering of massage care and only to other massage care providers involved in that care.

INVASION OF PRIVACY

Invasion of privacy is a tort that refers to several wrongs involving the use of otherwise private information. As relevant here, a tort may involve publishing or otherwise making known or using information relating to the private life or affairs of a person without that person's approval or permission; prying into private affairs; or appropriating the plaintiff's identity for commercial use.

To avoid this situation, you must remember that any information a client gives you or the massage office staff remains confidential within the office. No information about a client should be shared outside the office. When a client requests a transfer of massage treatment records, a signed authorization to transfer should be completed by the client. In the health care setting, the massage therapist must adhere to the regulations of the Health Insurance Portability and Accountability Act (HIPAA).

COMPUTER SECURITY

The massage therapist may be exposed to activities that may cause illegal or unethical activity while using a computer. *Computer security* refers to safeguards that are implemented to prevent and detect unauthorized access or deliberate damage to a computer system and data. A *computer crime* is the use of a computer to commit an illegal act.

In a massage office, the most common activity that can violate computer integrity is software theft, or *piracy*. Some people make an illegal copy of a disk or tape instead of paying for an authorized copy. Software theft is a violation of copyright law, and it is a crime. For large users, such as massage schools or other health care institutions, most software companies provide a site license and multiple-copy discounts.

Although most massage offices use personal computers rather than a mainframe, the potential for gaining unauthorized access to data still exists, especially in a hospital-type setting. If you inadvertently gain access on the computer to unauthorized or confidential data, you should exit the file, including the data, and report to the appropriate supervisor that you accidentally entered a confidential file. To make changes in a confidential file without authorized permission constitutes an unethical and possibly illegal act. Refer to the HIPAA standards in Chapter 7 to ensure information integrity.

Good Samaritan Law

During the past 3 decades in the United States, every state has passed some form of legislation that grants immunity for acts performed by a person who renders care in an emergency situation. This concept, called the Good Samaritan law, was considered necessary to create an incentive for health care providers to provide medical assistance to the injured in cases of automobile accidents or other disasters without the fear of possible litigation. This law is intended for individuals who do not seek compensation but rather are solely interested in providing care to the injured in a caring, safe manner, with no intent to do bodily harm. This law does not provide protection for a negligent health care provider who is being compensated for services.

Americans with Disabilities Act

In 1990, the federal government enacted legislation to ensure that persons with some degree of disability are not discriminated against. The Americans with Disabilities Act (ADA) affects the massage office in the area of prohibitions against employment discrimination and by requiring facilities to be accessible to physically and mentally compromised clients. This law identifies five categories of persons who are protected from discrimination. The categories protect individuals who have a physical or mental impairment that substantially limits one or more major life activities, those who have a record of such impairment, and those who are regarded as having such impairment:

1. Persons whose physical or mental impairment substantially limits one or more major life activities, such as seeing, hearing, speaking, walking, breathing, performing manual tasks, learning, caring for oneself, or working. Included in this category are persons who have disabling conditions such as acquired immunodeficiency syndrome (AIDS), human immunodeficiency virus (HIV) infections, heart disease, diabetes, cancer, learning disabilities, and mental retardation.
2. Persons who have a record of impairment, such as a history of heart disease or mental illness
3. Persons who, although fully functional and not disabled, are regarded as having such an impairment due to severe disfigurement
4. Persons who are discriminated against because they have a known association or relationship with a disabled individual
5. Persons who currently participate in or who have completed a drug or alcohol rehabilitation program

Box 4-2 lists Titles that describe the provisions of the ADA. This federal mandate is aimed at the elimination of discrimination against individuals with disabilities and clearly defines enforceable standards. It is wise to obtain a copy of this act for the office and routinely update the office policies as required. The address for the Office of Americans with Disabilities is listed in Chapter 6.

BOX 4-2	Provisions of the Americans with Disabilities Act

- Title I prohibits discriminating employment policies.
- Title II prohibits discrimination against disabled persons in the use of public transportation.
- Title III requires that public accommodations operated by private entities do not discriminate against persons with disabilities.
- Title IV prohibits discrimination against disabled individuals, especially hearing-impaired and speech-impaired individuals, in the area of communication.
- Title V contains miscellaneous provisions regarding the continued viability of other state or federal laws that provide disabled persons with equal or greater rights than the Americans with Disabilities Act. This section prohibits state or local governments from discriminating against individuals with disabilities.

Data from http://www.ada.gov/pubs/adastatute08.htm

Contracts

A *contract* is an agreement between two or more parties that creates an obligation to do or not do particular things. Contracts usually contain the following essential elements:

- Parties who are competent to enter into a contract. For example, a mentally disabled person cannot enter into a contract. Minors can enter into contracts, but they can void them in most cases before they reach majority age.
- Mutual agreement by all the parties (i.e., all parties have a meeting of the minds on a specific subject). Each party promises to perform an act that the party is not legally required to perform or promises to forego performing an act that it is legally entitled to perform.

Depending on the circumstances, a contract may or may not have to be put in writing and may or may not have to be signed. To be enforceable, some agreements must be in writing. The situations in which an agreement must be in writing are different among states but usually include transfers of real estate, sales of goods valued at more than $500, and contracts that require more than 1 year to perform.

The written agreement becomes your proof of what was agreed on and prevents someone from forgetting or changing the story later. Writing makes the parties focus on the essential points and come to a definite agreement.

Although you can write your own contracts, if there is much at stake or if the matter is complex, you should definitely use a lawyer. Your money may best be spent up front in preventing problems. If the amount is moderate or the terms are simple, you may use a legal form that both sides understand.

A contract may be unenforceable because it fails to contain an essential element outlined previously, there was fraud or mistake in the making of the contract, or the contract contains an illegal subject matter or is against public policy. When attempting to enforce a contract, it is important to consider the effect it will have on any long-term personal or professional relationship. It is often more beneficial to attempt to renegotiate a contract or let the situation go, which may even be financially wise considering the cost of a court battle.

Legal and Ethical Monetary Responsibilities

Money is one of the major reasons we pursue career success. In our society, money is necessary for a business to succeed. Money can become the vehicle for illegal and unethical practices because it is so important to the success of the business.

FRAUD

Fraud is a deception that is deliberately practiced to secure unfair or unlawful gain. One of the most common practices of fraud in health care is obtaining fees through third-party payments by misrepresentation. Third-party insurance reimbursement for massage services is not common, but the trend is increasing. It is therefore important to understand some of the problems that occur with health insurance reimbursement.

An example of a fraudulent action follows. A client had insurance coverage from July 1 of the past year until June 30 of the current year, after which time she would no longer receive this benefit. The client had a maximum benefit coverage of $1200 for the year and had used only $450 of the benefit. Toward the end of June, it was determined that the client would benefit from massage twice weekly instead of once weekly. The client was informed of the fees for the increase in service. The client was further informed that after June 30 the services would not be covered and that she would be responsible for payment. The client argued that it was the responsibility of the massage therapist to alter the date on the claim form, because she still had a $700 available benefit and in the future would bring her business to the massage therapist. It is fraud to change the date on the claim form to indicate that massage was provided before June 30 when the massage continued through mid-July.

Managed Care Legalities

Managed care refers to a cost-containment system of health care insurance that may direct use of health benefits by restricting the type, level, and frequency of treatment; limiting access to care to certain entities or practitioners; and basing the level of reimbursement for services on a capitation or other risk basis. Massage therapy is not typically involved in managed care systems, but this could change in the near future as more massage therapists work in the heath care setting. Limitations imposed by managed care companies generally are directed at payment for services, but the policies may also limit the actual services received by a client. In this way, managed care systems raise several legal and ethical issues for health care professionals. Clients may ask health care professionals to render only the treatment that is covered by the insurance plan, rather than the

necessary treatment. Insurance companies are profit driven and may not sufficiently consider the health care professional's responsibilities. Capitated plans can cause an ethical dilemma when, for example, a health care professional is paid for client care whether or not it is provided, because it is obvious that it is not in the short-term economic interest to provide that care. If certain care is not reimbursed, a client may forgo needed treatment due to financial concerns. For the client's interest to be protected, the massage therapist must be relied on to adhere to legal and ethical principles.

RECORDS MANAGEMENT

Nothing can be more valuable in defending against potential litigation than adequate records. These are a vital responsibility of the massage therapist. Although discussed in other areas of this text, the importance of including complete and thorough information in a client's record cannot be overemphasized. You should record the exact date, type of massage treatment, materials or adjunct methods used, unusual events (e.g., draping problems, allergic reaction to the lubricant), special notations about the treatment, and any incidence regarding the client's comments or reactions. The better the documentation is, the less the legal risk will be.

You should also document irregularities or unusual incidents occurring between clients, employees, and employers. All employee reports need to be retained in employee records. This documentation may include narratives of accidents that occurred. These incidents require a report that includes the name of the employee, the name of the client being treated, and the date and time of the injury. Incidents that may warrant documentation may include unusual behavior on the part of a client or a verbal confrontation between staff members. Thorough, accurate, and objective documentation is your best defense in litigation.

LITIGATION

Litigation is the process of a lawsuit. A *lawsuit* is a legal action in a court. The person or party that institutes the suit in court is the plaintiff. The person being accused of the wrongdoing is the defendant.

During malpractice litigation in a massage therapy practice, the client may be the plaintiff. The massage therapist or person who is being sued is the defendant. It is likely that other individuals in the massage office may be named as a defendant, fact witness, or an expert witness in the legal proceedings (Box 4-3).

A *fact witness*, when placed under oath, must provide only firsthand knowledge, not hearsay. A simple definition of hearsay is a statement other than one made specifically by a witness while testifying at the trial or hearing. The fact witness can describe only what he or she saw or did during a specific act.

BOX 4-3	Common Business Activities that Can Lead to Litigation

- Making false accusations about another person in verbal or written communications
- Providing another party or agency with confidential information without the client's consent
- Entering inaccurate data on clients' records
- Duplicating copyrighted material without permission
- Using unauthorized software
- Gaining illegal access to computer data
- Maliciously or deliberately damaging data in a computer
- Falsely entering data on insurance claims
- Failing to follow federal or state disease-transmission or waste-management regulations
- Failing to maintain accurate local, state, or federal governmental records

An *expert witness* is called to testify and explain to the judge and jury what happened based on the client's record and to offer an opinion about whether the massage care, as administered, met acceptable standards. Standards may vary by state. Often, a massage therapist may be called as an expert witness to testify in malpractice litigation because of his or her educational background and clinical expertise. A robust knowledge of massage law and massage standards, as well as an understanding of malpractice liability, is beneficial in such cases. Massage therapists should be insured against malpractice and premise liability, often called trip and fall insurance. The professional organizations that represent the massage professional provide these types of insurance coverage (see Box 4-3).

LEARNING ACTIVITY

Obtain copies of the insurance policies available from the American Massage Therapy Association and the Association of Massage and Bodywork Professionals. Compare and identify similarities and differences, and list at least three similarities and one difference in the space provided.

_____

_____

_____

_____

SELF-REFLECTION

How do I feel about the various laws that influence my business? Which type of law could I find myself breaking? Fraud? Negligence? Malpractice? Defamation of character? Invasion of privacy? Software theft or piracy? What makes me vulnerable to breaking this type of law?

MASSAGE PRACTICE ACTS AND CREDENTIALING

The legal requirements necessary to practice therapeutic massage and the scope of what can be practiced are developed through legislative action within the state and are typically identified as the state's Massage Practice Act. This act defines the minimum educational standards, requirements for credentialing, and the criteria for license revocation or suspension. Other legal requirements are enacted by the government in the form of rules and regulations. Unlike most health professions that have relatively standardized legislation, massage therapy legislation varies extensively. This makes it very difficult to discuss massage legislation specifically. However, there are enough similarities that can be described so that the general process of licensure can be understood (Box 4-4).

Many state Massage Practice Acts define conditions under which a massage therapist may perform specific duties. Each state provides a list of definitions within the law, and the descriptive language may vary significantly from state to state.

SELF-REFLECTION

What would I do and how would I feel if I were accused of malpractice or breaking some other law? What if I was at fault? What would I do and how would I feel if I were falsely accused of breaking a law? Have I ever reported someone for breaking a law? How did I feel? Proud, scared, nervous, or regretful? Have I ever falsely accused someone of anything? Was it an accident or mistake? Did I pass on wrong information? Was I being spiteful? How do I feel when I think about this?

The legal standards within various health professions' practice acts are for the protection of the general public, and interpretations of requirements for the protection of the general public may vary in different states. The license usually is granted after the person has met certain educational requirements and has completed some form of state testing. The tests used typically are the examinations from the National Certification Board for Therapeutic Massage and Bodywork (NCBTMB) (see "Voluntary Credentialing") or the FSMTB. A couple of states use examinations that have been developed by the state itself.

Federation of State Massage Therapy Boards and the Massage and Bodywork Licensing Examination

The FSMTB is an organization of states that have massage licensing, and it supports states seeking to license massage therapy. The mission of the FSMTB is to support its member

BOX 4-4 Excerpts of Representative Massage Practice Acts from Kentucky and Utah

KENTUCKY

(6) "Practice of massage therapy" means the application, by a massage therapist licensed by the board, of a system of structured touch, pressure, movement, and holding to the soft tissues of the human body with the intent to enhance or restore the health and well-being of the client. The practice includes the external application of water, heat, cold, lubricants, salt scrubs, or other topical preparations; use of electromechanical devices that mimic or enhance the actions of the hands; and determination of whether massage therapy is appropriate or contraindicated, or whether referral to another health care practitioner is appropriate.

UTAH

(6) "Practice of massage therapy" means:
- (a) The examination, assessment, and evaluation of the soft tissue structures of the body for the purpose of devising a treatment plan to promote homeostasis;
- (b) The systematic manual or mechanical manipulation of the soft tissue of the body for the therapeutic purpose of:
  - (i) promoting the health and well-being of a client;
  - (ii) enhancing the circulation of the blood and lymph;
  - (iii) relaxing and lengthening muscles;
  - (iv) relieving pain;
  - (v) restoring metabolic balance; and
  - (vi) achieving homeostasis;
- (c) The use of the hands or a mechanical or electrical apparatus in connection with this Subsection (6);
- (d) The use of rehabilitative procedures involving the soft tissue of the body;
- (e) Range of motion or movements without spinal adjustment as set forth in Section 58-73-102;
- (f) Oil rubs, heat lamps, salt glows, hot and cold packs, or tub, shower, steam, and cabinet baths;
- (g) Manual traction and stretching exercise;
- (h) Correction of muscular distortion by treatment of the soft tissues of the body;
- (i) Counseling, education, and other advisory services to reduce the incidence and severity of physical disability, movement dysfunction, and pain;
- (j) Similar or related activities and modality techniques; and
- (k) The practice described in this Subsection (6) on an animal to the extent permitted by;
  - (i) Subsection 58-28-307(12);
  - (ii) the provisions of this chapter; and
  - (iii) division rule.

WRITE YOUR OWN LAW

After reading through the Practice Acts from Kentucky and Utah above, take some time to research other states' massage practice acts online. Then, write your own massage practice act as you would like to see it enacted in your state. Share your thoughts with your class.

_____
_____
_____
_____
_____
_____
_____
_____
_____
_____
_____
_____
_____
_____
_____
_____
_____
_____
_____
_____
_____
_____
_____
_____
_____
_____

BOX 4-4	Excerpts of Representative Massage Practice Acts from Kentucky and Utah—cont'd

Kentucky information from http://www.lrc.state.ky.us/KRS/309-00/350.PDF *and* Utah information from http://www.dopl.utah.gov/laws/58-47b.pdf

boards in their work to ensure that the practice of massage therapy is provided to the public in a safe and effective manner.

The FSMTB has developed a model licensing examination for states and the structure to deliver the examination, relieving state boards of this task, which is burdensome and expensive. The development of this examination is to ensure the provision of a valid, reliable licensing examination to determine entry-level competence. For more information, you can contact the FSMTB (7111 W 151st Street, Suite 356, Overland Park, KS 66223; phone: 1-888-70-FSMTB).

Not all states use the FSMTB examination. Many use the examination from the NCBTMB. For more information, you can contact the NCBTMB (1901 South Meyers Road, Suite 240, Oakbrook Terrace, IL 60181; phone: 1-800-296-0664).

Voluntary Credentialing: Validation of Excellence

Credentialing is a generic term that refers to the ways in which educational programs and professionals can measure and maintain their competence. The voluntary processes used in credentialing include accreditation and certification.

Accreditation is the process by which an entity or educational program is evaluated and recognized by an outside agency for having attained a predetermined set of standards. *Certification* is a process by which an individual is evaluated and recognized by an outside agency for training beyond entry-level licensure requirements.

Accreditation is defined as granting approval to an institution of learning by an official review board after the school has met specific requirements. The accreditation process is a voluntary step that institutions, including massage and bodywork schools, may take to receive this additional endorsement beyond mandated licensing from the state department of education. The primary motivation for schools to seek accredited status is to assure prospective students that their programs have met quality and competency standards. These standards are identified by professional and educational organizations, including peer groups. Agencies recognized by the U.S. Department of

Education accredit the school as a whole. Students attending accredited schools may qualify for various types of government financial aid. Links to accrediting agencies are listed in the Evolve Annotated Web Links at the end of this chapter.

The Commission on Massage Training and Accreditation (COMTA) is one accrediting body responsible for accrediting educational programs in massage. The COMTA is a relatively new organization in the field of educational program accreditation. In 1989, the Commission on Massage Training Approval/Accreditation was founded to create standards for educational programs that offered massage therapy and bodywork training. The program changed its name to COMTA a few years later. Official U.S. Department of Education recognition of COMTA was granted in 2002. Accreditation validates that a specific educational program has met a set of standards to address the needs of the profession and the public.

For many professions, especially health professions, a criterion for obtaining a credential such as certification or licensure is contingent on successful completion of an accredited educational program. This is not the case for massage therapy. As a result, the educational standards are inconsistent.

Value of Credentialing beyond Licensure

Licensing determines the minimum qualifications to practice a profession or skill in a manner that protects the public health and safety. Licensing does not identify excellence. Individuals who seek credentials beyond what is legally mandated by becoming certified should seek additional training and increase their professional skills beyond the minimum requirements.

Credentialing is an important process. Massage therapists have the opportunity to become nationally certified by an independent, nonprofit, private organization, the NCBTMB. This board was established in 1992. The goals when established were to give massage professionals a way to demonstrate their desire for excellence in massage practice by establishing a credential beyond their education and experience and to provide consumers proof that they are receiving care from a massage professional who is committed to a high level of practice standards and ethical behavior.

The NCBTMB was accredited by the National Commission for Certifying Agencies in 1993. It is a member of the American National Standards Institute and the Coalition for Professional Certification.

To become a certified massage practitioner, a person must pass an examination and qualify to sit for this examination by meeting one of the following criteria:

- A certificate of achievement with a minimum of 500 in-class supervised hours from a qualified school
- A portfolio that shows training and experience that is equivalent to a formal 500-hour program

SELF-REFLECTION

If I have to be state licensed to practice massage therapy, why would I also want to be certified? What would motivate me to be certified? Would I ever practice massage without being licensed if licensing is required? How would I explain to someone else the importance of credentialing beyond the mandated licensure?

All information to become a certified massage therapist and the most current requirements to sit for the examination can be obtained by visiting the NCBTMB Web site. Those who graduated from a qualified program should request the candidate handbook, and those seeking portfolio approval should ask for the portfolio review handbook.

EDUCATIONAL STANDARDS FOR LEGAL AND ETHICAL MASSAGE THERAPY PRACTICE

The content outline in Box 4-5 is compiled from many sources, including the National Certification Examination (NCE), the National Certification Examination for Therapeutic Massage and Bodywork (NCETMB), the FSMTB, the MBLEx, the COMTA, and the National Accrediting Commission of Cosmetology Arts and Sciences (www.naccas.org).

It is important to not become overwhelmed as you review the content outline. Although it is comprehensive, it is not insurmountable. You should have all this information during your schooling and in your textbooks. The outline is provided so you understand the information that is tested on various licensing and certification examinations. As you read through the comprehensive content outline in Box 4-5 notice that each area relates to the mandates of licensure (e.g., protect the public health, welfare, and safety) or to excellence in professional practice validated by certification.

LEARNING ACTIVITY

Using Box 4-5, compare the content of your textbooks, lecture notes, instructor information, clinic experience, and other aspects of your education, and list areas you think need more study in the space provided.

_____

_____

_____

ETHICS

Ethics is a branch of philosophy and is a systematic, intellectual approach to the standards of behavior. The purpose of a professional code of ethics is to help members of the profession achieve high levels of behavior through moral consciousness, decision making, and practice. Ethics in daily professional practice challenges a practitioner to differentiate between right and wrong. _Morals_ are considered voluntary personal commitments to a set of values. _Values_ are the standards used for decision making that endure over a significant period. The expected behaviors of the massage professional are based on a set of standards derived from acceptable and exemplary behaviors. Every health professional must realize that there is right and wrong and that there is no right way to do a wrong thing (Fig. 4-2).

Ethics in Massage Therapy

Each organized group within the profession of massage has a code of ethics for its members. These codes of ethics are based on moral principles that reflect concern for the care of the client.

Each individual involved in the practice of massage assumes the obligation of maintaining and enriching the profession. The massage therapist may choose to meet this obligation according to the dictates of personal conscience based on the needs of the human beings the profession of massage is committed to serve. The Golden Rule is the basic guiding principle. The massage professional must strive at all times to maintain confidentiality, exhibit respect for the client and coworkers, and refrain from performing any professional service that is prohibited by state law. He or she has the obligation to prove competence before providing services to any client. The massage professional shall constantly strive to upgrade and expand technical skills for the benefit of the consumer public (Box 4-6).

Maintaining Quality Service

Although not necessarily mandated by licensure, it is ethically necessary to maintain high standards of care. The massage professional can continue to improve the quality of care

BOX 4-5	Comprehensive Compiled Licensing and Certification Examination Content Outline

Because the massage profession has not yet formalized a body of knowledge, many sources were compiled to produce this content outline. Sources include state licensing documents, accreditation bodies, professional organizations, test administration organizations, textbook instructor manuals, and textbook content outlines. The materials were compared and evaluated for similarities and differences. The overlapping content was targeted for developing the outline.

ETHICS, PROFESSIONALISM, BUSINESS PRACTICES, AND LEGAL ISSUES

Professional ethics
Standards of practice
Scope of practice
Documentation
Business practices
Client education and wellness practices

HYGIENE AND SANITATION

Standard precautions
Therapeutic environment

MASSAGE PROCEDURES

Massage methods
Physiologic effects of massage methods
Therapeutic applications
Applied structure and function and indications and contraindications for massage therapy

HYDROTHERAPY

PHARMACOLOGY

ANATOMY AND PHYSIOLOGY

The chemical level
The cellular level
The tissue level
The integumentary system
Bone tissue
The axial skeleton
The appendicular skeleton
Articulations
Muscle tissue
The muscular system
Nervous tissue
The spinal cord and spinal nerves
The brain and cranial nerves
The sensory, motor, and integrative systems
The special senses
The autonomic nervous system
The endocrine system
The blood
The heart
Blood vessels and hemodynamics
The lymphatic system
The respiratory system
The digestive system
The urinary system
The reproductive systems

PATHOLOGY

through education, training, research, and maintenance of a stringent code of ethics and professional conduct.

Supervision is an area that the massage therapist may encounter if working for another type of licensed professional, such as a physical therapist. One type of supervision is referred to as direct supervision. It means that the health care professional (e.g., physical therapist) has designated a client of record on whom services are to be performed and has described the procedure to be performed. Continuing with the example, the physical therapist examines the client before prescribing the procedures to be performed and again on completion of the procedure. Under the definition of direct supervision, the physical therapist (or other professional) must be physically present in the office at the time the procedures are being performed.

Consent

It is ethical and legally mandated to obtain consent from the client before providing massage. *Consent* is the voluntary acceptance or agreement to what is planned or done by another person. To massage a client without consent constitutes unauthorized touching and makes the person committing the act guilty of battery, as discussed earlier in this chapter. Two forms of consent exist in the delivery of massage care: informed and implied.

INFORMED CONSENT

Informed consent is a concept that has evolved over decades as courts and legislatures have demanded more disclosure on the part of the provider of care to a client. The idea behind informed consent is that every adult of sound mind has the right to determine what can and cannot be done with his or her body. For that person to make a proper judgment, he or she must be given information by the health care provider. The client must be given enough information about the proposed treatment, in understandable language, to make an intelligent decision about whether to proceed with the treatment. Moreover, the client must have ample opportunity to ask questions and have them answered.

In general, courts and legislatures have defined specific elements that describe informed consent. These elements state that consent must be given freely; treatment and outcomes must be described in understandable language; risks, benefits, and estimate of the success of treatment must be described; prognosis if no treatment is elected and alternative treatment plans must be explained; and the client must be given the right to ask questions and have them answered.

If these conditions are not met, the courts may conclude that the client did not consent to the procedure. In that case, the massage therapist may be liable for actions such as battery or negligence (depending on the individual state).

For consent to be legally valid, it must be informed and given freely, and the client must be an adult of sound mind. Clients under the influence of alcohol, drugs, or severe stress

Code of Ethics and Standards of Practice

Ethical Principles

- *Respect for the dignity of people*—Massage professionals will maintain respect for the interests, dignity, rights, and needs of all clients, staff, and colleagues.
- *Responsible caring*—Competent, quality client care will be provided at the highest standard possible.
- *Integrity in relationships*—At all times the professional will behave with integrity, honesty, and diligence in practice and duties.
- *Responsibility to society*—Massage professionals are responsible and accountable to society and shall conduct themselves in a manner that maintains high ethical standards.

Standards of Practice Based on Ethical Principles

In compliance with the principles of the code of ethics, massage professionals will perform the following:

1. Respect all clients, colleagues, and health professionals through nondiscrimination regardless of age, gender, race, national origin, sexual orientation, religion, socioeconomic status, body type, political affiliation, state of health, personal habits, and life-coping skills.

2. Perform only those services for which they are qualified and honestly represent their education, certification, professional affiliations, and other qualifications. The massage professional will apply treatment only when a reasonable expectation exists that it will be advantageous to the client's condition. The massage professional, in consultation with the client, will continually evaluate the effectiveness of treatment.

3. Respect the scope of practice of other health care and service professionals, including physicians, chiropractors, physical therapists, podiatrists, orthopedists, psychotherapists, counselors, acupuncturists, nurses, exercise physiologists, athletic trainers, nutritionists, spiritual advisors, and cosmetologists.

4. Respect all ethical health care practitioners and work with them to promote health and healing.

5. Acknowledge the limitations of their personal skills and, when necessary, refer clients to an appropriately qualified professional. The massage professional will require consultation with other knowledgeable professionals when:

   - A client requires diagnosis and opinion beyond a therapist's capabilities of assessment
   - A client's condition is beyond the scope of practice
   - A combined health care team is required

   If referral to another health care provider is necessary, it will be done with the informed consent of the client.

6. Refrain from working with any individual who has a specific disease process without supervision by a licensed medical professional.

7. Be adequately educated and understand the physiologic effects of the specific massage techniques used to determine if any application is contraindicated and to ensure that the most beneficial techniques are applied to a given individual.

8. Avoid false claims about the potential benefits of the techniques rendered, and educate the public about the actual benefits of massage.

9. Acknowledge the importance and individuality of each person, including colleagues, peers, and clients.

10. Work only with the informed consent of a client and professionally disclose to the client any situation that may interfere with the massage professional's ability to provide the best care to serve the client's best interest.

11. Display respect for the client by honoring a client's process and following all recommendations by being present, listening, asking only pertinent questions, keeping agreements, being on time, draping properly, and customizing the massage to address the client's needs.

FIGURE 4-2. Code of ethics and standards of practice for massage therapists. *(From Fritz S: Mosby's Fundamentals of Therapeutic Massage, ed. 4, St. Louis, 2009, Mosby.)*

Note: Draping is covered in Chapter 8. The Ontario guidelines give these requirements for
draping:

- It is the responsibility of the massage professional to ensure the privacy and dignity of
the client and to determine if the client feels comfortable, safe, and secure with the
draping provided.
- The client may choose to be fully draped or clothed throughout the treatment.
- The female client's breasts are not undraped unless specified by referral from a
qualified health care professional and the massage professional is working under the
supervision of such a health care professional.
- The genitals, perineum, and anus are never undraped.

The consent of the client is required for work on any part of the body, regardless of whether the
client is fully clothed, fully draped, or partly draped.

12. Provide a safe, comfortable, and clean environment.

13. Maintain clear and honest communication with clients and keep client communications
confidential. Confidentiality is of the utmost importance. The massage professional must
inform the client that the referring physician may be eligible to review the client's records
and that records may be subpoenaed by the courts.

14. Conduct business in a professional and ethical manner in relation to clientele, business
associates, acquaintances, governmental bodies, and the public.

15. Follow city, county, state, national, and international requirements.

16. Charge a fair price for the session. Gratuities are appropriate if within reasonable limits
(similar to percentages for other service providers [i.e.,10-20%]). A gift, gratuity, or benefit
that is intended to influence a referral, decision, or treatment may not be accepted and
must be returned to the giver immediately.

17. Keep accurate records and review the records with the client.

18. Never engage in any sexual conduct, sexual conversation, or any other sexual activities
involving clients.

19. Avoid affiliation with any business that uses any form of sexual suggestiveness or explicit
sexuality in advertising or promoting services or in the actual practice of service.

20. Practice honesty in advertising, promoting services ethically and in good taste, and
advertising only techniques for which the professional is certified or adequately trained.

21. Strive for professional excellence through regular assessment of personal strengths,
limitations, and effectiveness and through continuing education and training.

22. Accept the responsibility to oneself, one's clients, and the profession to maintain physical,
mental, and emotional well-being, and to inform clients when the professional is not
functioning at best capacity.

23. Refrain from using any mind-altering drugs, alcohol, or intoxicants before or during
professional massage sessions.

24. Maintain a professional appearance and demeanor by practicing good hygiene and
dressing in a professional, modest, and nonsexual manner.

25. Undergo periodic peer review.

26. Respect all pertinent reporting requirements outlined by legislation regarding abuse.

27. Report to the proper authorities any accurate knowledge and its supportive documentation
regarding violations by massage professionals and other health or service professionals.

28. Avoid interests, activities, or influences that might conflict with the obligation to act in the
best interest of clients and the massage therapy profession and safeguard professional
integrity by recognizing potential conflicts of interest and avoiding them.

FIGURE 4-2, cont'd

BOX 4-6   Overview of Principles of Ethics and Code of Professional Conduct

SECTION 1. PRINCIPLE: CLIENT AUTONOMY (SELF-GOVERNANCE)
- The massage therapist has a duty to respect the client's rights to self-determination and confidentiality.
- Professionals have a duty to treat the clients according to their desires, within the bounds of accepted treatment, and to protect the clients' confidentiality. Under this principle, the massage therapist's primary obligations include involving clients in treatment decisions in a meaningful way, with due consideration given to the client's needs, desires, and abilities, and safeguarding the client's privacy.

SECTION 2. PRINCIPLE: NONMALFEASANCE (DO NO HARM)
- The massage therapist has a duty to refrain from harming the client.
- Professionals have a duty to protect the client from harm. Under this principle, the massage therapist's primary obligations include keeping knowledge and skills current, knowing their own limitations, knowing when to refer to a specialist or other professional, and knowing when and under what circumstances delegation of clients' care to auxiliaries is appropriate.

SECTION 3. PRINCIPLE: BENEFICENCE (DO GOOD)
- The massage therapist has a duty to promote the client welfare.
- Professionals have a duty to act for the benefit of others. Under this principle, the massage therapist's primary obligation is service to the client and the general public. The most important aspect of this obligation is the competent and timely delivery of massage care within the bounds of clinical circumstances presented by the client, with due consideration given to the needs, desires, and values of the client. The same ethical considerations apply whether the massage professional engages in fee-for-service, managed care, or other practice arrangements.

SECTION 4. PRINCIPLE: JUSTICE (FAIRNESS)
- The massage therapist has a duty to treat people fairly.
- Professionals have a duty to be fair in their dealings with clients, colleagues, and society. Under this principle, the massage therapist's primary obligations include dealing with people justly and delivering massage care without prejudice. In its broadest sense of this principle, the massage profession should actively seek allies throughout society on specific activities that will help improve access to care for all.

SECTION 5. PRINCIPLE: VERACITY (TRUTHFULNESS)
- The massage therapist has a duty to communicate truthfully.
- Professionals have a duty to be honest and trustworthy in their dealings with people. Under this principle, the massage therapist's primary obligations include respecting the position of trust inherent in the massage therapist–client relationship, communicating truthfully and without deception, and maintaining intellectual integrity.

---

may not have sufficient mental capacity to grant permission for treatment. When a massage therapist treats a minor, only the parent or guardian of the minor may grant consent. This excludes grandparents, babysitters, and siblings. However, parents may authorize another party to grant consent for treatment during the parents' absence. Such authorization must be signed before treatment consent. A variety of consent forms are available. Figure 4-3 shows an example of a common form for a general practice. These forms must be signed, dated, and retained in the client's record.

IMPLIED CONSENT

Other agreements that flow automatically from the relationship between the client and the massage professional are in the category of implied consent. These agreements trigger responsibilities that work in two ways: those that the massage therapist owes to the client and those that the client owes to the massage therapist. Accepting a client for treatment implies that the massage therapist agrees to accept certain responsibilities for that client's massage care. Likewise, if a client agrees to accept treatment by the massage therapist, the client assumes certain responsibilities.

Boxes 4-7 and 4-8 list implied responsibilities for each of these parties.

   SELF-REFLECTION

How ethical am I? When I measure my professional behavior against the list in Box 4-8, in which areas I am most likely to have difficulty? What makes me vulnerable to unethical behavior? How do I feel when I am treated in a disrespectful way? When was the last time I was disrespectful to someone? What factors led to that behavior? What did I learn from it?

Making Ethical Decisions

The massage therapist has much to consider when carrying out routine duties in the massage business office. During all activities, you must keep in mind questions about the tasks being performed. Routinely ask yourself the questions in Box 4-9.

Combined Massage Therapy Intake and Consent Form
THIS FORM MUST BE COMPLETED AND SIGNED BEFORE RECEIVING A MASSAGE.

Forms of payment accepted
Cash, checks, or money orders are accepted. Credit cards are not.
Travel to client
There is an additional charge for any travel to the client depending on time and distance. The minimum additional charge is $30.
Contraindications (situations where massage is not indicated)
Under certain medical conditions, massage/bodywork may not be advised (e.g., when a fever is present, indicating an infection). If a massage could be potentially harmful to a client's condition, the massage therapist has the right to decline to do the massage.
Insurance claims
I do not handle insurance forms, but I will be glad to give you a receipt for you to submit to your insurance company for possible reimbursement.

Medical Information

Have you ever experienced a professional massage? _____

Which areas would you like to focus on during this massage? _____

Do you have any of the following conditions? If yes, please explain below as clearly as possible.

_____ Stress	_____ Allergies	_____ Contagious disease
_____ Diabetes	_____ Wear contact lenses	_____ Back pain
_____ Pregnancy	_____ Cancer	_____ Cardiac/circulatory problems
_____ Arthritis	_____ Sensitive to touch or pressure	_____ Frequent headaches
_____ Osteoporosis	_____ Epilepsy or seizures	_____ Bruise easily
_____ Joint swelling	_____ Varicose veins	_____ Depression

_____ Numbness or stabbing pains? Explain below.
_____ High blood pressure. If yes, are you taking medication for this? Explain below.
_____ Surgery in the past 5 years? Explain below.
_____ Accident or suffered any injuries in the past 2 years? Broken bones, etc. Explain below.
_____ Other medical conditions not listed. Explain below.
_____ Medications (prescribed or over-the-counter)

Comments: _____
_____
_____
_____

I understand that the massage I receive is provided for the basic purpose of relaxation and relief of muscular tension. If I experience any pain or discomfort during the session, I will immediately inform the therapist so that the pressure and/or strokes may be adjusted to my level of comfort. I further understand that massage should not be construed as a substitute for medical examination, diagnosis, or treatment. I understand that massage therapists are not qualified to perform spinal or skeletal adjustments; diagnose, prescribe, or treat any physical or mental illness; and that nothing said in the course of the session given should be construed as such. Because massage should not be performed under certain medical conditions, I affirm that I have stated all my known medical conditions and answered all questions honestly. I agree to keep the massage therapist updated as to any changes in my medical profile during the session and understand that there shall be no liability on the massage therapist's part should I fail to do so. I understand that any illicit or sexually suggestive remarks or advances made by me will result in immediate termination of the session. I also understand that the Licensed Massage Therapist reserves the right to refuse to perform massage on anyone whom he/she deems to have a condition for which massage is contraindicated.

Client signature _____ Date _____

NAME: _____ PHONE: _____

E-MAIL: _____ THERAPIST'S NAME: _____

FIGURE 4-3. Informed consent form.

BOX 4-7 **Implied Duties Owed by the Massage Therapist to the Client**

- Use reasonable care in the provision of services as measured against acceptable standards set by other practitioners with similar training in a similar community.
- Be properly licensed and registered, and meet all other legal requirements to engage in the practice of massage.
- Obtain an accurate health history of the client before massage treatment begins.
- Employ competent personnel and provide for their proper supervision.
- Maintain a level of knowledge in keeping with current advances in the profession.
- Use methods that are acceptable to most similar practitioners in the community.
- Refrain from performing invasive procedures.
- Obtain informed consent from the client before massage treatment.
- Charge a reasonable fee (by community standards) for services.

- Refrain from exceeding the scope of practice authorized by your license or permitting those acting under your direction to engage in unlawful acts.
- Keep the client informed of his or her progress.
- Refrain from undertaking any procedure for which you are not qualified.
- Complete care in a timely manner.
- Keep accurate records of the massage application rendered to the client.
- Maintain confidentiality of information.
- Inform the client of any untoward occurrences in the course of treatment.
- Make appropriate referrals, and request necessary consultations.
- Comply with all laws regulating the practice of massage.
- Practice in a manner consistent with the codes of ethics of the profession.
- Use standard precautions in the treatment of all clients.

BOX 4-8	Implied Duties Owed by the Client to the Massage Professional

- Keep appointments, and notify the office of cancellations or appointment delays.
- Provide honest answers to questions asked on the history form and by the massage therapist.
- Notify the office staff or massage therapist of any change in health status.
- Pay a reasonable fee for the service if no fee is agreed on in writing or orally.
- Remit the fee for services within a reasonable time.

BOX 4-9	Nine Steps to Making Ethical Decisions

1. Is the task I am performing legal?
2. Do I have the necessary credentials to perform this task?
3. Am I physically and emotionally competent to perform this task?
4. Am I performing this procedure in a safe working environment?
5. Has the client been informed about his or her massage session?
6. Am I respecting the client's rights to privacy and confidentiality?
7. Do I maintain complete and accurate records, and have I documented special problems arising with clients, employees, or an employer?
8. Do I maintain professional liability insurance?
9. Do I actively participate in my professional organization and contribute to community awareness of therapeutic massage?

 Good Stuff from the Government

BUSINESS ETHICS: THE FOUNDATION OF EFFECTIVE LEADERSHIP

Business ethics are a hot topic. With everything from insider trading to employee theft on the rise, it is no wonder that businesses are beginning to focus on the impact of ethical leadership. However, along with this new focus comes gray areas. Managers often are forced to decide on issues for which there are arguments on both sides, making ethical decisions very difficult. The Evolve site has links to the small business planner with information about professional ethics.

HANDLING LEGAL CONCERNS

It makes good business sense to know how to handle legal issues that affect your business. Not all legal matters require a lawyer, but they do require understanding. Sometimes, the best way to protect yourself and your business is to know where to go for assistance. For example, the Small Business Association Web site provides information on finding the following legal information at http://www.sba.gov.

American Bar Association (ABA) lawyer referral service: Find a lawyer in your state who's prepared to help you.

Tips on hiring an attorney presented by the National Federation of Independent Business (NFIB): One of the best ways to find the right lawyer for your business is to ask people you trust for referrals.

Your state bar association: Link to the ABA's guide to finding bar associations in your state.

Fees and expenses: It is important to negotiate legal fees when first visiting a lawyer. You have a right to know how you will be charged, how much the case is likely to cost, and when you have to pay.

Small claims court is usually the best option if the size of the case does not justify the cost of hiring a lawyer.

International Center For Dispute Resolution (ICDR) is a resource for business, organizations, government agencies, and communities seeking to manage human relations issues and harmonize relationships that threaten productivity and performance, especially in the workplace.

Arbitration provides a quicker and less expensive method for resolving disputes.

Plain English Guide to Contracts provides a simple, easy explanation about contracts.

Legal FAQs: Answers to common questions about the legal aspects of running a business.

Hiring a lawyer FAQs: Commonly asked questions about hiring a lawyer.

SCORE Legal Questions: Legal questions regarding business as answered by the SCORE organization.

SUMMARY

There are legal requirements regarding the standards of care in the delivery of massage treatment, especially when it comes to ethics. Ethical standards are involved in your speech, your demeanor, possibly your clothing, or even your massage office. As a massage therapist, you must always be aware of the ethical implications of your actions. Whether you are working at your office, making a house call, or working at a medical facility, the same correct ethical behavior and responses need to be second nature.

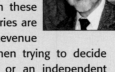

| EXPERT Outlook | **THREE ISSUES INVOLVING ETHICS AND LAW** |

BRUCE FROELICH, JD, NCTMB
WHAT CHOICE OF LEGAL ENTITY DO WE USE TO SET UP OUR BUSINESS?

Ethically and legally, massage therapists (MT) have a limited scope of practice. Legally, we should be concerned to maintain a limited liability, which both protects our personal property and the financial integrity of our business. Each state has different business entities we can choose among, such as corporations or partnerships. Most states allow us another choice: the Limited Liability Company, or LLC, as it is known here in Michigan.

For most MTs, LLC is the option I would recommend. However, it is not "one size fits all"; remember that each person has to select and design the best business entity for his or her circumstances. There are no solo acts; we each need competent advice to make the best choices for ourselves, so get a good tax advisor and lawyer before you start out.

Most MTs have to start out small and hope to grow their practice. Consider these business factors: LLC has flexibility and informality, limited liability, and broad powers and purposes; allows for single or multiple owners; helps us structure our capital investment, profits, and business management rights; allows us to buy or sell ownership interests; and gives the business legal continuity. There is flexibility for tax planning, allocation of profits and losses to owners, deductibility of expenses, and so on. Owners can sell or liquidate the business, too. The LLC can be used for large privately held corporations or small and medium-sized closely held businesses, and can be a tool to assist planning for estates and preserving family wealth.

EMPLOYEE OR INDEPENDENT CONTRACTOR?

Ethical and legal duties arise when we grow our business enough to require hiring additional people, whether those are employees or independent contractors. Circumstances may make either choice preferable. Owners wanting to

know where the limits are between these choices must first realize the boundaries are not always clear. Even the Internal Revenue Service looks at multiple factors when trying to decide whether a person is an employee or an independent contractor. So we have to become informed and then from the start communicate clearly with the persons we hire.

BUSINESS POLICIES AND PROCEDURES?

Massage therapists' business policies and procedures involve both ethics and legal requirements, whether we are working alone or have hired other persons. What policies and procedures do we adopt in our business, either internally or for presentation to our clients? Do we want to simply post them in our lobby; or do we require clients to read them, offer to answer their questions, and then require the client to sign them? Hint: clear communication, both with clients and persons we hire, helps establish mutual expectations and prevents problems from occurring.

My clients are handed a policies and procedures document to read, given an opportunity for asking questions face-to-face, and required to sign and date the document—all *before* they disrobe or get on the massage table. Topics covered include: scope of practice, first and subsequent visits, paperwork expected, contraindications, clients' goals and preferences, draping, inviting clients to ask any questions they may have, scheduling appointments and giving notice for canceling them, fee structure and methods of payment, mutual right of refusal, consequences if the therapeutic massage is sexualized, and informed consent. The informed consent paragraph indicates they have read the document, discussed it, asked questions, understood the document, and agreed to comply. They also promise to promptly raise any questions they may have in the future, and keep their MT informed about any changes in their health status.

Employees must also be aware of the laws and ethical standards that affect their profession. An understanding of the legal principles involved can help employees to support decisions that the business owner must make and can help to protect everyone's livelihood. To have knowledge is priceless, and to use your knowledge is called success. The knowledge gained in this textbook should be used wisely and with the intention of making yourself a successful, law-abiding massage therapist.

Bibliography

Americans with Disabilities: *ADA Principles of Ethics and Code of Professional Conduct*, Chicago, 2005, American Massage Association.

Davison JA: *Legal and Ethical Considerations for Dental Hygienists and Assistants*, St. Louis, 2000, Mosby.

Johnson CE: *Meeting the Ethical Challenges of Leadership: Casting Light or Shadow*, ed 2, Thousand Oaks, CA, 2005, Sage Publications.

Evolve Annotated Web Links
http://evolve.elsevier.com/Fritz/Links

U.S. Small Business Association: www.sba.gov

Associated Bodywork & Massage Professionals (www.Massagetherapy.com), State Boards and Requirements: www.massagetherapy.com/careers/stateboards.php

Associated Bodywork & Massage Professionals (Massagetherapy.com), Massage State Regulation Guide: www.massagetherapy.com/_content/careers/MTreg.pdf

Americans with Disabilities: www.usdoj.gov/crt/ada/

Commission of Massage Therapy: www.comta.org

National Certification Examination for Therapeutic Massage and Bodywork: www.ncbtmb.org

U.S. Department of Education Accrediting Agencies:

Accrediting Bureau of Health Education Schools: www.abhes.org

Accrediting Council for Continuing Education and Training: www.accet.org

Accrediting Commission for Career Schools and Colleges of Technology: www.accsct.org

Accrediting Council of Independent College and Schools: www.acics.org

Council on Occupational Education: www.council.org

Distance Education and Training Council: www.detc.org

National Accrediting Commission of Cosmetology Arts and Sciences: www.naccas.org

North Central Association of Colleges and Schools: www.ncacihe.org

Workbook

1. Explain the application of the two forms of consent that apply to the delivery of massage care.

_____
_____

2. What four questions should be asked to determine an unintentional tort of negligence in massage care?

_____
_____
_____
_____

3. Identify 10 steps that should be followed when making ethical decisions.

_____
_____

4. Identify 10 implied duties that a massage therapist owes a client.

_____
_____
_____
_____

5. List five business office activities that may lead to potential litigation.

_____
_____
_____

6. Explain the element of informed consent.

_____
_____

7. Explain the function of a state Massage Practice Act and its impact on a consumer.

_____
_____

8. Describe the role of the massage therapist in the state in which you practice.

_____
_____

9. Search the Americans with Disabilities Act Web site to determine how this act would affect the renovation of a massage office building built in 1995.

_____
_____

TECHNOLOGY IN THE MASSAGE PRACTICE

OUTLINE

KEY TERMS

Computers
Data
Dumb terminals
Electronic spreadsheet

Feasibility study
Impact printer
Information system
Intelligent terminals

Mosaic Netscape
Nonimpact printer
Software
Technology

LEARNING OUTCOMES

Mastery of the content in this chapter will enable the reader to:

- Define glossary terms
- Differentiate between a manual massage practice and a massage practice using new technology
- List types of electronic massage practice equipment considered to be new technology
- Describe the elements of information systems
- Explain the four operations of a computer
- Explain how technology can be used to increase profitability
- Describe the application of technology to a massage practice

- Explain the purpose of a feasibility study
- Explain the difference between general and specific task software
- Discuss software, word processing, electronic spreadsheet, database, graphics, and Internet software
- List guidelines to follow when selecting software
- Explain why implementing a change to a computer system is important to all staff members

e Guidelines for the Learning Activities and answers to the Workbook questions are located on Evolve at http://evolve.elsevier.com/Fritz/business.

BOX 5-1	Applications of New Technology in the Business Massage Practice

- Electronic charting
- Computerized scheduling
- Online massage practice procedures manuals
- Add progress notes to online records
- Automated insurance claims
- Buying supplies from online supply warehouses
- Telemarketing with Web pages
- E-mail staff and clients
- Enrolling in online college courses
- Providing a means for continuing education
- Allowing for virtual group practices in which solo practitioners share one set of records
- Consulting with experts from all over the world

Modified from Finkbeiner BL, Finkbeiner CA: *Practice Management for the Dental Team,* ed 6, St. Louis, 2006, Mosby.)

Products and services can be low tech or high tech. *Low tech* refers to a design or development that typically occurred before the availability of electricity. Because massage has a history that is centuries old, massage is low tech, and that is a great thing. Just like yin and yang, there needs to be a balance in life. We have become so high tech that basic things such as gardening and massage are even more important to establish a balance. Although the practice of massage therapy is considered to be low tech, the business of massage is benefiting by high-tech advances in communication systems, computer hardware and software, Web sites and Web networks, and communities such as Facebook, MySpace, and more. Technology advances help the large, multidisciplinary practice and in many ways allow the sole practitioner of massage to streamline and optimize their business responsibilities.

Technology is advancing at a rate so fast that it is almost impossible to keep current. A smartphone today can do what a full computer system could do 2 years ago. It boggles the mind. It is unrealistic to expect that the most current information will be presented in this chapter. Instead, the content focuses on basics, what is currently familiar, and what can help to prepare you to learn how to remain aware of all the technologic advances of the future.

Just 10 years ago in the traditional massage practice, computers were seldom used. Today, technology has replaced manual systems with online, interconnected commerce. New technology in the massage practice is the application of computers and associated electronic equipment to prepare and distribute information. The computer has made an impact on the profession of massage therapy and is now used routinely in the clinical and business applications of the massage practice.

Few businesses can avoid the need for more information. The prudent selection of technology equipment is a major component of massage practice productivity and efficiency.

The use of a Web site is more than a mode of advertising. The platform can be used for distributing information, client education, networking, appointments, and more functions.

The electronic massage practice is a workplace where sophisticated computers and other electronic equipment carry out many of the massage practice's routine tasks and provide more options for gathering, processing, displaying, and storing information. Some applications of technology in the electronic massage practice are outlined in Box 5-1.

The technologic revolution that led to the information age has had a profound effect on the massage practice. The use of electronic technology in the massage office assists with organization and efficiency. It can help to automate routine massage practice tasks such as appointment reminders, improve cash flow, and increase accuracy.

INFORMATION SYSTEMS

An *information system* is a collection of elements that provides accurate, timely, and useful information. To understand the procedure of an information system, the massage therapist must understand basic terminology related to this concept. A glossary of terms and definitions can help the novice understand the terminology of the modern electronic massage practice and is useful in selecting contemporary massage practice equipment. Box 5-2 contains a detailed list of basic information system terms.

Figure 5-1 depicts the five elements that make up the information system:

- Hardware (equipment)
- Software (programs)
- Data
- Personnel
- Procedures

Hardware

Hardware is the information system's physical equipment. The central piece of hardware in the information system is the computer. A computer is a device that electronically accepts *data,* processes the data arithmetically and logically, produces output from the processing, and stores the result for future use. Computers usually are classified in three categories: mainframe, minicomputers, and microcomputers.

The mainframe computer is a large system that handles numerous users, stores large amounts of data, and processes data at very high speeds. This type of system may be found, for example, in an insurance company in which the mainframe computer is used to process many claim forms with large amounts of data that must be processed quickly.

A midrange system, or minicomputer, is compact and has a slower processing speed and more limited storage capacity than the mainframe system, but it is more powerful than

BOX 5-2   Technology Terms

CD/DVD drives: Most computers come with a 32× to 48× speed CD-ROM drive that can read CDs. If you plan to write music, audio files, and documents on a CD or DVD, you should consider upgrading to a CD-RW. A better alternative is to upgrade to a DVD-R/RW combination drive. It allows you to read DVDs and CDs and to write data on (burn) a DVD or CD. A DVD has a capacity of at least 4.7 GB, compared with the 650-MB capacity of a CD.

Card reader/writer: A card reader/writer is useful for transferring data directly to and from a removable flash memory card, such as the ones used in your camera or music player. Make sure the card reader/writer can read from and write to the flash memory cards that you use.

Digital camera: Consider an inexpensive point-and-shoot digital camera. They are small enough to carry around, usually operate automatically in terms of lighting and focus, and contain storage cards for storing photographs. A 1.3- to 2.2-megapixal camera with an 8-MB or 16-MB storage card is fine for creating images for use on the Web or to send by e-mail.

Digital video capture device: A digital video capture device allows you to connect your computer to a camcorder or VCR and record, edit, manage, and then write video back to a VCR tape, a CD, or a DVD. The digital video capture device can be an external device or an adapter card. To create quality video (true 30 frames/second, full-sized TV), the digital video capture device should have a USB 2.0 or FireWire port. You will find that a standard USB port is too slow to maintain video quality. You will also need sufficient storage: an hour of data on a VCR tape takes up about 5 GB of disk storage.

Hard disk: It is recommended that you buy a computer with a 40- to 60-GB hard disk if your primary interests are browsing the Web and using e-mail and massage practice suite–type applications; 60 to 80 GB if you also want to edit digital photographs; 80 to 100 GB if you plan to edit digital video or manipulate large audio files even occasionally; and 100 to 160 GB if you will edit digital video, movies, or photography often; store audio files and music; or consider yourself to be a power user.

Joystick/wheel: If you use your computer to play games, you will want to purchase a joystick or wheel. These devices, especially the more expensive ones, provide for realistic game play with force feedback, programmable buttons, and specialized levers and wheels.

Keyboard: The keyboard is one of the more important devices used to communicate with the computer. For this reason, make sure the keyboard you purchase has 101 to 105 keys, is comfortable, easy to use, and has a USB connection. A wireless keyboard should be considered, especially if you have a small desk area.

Modem: Most computers come with a modem so that you can use your telephone line to dial out and access the Internet. Some modems also have fax capabilities. Your modem should be rated at 56 kbps.

Monitor: The monitor is where you will view documents, read e-mail messages, and view pictures. A minimum of a 17-inch screen is recommended, but if you are planning to use your computer for graphic design or game playing, you may want to purchase a 19- or 21-inch monitor. The LCD flat panel monitor should be considered, especially if space is an issue.

Mouse: As you work with your computer, you use the mouse constantly. Spend a few extra dollars if necessary, and purchase a mouse with an optical sensor and USB connection. The optical sensor replaces the need for a mouse ball, which means you do not need a mouse pad. For a PC, make sure your mouse has a wheel, which acts as a third button in addition to the top two buttons on the left and right. An ergonomic design is also important because your hand is on the mouse most of the time when you are using your computer. A wireless mouse should be considered to eliminate the cord and allow you to work at short distances from your computer.

Network card: If you plan to connect to a network or use broadband (cable or DSL) to connect to the Internet, you will need to purchase a network card. Broadband connections require a 10/100 PCI Ethernet network card.

Printer: Your two basic printer choices are inkjet and laser. Color inkjet printers cost on average between $50 and $300. Laser printers cost $300 to $2000. In general, the cheaper the printer, the lower the resolution and speed, and the more often you are required to change the ink cartridge or toner. Laser printers print faster and with a higher quality than inkjet printers, and their toner on average costs less. If you want color, go with a high-end inkjet printer to ensure quality of print. Duty cycle (i.e., number of pages you expect to print each month) also should be a determining factor. If your duty cycle is on the low end—hundreds of pages per month—stay with a high-end inkjet printer rather than purchasing a laser printer. If you plan to print photographs taken with a digital camera, you should purchase a photo printer. A photo printer is a dye-sublimation printer or an inkjet printer with higher resolution and features that allow you to print quality photographs.

Processor: For a PC, a 2.0-GHz Intel or AMD processor is more than enough processor power for application home and small massage practice or home massage practice users. Game home users, large businesses, and power users should upgrade to faster processors.

RAM: RAM plays a vital role in the speed of your computer. Make sure the computer you purchase has at least 256 MB of RAM. If you have extra money to invest in your computer, consider increasing the RAM to 512 MB or more. The extra money for RAM will be well spent.

Scanner: The most popular scanner purchased with a computer is the flatbed scanner. When evaluating a flatbed scanner, check the color depth and resolution. Do not buy anything less than a color depth of 48 bits and a resolution of 1200 × 2400 dpi. The higher the color depth, the more accurate the color. A higher resolution picks up the more subtle gradations of color.

Sound card: Most sound cards support the Sound Blaster and General MIDI standards and should be capable of recording and playing digital audio. If you plan to turn your computer into an entertainment system or are a game home user, you will want to spend the extra money and upgrade from the standard sound card.

(Continued)

BOX 5-2	Technology Terms—cont'd

Speakers: After you have a good sound card, quality speakers and a separate subwoofer that amplifies the bass frequencies of the speakers can turn your computer into a premium stereo system.

Video graphics card: Most standard video cards satisfy the monitor display needs of application home and small massage practice users. If you are a game home user or a graphic designer, you will want to upgrade to a higher-quality video card. The higher refresh rate will further enhance the display of games, graphics, and movies.

PC video camera: A PC video camera is a small camera used to capture and display live video (in some cases with sound), primarily on a Web page. You also can capture, edit, and share video and still photos. The camera sits on your monitor or desk. Recommended minimum specifications include 640 × 480 resolution, a video with a rate of 30 frames per second, and a USB 2.0 or FireWire connection.

USB flash (jump) drive: If you work on different computers and need access to the same data and information, this portable mobile storage device that can fit on your key chain is ideal. USB flash drive capacity varies from 128 MB to 4 GB.

Wireless LAN Access Point: A wireless LAN Access Point allows you to network several computers so they can share files and can access the Internet through a single cable modem or DSL connection. Each device that you connect requires a wireless card. A wireless LAN Access Point can offer range of operation up to several hundred feet, so be sure the device has a high-powered antenna.

Zip drive: Consider purchasing a Zip disk drive to back up important files. The Zip drive, which has a capacity of up to 750 MB, is sufficient for most users. An alternative to purchasing a backup drive is to purchase a CD-RW or DVD-R/RW and burn backups of key files on a CD or DVD.

From Shelly GB, Cashman TJ, Vermaat ME: *Discovering Computers: Fundamentals Edition.* Boston, 2004, Course Technology.

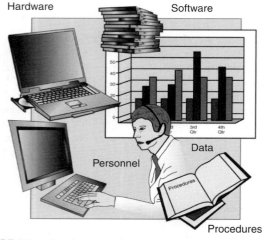

FIGURE 5-1. Five elements of an information system. *(From Finkbeiner BL, Finkbeiner CA:* Practice Management for the Dental Team, *ed 6, St. Louis, 2006, Mosby.)*

the microcomputer. This type of system is often found in large health care practices in which computer resources are shared. A centralized processing area may be implemented with this system, and processing can be done for several massage therapists in one practice or different health professionals including the massage therapist throughout a large establishment.

The microcomputer, also called a *personal computer,* is the smallest computer of the systems described and is self-contained with regard to the circuitry and components for arithmetic, logic, and control operations. These machines usually are priced at less than $2000, and the cost continues

to decrease. This kind of system is becoming increasingly popular in many small massage therapy practices and can be connected together to form a local area network (LAN).

In addition to the computer system previously described, other technologies prevalent in massage practice include telephone systems with the capacity for voicemail or paging, fax (facsimile) machines, copy machines, calculators, and scanners.

- Voicemail allows incoming and outgoing telephone messages to be recorded and processed.
- Pagers or cell phones carried by members of the massage practice staff allow them to be signaled when needed.
- Fax machines send and receive documents or other graphic images over telephone systems.
- Copy machines reproduce letters, charts and drawings, financial reports, clinical records, and statements from the clients' ledger cards. Box 5-3 describes features of copiers.
- Calculators found in computer *software* or those purchased separately are a great help to massage therapists with many routine duties that require mathematical skill. Except for the computer calculators, many are inexpensive enough to be sold at department and discount stores. The price of a calculator is not determined entirely by the number of its functions, although this is an important factor. The types of components and materials used to produce the machine also affect the price (Box 5-4 and Fig. 5-2).
- Scanners input text or graphic data directly into computer storage without keying. Any of these devices may be directly connected to the computer system and provide a centralized source for information. Chapter 10 includes detailed descriptions of telecommunications systems and techniques.

BOX 5-3	Features to Consider When Selecting or Using Copiers

1. Style of copiers: tabletop size or stand-alone floor models
2. Volume of work to be done: low-volume, mid-volume, high-volume work
3. Quality of copy desired: clear and sharp
4. Selection of paper size for reports, ledger cards, and letters
5. Ability to reproduce from a colored original or colored ink
6. Speed and output: number of copies per minute
7. Capability to make copies on regular massage practice forms and paper
8. Availability of outside copying business to handle a large volume of documents (e.g., new massage practice policy) or other specialized copying services

See Figure 5-6.
From Finkbeiner BL, Finkbeiner CA: *Practice Management for the Dental Team*, ed 6, St. Louis, 2006, Mosby.

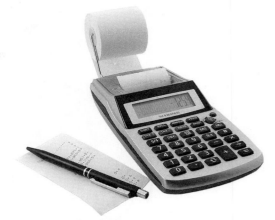

FIGURE 5-2. Calculator. *(2007 © Brent Hathaway. Image from BigStockPhoto.com.)*

BOX 5-4	Features to Consider When Selecting a Calculator

1. Type of display
2. Printing capabilities
3. Quality of keyboard
4. Type of batteries: On portable models, are they easily obtained? Are they throwaway or rechargeable?
5. The durability of components and materials: Factors other than cost will influence the selection of a calculator.
6. Ease of operation: The calculator should allow for the basic computations of addition, subtraction, multiplication, and division. Some machines can solve difficult trigonometry problems that only an accomplished mathematician could answer accurately.
7. Decimal functions: A fixed decimal restricts the number of decimals; a floating decimal puts no restriction on the position of the decimal point.
8. Repeat and constant operations: This feature allows the operator to add or subtract a series of identical numbers by depressing the *add* or *subtract* function key repeatedly.
9. Memory register: Figures can be added to or subtracted from and are available until the register is cleared.

From Finkbeiner BL, Finkbeiner CA: *Practice Management for the Dental Team*, ed 6, St. Louis, 2006, Mosby.

Software

The computer system is directed by a series of instructions called a *computer program,* or *software,* which directs the sequence of operations the system is to perform. Software in the massage practice may include general purpose software, such as word processors, spreadsheets, or database systems, or it may include software specifically designed for massage practice management. Software may be provided with the computer system or be purchased as individual or bundled packages. The parts of the desktop window that need to be identified are shown in Figure 5-3. The CD with this textbook contains massage business practice software for you to practice with and learn about the various functions. As mentioned previously, you will be instructed when to activate your CD. There are many screen shots of the software on Evolve site for you to view before using the actual software.

Data

The term *data* refers to the facts or figures that the information system needs to produce accurate and timely information. Data are the raw material of the information system and are manipulated or processed by the computer to produce the finished product: information. For instance, the massage therapist enters data such as fees and payments on a financial record if the practice bills clients for services. The finished product can result in a statement for the client. If the data are incorrect, the resulting information will be incorrect: garbage in; garbage out.

Procedures

Procedures are the written documentation or policies that help maintain the information system efficiently. Specialized manuals can be assembled, or these procedures may be included in the massage practice procedures manual described in Chapter 2.

SELF-REFLECTION

How comfortable and capable am I with technology? Do I need to take some additional training to be more efficient? Am I nervous or excited about technology? How can I incorporate technology into my massage practice?

FIGURE 5-3. Parts of a typical desktop window. *(Microsoft product screen shot reprinted with permission from Microsoft Corporation.)*

If any of the elements—hardware, software, data, personnel, or procedures—are missing or flawed, the entire information system may be affected.

OPERATIONS OF AN INFORMATION SYSTEM

Regardless of the model that is selected for the massage practice, computers are capable of performing four general operations known as the *information processing cycle.* The four operations are input, process, output, and storage. By using these four operations, the computer can process the data into information.

Parts of a Computer

INPUT DEVICE

The most common means of entering information and instructions into the computer is the keyboard (Figs. 5-4 and 5-5). Special keys on the enhanced 101-key keyboard may include a numeric keypad, cursor control keys, and function keys. In addition to the keyboard, other data collection devices include the mouse or trackball, touch screens, graphic input devices, scanners, and voice input. These devices may input data directly without any keystrokes.

PROCESSOR

The processor is the controlling unit of the system that contains the electronic circuitry to manipulate data. This unit is known as the *central processing unit* (CPU) (see Fig. 5-4), and it directs and controls all of the computer's activities. As the data are accepted from the input device, they are processed according to the program. The *program* is a series of instructions directing the computer to perform a sequence of tasks. The number of programs and data that can be stored in the

processing unit depends on the main memory of the system. The memory capacity of computers varies, but the computer has a fixed memory capacity. One byte of computer memory can be considered equivalent to one character of storage. The memory capacity is expressed in terms of kilobytes, megabytes, or gigabytes, which roughly represent 1 thousand, 1 million, or 1 billion bytes of storage, respectively. The typical massage practice system may have 8 megs (megabytes) of main memory and a 4-gig (gigabytes) hard drive for storing client records.

OUTPUT DEVICE

The printer and the monitor are the two most commonly used output devices (see Fig. 5-4). If a paper copy (hard copy) is needed, the computer is directed to print a copy. When no permanent record is needed, the output is displayed on the monitor (soft copy).

There are two classifications of printers: impact and nonimpact. The *impact printer* creates images on the paper as the mechanism strikes the paper, ribbon, and characters together. The two most common impact printers are the dot matrix and letter-quality printers.

The *nonimpact printer* creates images on the paper without characters striking the sheet of paper. Nonimpact printers are almost noiseless, because the characters are shaped with the use of light or a spray of ink. The two most common nonimpact printers are inkjet and laser printers. The laser printer, often called an *intelligent printer,* combines printing and photocopying features to make it the most economical choice. The intelligent printer is able to collate, stack, and place images on both sides of the paper. The cost of these printers has decreased, and they now produce multiple copies more economically. Some printers in both categories are able to print color images, which greatly enhances the visual effect of the output (Fig. 5-6).

As the information is entered, it is displayed on the video display screen, also known as a *monitor.* Terminals are

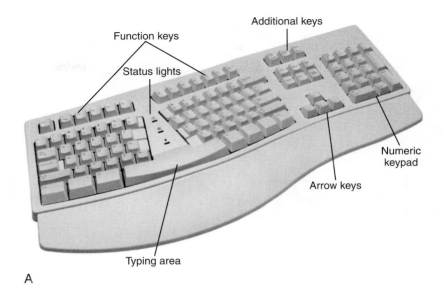

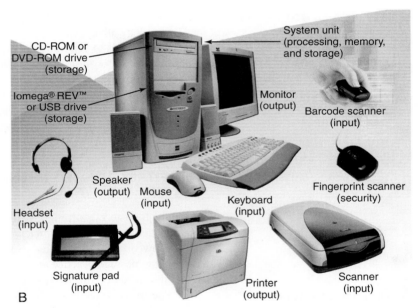

FIGURE 5-4. **A**, Computer keyboard. **B**, Components of an office computer. *(Modified from Finkbeiner BL, Finkbeiner CA:* Practice Management for the Dental Team, *ed 6, St. Louis, 2006, Mosby.)*

classified as *dumb terminals* or *intelligent terminals.* Dumb terminals depend on the system to which they are connected for memory and processing circuitry. Intelligent terminals have their own processing capabilities (see Fig. 5-5).

STORAGE MEDIA

Auxiliary storage is used to store data and programs that are not being processed on the computer. Types of storage include hard disk, tape cartridge, compact disk, flash drive, and jump drive (Fig. 5-7). Other devices for storage are used, but they usually require a large computer system. The hard disk is a rigid metal disk coated with magnetic material that

makes it suitable for recording and storing data. The optical compact disk system uses a laser to burn microscopic holes on the surface of a hard plastic disk. The most popular optical disk formats used for data storage are the recordable compact disk (CD-R) and rewritable compact disk (CD-RW). Another small optical disk format used for storage is the compact disk read-only memory (CD-ROM). Most software is distributed on the CD-ROM format. Other types of popular storage devices are jump, thumb, or flash drives, which are portable storage devices that plug directly into computers, hold large amounts of data, and do not require any type of disk.

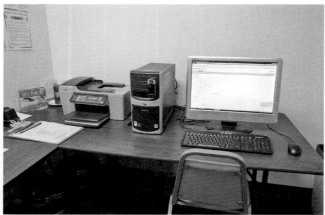

FIGURE 5-5. Workstation with a keyboard and monitor.

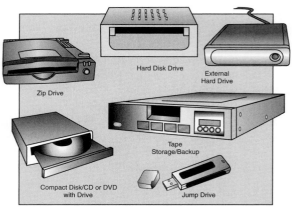

FIGURE 5-7. Different types of storage media. *(From Finkbeiner BL, Finkbeiner CA:* Practice Management for the Dental Team, *ed 6, St. Louis, 2006, Mosby.)*

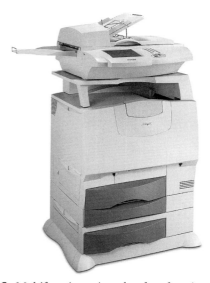

FIGURE 5-6. Multifunction printer has four functions: color printer, scanner, plain-paper fax, and copier. *(Courtesy of Lexmark International.)*

LEARNING ACTIVITY

Research the various anticipated advances in technology, such as increased satellite transmission for wireless Internet connection. List at least three expected advances in technology that you think will benefit the massage therapy business operations.

_____

_____

_____

Technology advancements are progressing at a rate that makes it difficult to remain current. Some of the information in this chapter soon will be obsolete. For example, tape backup for computers is quickly being replaced by other, more efficient backup devices, but the fundamental principles remain valid. The use of technology for massage practice will continue to increase.

PROFITABILITY OF THE INFORMATION SYSTEM

All of the high-tech equipment available today will not make the massage practice more efficient if proper procedures are not followed before investing in the information system. Before the massage practice acquires new equipment of any kind, the needs of the massage practice should be identified. The major categories of equipment you may need to consider include computers dedicated to tasks such as word processing, records management, and accounting; copying machines; and calculators. Other specific types of equipment used to handle mail and telephone systems are discussed in other chapters.

A *feasibility study* is one of the most reliable ways to determine what type of computer system would best serve the massage practice. A feasibility study must involve everyone who will use the system and other support staff. Some factors to consider when doing the feasibility study include type and size of the practice, cost, ability of the staff, and training requirements. A massage practice is prepared for automation if the questions in Box 5-5 can be answered in the affirmative. After the need for a system has been established, it is time to begin selecting equipment and software, setting up the procedures for using the equipment, training personnel, and entering the initial data.

SOFTWARE SELECTION

The first part of the chapter can be used as a guideline in selecting the hardware components of the information system for the massage practice needs, with the help of equipment manufacturers. The next task is the selection of software. Software is the computer program written to meet specific user needs.

Selecting software that will perform the jobs specific to your massage practice is important. Software is available that can perform a general task such as word processing and generate spreadsheets, databases, graphics, and electronic and desktop publishing. Software can also perform specific tasks for massage practices, including account reports, client reports, client history, insurance claim processing, appointment scheduling, treatment planning, summary reports, billing and receivables, referral tracking, income analysis, recall, and inventory management. Figures 5-8 through 5-10 show some of the screens that can be accessed in Massage Office Professional on the CD-ROM at the back of this book.

- The *client information screen* (see Fig. 5-8) includes comprehensive client information. The accounts screen includes accounts payable information (see Fig. 5-9). A variety of payment and remittance information is found on this screen, including the minimum monthly payment, date of the last statement, current account balance, and outstanding insurance or budget plan balances.
- The *client master report* (see Fig. 5-10) can be filtered or sorted using different criteria, such as client zip codes, birthdays, phone numbers, or insurance coverage.
- The *treatment plan screen* enables you to produce a treatment plan for the client and to track all of the planned treatment to completion.
- The daily *appointment screen* with an expanded view can indicate various treatment rooms.
- A *tickler file* is provided in the appointment section of the program to collect and store information on clients who have missed, canceled, or broken appointments.
- *Clinical charting* may be linked to the software system. Charting can be done in the treatment room using a graphic format. Charting can be done in a basic format or may include complex charts for test results or specialty areas. This chart can even be e-mailed to another massage therapist for evaluation.
- The *daily treatment room schedule* includes the amount of time and type of treatment to be rendered.
- The *day sheet report* summarizes practice activity for a period of time.
- *Annual graphic reports* are generated to illustrate categorical treatment production.

BOX 5-5	Questions to Consider When Preparing to Automate

1. Is there a manual system in place that gives all the data needed to evaluate the practice monthly?
2. Does the massage therapist and staff understand the significance of the data?
3. Is the staff organized?
4. Does the work get done in a timely manner?
5. Do the clients receive current and accurate information?
6. Is the staff stable and team oriented?

Modified from Finkbeiner BL, Finkbeiner CA: *Practice Management for the Dental Team,* ed 6, St. Louis, 2006, Mosby.

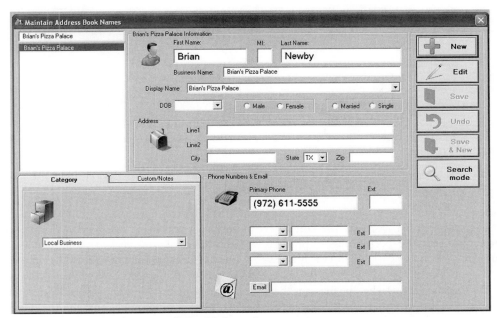

FIGURE 5-8. Client information screen. *(Courtesy of Island Software.)*

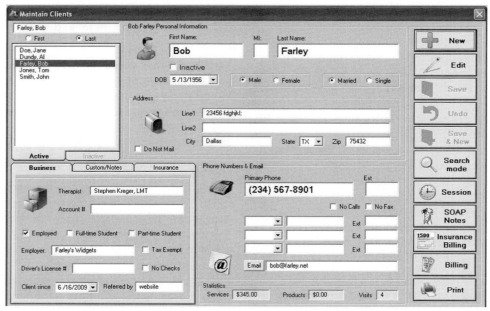

FIGURE 5-9. Client accounts screen. *(Courtesy of Island Software.)*

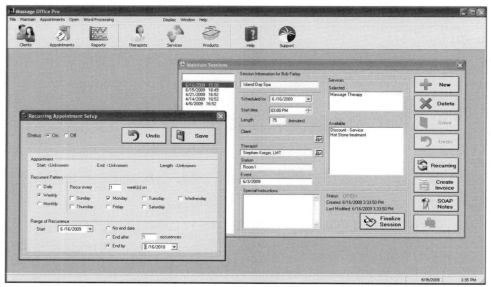

FIGURE 5-10. The client master report can be filtered or sorted using a variety of criteria: client zip code, birthday, phone number, insurance status, and other delimiters. *(Courtesy of Island Software.)*

Appropriate selection of a software package is extremely important. For the software to be effective, the computer functions must be applicable to the specific massage practice. Stored data and information must be usable and easily accessible. The required applications should be presented to the vendor rather than asking the vendor what the massage therapy practice should do. Take a routine accounts receivable task and have the vendor explain how it would be processed with that company's equipment and software. Inquire how different procedures (e.g., billing, payments, appointment notification) can be combined. Another option is starting with basic software packages and then adding appointment tracking, treatment planning, marketing, and payroll.

The word processing function is invaluable to the business, and it can be integrated with the information system to improve communications with the clients. The computer, when used to produce welcome letters, newsletters, and special greetings, can be a very effective marketing tool.

When using word processing software on the computer, the document is prepared electronically, and the text is entered on the computer keyboard in the same manner as on a typewriter. As the text is entered, it is displayed on the screen (monitor) and stored in the computer's memory. This is an electronic format, and it is easy to edit a document by making changes in the text. Text can be corrected by using a backspace or delete key. Words, sentences, paragraphs, or pages may be added or deleted from a document. Text can be moved from one section to another. The document is formatted according to your specifications. For example, margins, type style, double or single spacing, underlining, boldface or italics, and page length are determined by the user. When the document is finalized and all corrections made, a command is made to print the document. You can have more than one copy printed, and each copy is an original. These documents are stored in the computer's memory, and they can be used again in their original form or edited and brought up to date.

Most word processing packages include features such as spell check, grammar check, and a thesaurus. Some spell-check software allows you to add words specific to massage therapy and medical terminology. Word processing software can be a very productive tool for the massage practice and should be selected wisely. Box 5-6 lists common features of word processing software packages. Software that has been written specifically for the massage practice may include the capabilities of electronic spreadsheet calculations, databases, and graphics. If these functions are not included but are needed, additional commercial software packages may be another option.

An electronic spreadsheet software package allows the user to organize numeric data in a worksheet or table format. The user enters the data into the formula that has been typed in specific rows and columns, known as *cells*. As the data are entered in the proper cells, the electronic calculations are performed automatically. Daily postings and updates can be made very easily. An electronic spreadsheet's ability to recalculate data makes this an invaluable tool for business massage practice management.

Database software allows the user to create electronic files that can be retrieved, manipulated, and updated as necessary. A database is a collection of data that is stored in multiple files. Database software features include operations to create the database, copy, delete, and sort the data; data editing and updating capabilities; mathematical functions; and the ability to retrieve data and produce a report. This type of software package is a valuable tool in an inventory control or recall system.

A graphics software package allows the user to create graphs from numeric data; this is sometimes part of the spreadsheet software package. The most common forms of graphics are pie charts, line diagrams, and bar graphs. Graphs are good management tools for reviewing information and helping to communicate information more effectively. When using graphics in a presentation, select the type of graph that is most appropriate for your purpose. Do not try to present too much information, use few words, be consistent, and keep the graphics simple.

BOX 5-6	Common Features of Word Processors

INSERT
Insert characters
Insert words
Insert lines
Insert documents
DELETE
Delete characters
Delete words
Delete sentences
Delete paragraphs
Delete pages
Delete entire document
KEYBOARD AND SCREEN CONTROL PRINTING
Cursor movement
Page up and down
Word wrap
Upper- and lower-case display
Function keys
Control keys
Status line
Line
Column
FORMAT
Top and bottom margins
Left and right margins
Tab stops
Single and double spacing
MOVE
Move sentences
Move paragraphs
Move blocks
SEARCH AND REPLACE
Search to specific text
Search and replace word
Search and replace character strings
PRINTING
Print columns
Subscripts
Superscripts
Underline
Boldface
Headers
Footers
Page numbering
Document title

Modified from Finkbeiner BL, Finkbeiner CA: *Practice Management for the Dental Team,* ed 6, St. Louis, 2006, Mosby.

Integrated Applications

Electronic spreadsheet software and word processing typically are used independently of each other, but what if you wanted some of the information from the spreadsheet in a word processing document? Integrated software combines these applications into a single set of programs that allow the user to share data between applications.

Clinical Records Applications

Although it may appear that the bulk of record management is generated only in the business aspect of the massage practice, you should not overlook the computer as a communication tool between the treatment room and the business office. Systems are available for client histories, general and specialty charting, and treatment-completed records. Such a system also eliminates record contamination, because barrier covers may be placed over the keyboard, and the chances of disease transmission through record management are decreased.

Guidelines for Selecting Software

Choosing the right software for the specific need of the massage practice can be difficult. The information in Box 5-7 should help.

IMPLEMENTING THE CHANGE TO COMPUTERIZATION

Establishing Procedures

Establishing procedures is necessary to make sure that work flows smoothly through the entire process of origination to completion. A procedures manual for computer tasks

---

BOX 5-7 Guidelines for Choosing the Right Software

1. Determine the needs of the massage practice: type of practice, size of practice, ability of staff, cost, and training required for the physician and support staff.
2. Select a vendor who is reputable and provides fast and efficient support when you have questions. Ask about other massage practices that use the system. How many systems have they installed within your geographic area? Are the insurance forms that are processed through the system accepted by participating insurance companies?
3. Know what you want the computer to do: improve billing, improve practice management, improve massage practice efficiency, track delinquent accounts, compute monthly finance charges, and aid in communications as a marketing device.
4. What type of backup does the system have in case of computer failure?
5. If security of information is a concern, how is it managed?
6. Know what type of training is available from the vendor. Systems are available that have tutorial software. Does the software have a written paper text and recorded instructions for the learner?
7. The computer and software selection process requires a great deal of thought and time, so make the selection carefully. Everyone will have to live with the decision that is made.

Modified from Finkbeiner BL, Finkbeiner CA: *Practice Management for the Dental Team*, ed 6, St. Louis, 2006, Mosby.

---

is beneficial for all staff members. This manual provides detailed information about how various tasks are completed and by whom, as well as the purpose of each task.

Software manuals that are provided with the software should be carefully evaluated. If the documentation and instructions are difficult to follow or understand, the individual will not use the system properly and efficiently.

UNDERSTANDING THE INTERNET

If you are using the Internet to gather information, to shop, or for entertainment, you are probably familiar with the process of logging in and moving from one Web site to another. However, do you really understand how you are doing what you are doing as you move from one Web location to another? How did the Internet get started?

The Internet began in the late 1960s as an experiment by the U.S. Department of Defense to see if a noncentralized network could be built to withstand the destruction of one or more of its parts. Unlike previous networks, this new network did not have a single central point. Instead, all sites on the network were interconnected.

Out of this network came a protocol for linking computers together. A *protocol* is a set of standards for how network communication takes place. The protocol is called the Transmission Control Protocol/Internet Protocol (TCP/IP). This protocol is the standard that makes it possible for different computers all over the globe to talk to each other. The TCP/IP protocol is the foundation of the Internet.

At first, the Internet was used solely by the government, but universities and other institutions soon connected themselves to the Internet to communicate with one another and collaborate on projects. The Internet grew to connect hundreds of different sites all across the world. Each organization on the Internet was responsible for maintaining its part of the network, so the Internet was not owned or controlled by any one organization. The Internet now connects up to 40 million people around the globe, and it is growing by as much as 10% per month.

The Internet is like a system of roads, freeways, and bridges. Internet access companies, or Internet service providers (ISPs), provide "onramps" to the information superhighway—physical connections that allow you to access the Internet. These onramps are called *POPs*, or points of presence. Dial-up service used to be the only way for many computer users to access the Internet. Luckily, that has changed, and there are options for getting online. The main disadvantage of dial-up is that it is very slow. It takes much longer to navigate the Web or download a file when you are using a dial-up connection. A wireless network uses radio waves, just like cell phones, televisions, and radios do. Communication across a wireless network is like two-way radio communication. Cable modems can provide your computer with Internet connectivity by means of your television's cable connection if you are a cable television subscriber. DSL is another option that is comparable to the speeds of cable, but DSL subscribers do not need to have cable television in their homes. A T3 connection is another high-tech option, and it is usually too expensive for personal use. However, if you run a business from home and the benefits warrant the cost, you may want to consider the T3 option for your computer. High-speed Internet is unavailable in some parts of the country without the use of a satellite connection. The cost of satellite Internet service is comparable to cable service in more populated areas, although it is a little less reliable. The term *broadband* is used to describe almost any always-on, high-speed connection to the Internet.

After you are connected to a POP, you have access to all the resources of the Internet. Most ISPs supply you with software for surfing the Internet: a Web browser.

The Birth of Domain Names

In the 1980s, a major shift occurred as a result of the increase in scale of the Internet and its associated management issues. To make it easy for people to use the network, hosts were assigned names so that it was not necessary to remember the numeric addresses. Originally, there were a fairly limited number of hosts, and it was feasible to maintain a single table of all the hosts and their associated names and addresses. The shift to having a large number of independently managed networks (e.g., LANs) meant that having a single table of hosts was no longer feasible, and the Domain Name System (DNS) was established. The DNS permitted the conversion of a numeric host address (e.g., 215.72.87.66) to an easier to remember name address (e.g., somesite.com). A domain name is the name of a Web site that you place in the hypertext window (where the http:// is seen).

The Birth of the Web Browser

In October 1994, Mosaic Communications Corporation (renamed Netscape Communications on November 11, 1994) introduced the first public beta of their browser, Mosaic Netscape. This was one of the first Web browsers to be freely distributed across the Internet.

How Does E-mail Work?

Let's say you are sending mail to joy@aol.com. When you have finished composing your e-mail, your mailer (i.e., e-mail software) performs a gethostbyname system call to look up the IP address of the remote host (e.g., aol.com). Normally, the host would be looked up from /etc/hosts, but because you are on the Internet, your system queries an Internet name server to find the address of aol.com.

Your mailer opens a virtual circuit over the Internet to "joy's" mailer. It communicates with the remote mailer by using the Simple Mail Transfer Protocol (SMTP). If all goes well, the mail is usually delivered within a few seconds, even if the recipient's machine is on the other side of the world. If the remote site is down, your mailer will keep trying every hour or so, usually for a couple of days. If the site still cannot be reached, the mail will be returned to you as "undeliverable."

The Web Site

The Internet, particularly in its graphic interface known as the World Wide Web, is probably the most important communication vehicle developed since the telephone. More importantly, the Web levels the playing field between small business and big business.

The Web is the newest medium for advertising and is dynamic, interactive, and inexpensive. As the Web matures, advertising rates for the most popular sites will increase.

The Web is an important customer service tool. The Web allows you to communicate with your customers at their convenience.

GETTING A WEB SITE

To have a Web site, you need a domain name. There are a couple of ways to do this:

■ Go online to InterNIC (www.internic.com) or a name registration service such as www.register.com, and perform a name search to make sure the domain you want to establish is available. After confirming the availability of your domain name, complete the online registration form to secure your name.
■ You select an ISP to host your Web site. The service provider registers your company with the InterNIC—the Internet's Network Information Center.

A unique domain name of your choosing is assigned to your business or organization, such as sun.com, indiana.edu, nasa.gov, or neosoft.com. One or more IP network numbers are assigned to you, such as 198.64.6. Internet zone tables are updated to include your domain name, the mapping between your domain name and network numbers, and to show that the route to your network is through your service provider.

COST OF A WEB SITE

Hosting fees are based on your individual need for space, download capacity, security, and special programming requirements. In general, the monthly hosting fee for a basic Web site account should cost between $25 and $50. There are many places on the Internet that offer hosting at no charge. Before you decide to host your Web site with one of these services, be sure you understand the fine print of your hosting agreement. In general free hosting services are free because of the following:

- You will be required to place banner advertisements on the top or bottom of each page of your Web site. In some cases, you will be required to place banner advertisements on the top and the bottom of your Web pages.
- The activities of visitors to your Web site will be tracked by means of cookies or other online software. Their activities on the Internet will be monitored, and the data collected will be sold to marketing services.

Good Stuff from the Government

SMALL BUSINESS ASSOCIATION
The very competitive business climate demands that business owners understand and use advanced technologies. Technology is an enabler; it can help a business improve efficiencies and expand operations. However, the use of technology should be balanced with business needs and practicality. The SBA's Web site (http://www.sba.gov) is a source of information:

Understanding the Internet: A brief history and discussion of the Internet.

Glossary of Internet terms: The meanings of terms used about the Internet.

Getting on the Web: Explanation about how to get your business on the Web.

eCommerce resources: A list of resources about eCommerce, provided by the SBA.

Online advertising: U.S. Department of Commerce's guide to the regulations of online advertising.

Online advertising regulations: Guide to the Federal Trade Commission's rules and regulations on online advertising.

TECH-Net: Sponsored by the SBA, TECH-Net provides a network for small businesses to find innovation and research grant opportunities.

FREE ONLINE COURSES
The SBA Web site also offers free online courses. The course called Technology 101 is especially relevant to the content in this chapter.

SUMMARY

A computer's primary advantage is the accuracy and quality of its finished results, but without proper management and usage, the computer becomes a costly investment with poor returns. A well-planned information system can help to make the massage practice more efficient, and the combination of an experienced staff and high-technology equipment can result in higher productivity, better client relations, and a happier staff. Advances in technology are occurring at such a rate that it is impossible to remain current in a written textbook. Implementation of time-saving and communication technologies will continue to grow in the future and will allow the massage therapist to streamline many of the business tasks, freeing more time for doing what we love—massage therapy.

Bibliography

Lavine L: Proper positioning of monitors, *Dent Econ* 99:102, 2004.

Neilburger EJ: Computers: 10 rules for selecting a computer system, *Dent Econ* 8:96, 1998.

Shelly GB, Cashman TJ, Vermat ME: *Discovering Computers 2006: A Gateway to Information*, Boston, 2005, Course Technology.

Shelly GB, Cashman TJ, Vermaat ME: *Discovering Computers: Fundamentals Edition*, Boston, 2004, Course Technology.

Evolve Annotated Web Links
http://evolve.elsevier.com/Fritz/business

InterNIC offers public information regarding Internet domain name registration services. It is a registered service mark of the U.S. Department of Commerce, and it is licensed to the Internet Corporation for Assigned Names and Numbers (http://www.icann.org/).

InterNIC: www.internic.com

Register.com (register domain names): www.register.com

Small Business Association free online courses: http://www.sba.gov/services/training/onlinecourses/TRANING_ATC_BUS.html

Small Business Association: http://www.sba.gov/smallbusinessplanner/manage/technology/index.html

Technology 101: A Small Business Guide: http://web.sba.gov/sbtn/registration/index.cfm?CourseId=60

1. Describe the importance of an information system to massage therapy.

_____

_____

_____

_____

_____

_____

_____

2. List and explain the operations a computer can perform.

_____

_____

_____

_____

_____

_____

_____

3. Explain the difference between an impact and a nonimpact printer.

_____

_____

_____

_____

_____

_____

_____

4. Describe how a feasibility study aids in determining the need for automation.

_____

_____

_____

_____

_____

_____

_____

5. Describe computer software.

_____

_____

_____

_____

_____

_____

_____

6. Explain the difference between general-task and specific-task software.

_____

_____

_____

_____

_____

7. Describe how word processing, electronic spreadsheet, database, and graphics software can be used effectively in the massage practice.

_____

_____

_____

_____

_____

_____

_____

_____

8. List six guidelines used in making the right software selection.

_____

_____

_____

_____

_____

_____

_____

9. Explain why computer procedures are important when setting up a new computer system within the massage practice.

_____

_____

_____

_____

_____

_____

_____

10. Select an activity such as accounts receivable or letter writing and determine an approximate time saving that can be achieved from using the computer instead of producing the end result in a traditional manual manner.

_____

_____

_____

_____

_____

_____

_____

MASSAGE THERAPY BUSINESS OFFICE DESIGN

KEY TERMS

Ergonomics
Reception room
Time and motion

LEARNING OUTCOMES

Mastery of the content in this chapter will enable the reader to:

- Define glossary terms
- Define ergonomics as it applies to the massage business office
- Describe classifications of motion
- Describe the implementation of time and motion in a massage business office
- Describe seasonal affective disorder

- Explain the effect of the Americans with Disabilities Act on office design
- Identify criteria for reception room design
- Identify criteria for business office design
- Describe factors involved in office design that relate to the Americans with Disabilities Act
- Describe the arrangement of common business equipment

Ⓔ Guidelines for the Learning Activities and answers to the Workbook questions are located on Evolve at http://evolve.elsevier.com/Fritz/business.

In the past, more emphasis was placed on the design of the massage treatment rooms than on the design of the business office. However, planning of the business office workspace is important. This area should be ergonomically designed so business tasks are performed with the greatest efficiency. *Ergonomics* is the science that studies the relationship between people and their work environments. Interrelated physical and psychological factors are involved in the creation of a stress-free work environment. By understanding the abilities that people have and their work patterns, it is possible to design work environments that conform to the abilities and work needs. Just as when giving a massage, the appropriate use of ergonomics can make the job more productive and efficient and can reduce work-related discomfort and injuries. There are many formal ergonomics studies about office tasks, but formal studies on the ergonomics of how to best perform massage are lacking. The good news is that the information for use of the computer, telephone, and other devices is well documented. This chapter is based on current understanding of ergonomics in the workplace. Ongoing research should improve our understanding of this important topic.

PHYSICAL ENVIRONMENT

Physiologic factors include color, lighting, acoustics, heating, air conditioning, space, furniture, and equipment. Color plays a major role in how a client perceives a practice, the massage therapist, health, productivity, and morale. An attractive, cheerful, and efficient office inspires confidence and comfort in the client. A drab, dirty, or untidy office can create an attitude of doubt or mistrust. Light colors are more appealing than dark colors. Some decorators work with dark colors for walls but use lighter accent colors to downplay the dark base color. Grays are often used with tones of mauves. Certain tones of gray can be tiring, and they tend to put workers to sleep. Light hues of warm colors can create cheerful surroundings. Cool colors, such as light greens and blues, can produce a tranquil atmosphere.

Massage offices do not need to present a stark, sterile image, but they should have a neutral atmosphere. It is best to avoid specific references to political, cultural, lifestyle, or religious preferences, although there are exceptions. A theme for the massage environment may be based on a specific geographic location, such as the ocean or mountain setting. If a specific cultural style of massage is offered, such as Shiatsu, the décor may reflect a Japanese landscape. Massage therapy supports healthy lifestyles but not typically a specific path to health, such as a vegan diet or a line of herbal supplements. Individual's religious or spiritual beliefs need to be respected, and someone may be offended by a specific reference to another religion. If you have a strong desire to express your beliefs in the professional environment, be aware that this may limit the clients who are comfortable in the environment. This situation has pros and cons, depending on how you want your massage client base to develop. The more neutral the environment and your professional presentation, the more comfortable will be a diverse population.

Designs for massage clinics or offices are adding warmth and beauty to the office while providing comfort and efficiency. A comfortable client is a happier client. Moreover, productivity is likely to be greater in a pleasant working environment. Many office plans are available; the one chosen should satisfy the needs of the massage therapists, colleagues, and clients.

SELF-REFLECTION

What are my favorite colors? What type of atmosphere do these colors create? What is my style—cozy and comfortable, clear glass and chrome, outdoors, or cultured? What type of decorating schemes are attractive—fun, tranquil, clinical, casual, or industrial? How can I develop an environment that is pleasing to me and to clients?

LEARNING ACTIVITY

In the space provided on p. 101 and using the graph, design a reception area and business office, keeping in mind the requirements of the Americans with Disabilities Act.

Seasonal Affective Disorder

In geographic locations where there are extremes of sunshine and darkness, clients or coworkers may experience seasonal affective disorder (SAD). Sunlight keeps the body's internal circadian clock in sync, so a person is alert and awake during the day and ready to sleep at night. A person's health, mood, and behavior can be affected when the quality and quantity of sunlight is diminished. A direct consequence of SAD can be winter depression or sleep disorders.

Many companies provide lighting systems to overcome SAD. Most of the lights are designed for the brightness needed for light therapy. With a brightness level of 10,000 lux at 24 inches, these lights have proved to be a fast and effective therapy at a comfortable distance. Most lights are easy to use and safe (no harmful UV rays). This type of lighting is recommended for the massage office.

Office Design and the Americans with Disabilities Act

Some clients have had difficulty gaining access to massage treatment rooms. The Americans with Disabilities Act of 1990 has affected the design public accessible facilities.

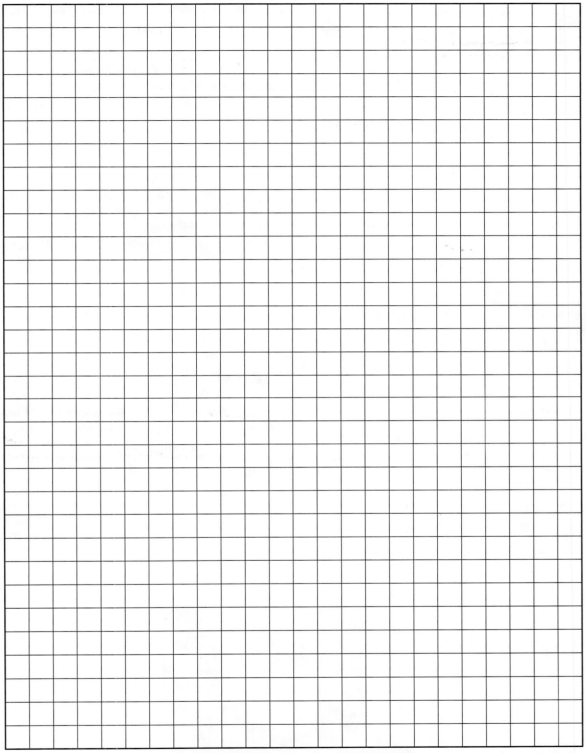

Using the sample graph paper above, design a reception area and business office. As you draw, keep in mind the requirements of the Americans with Disabilities Act. Use this scale: each quarter-inch line is equivalent to a foot of actual space.

BOX 6-1 Design Features of a Barrier-Free Office

The following modifications for creating a barrier-free environment comply with the Americans with Disabilities Act:
- Designate handicapped parking areas.
- Install sidewalk and curb access to accommodate wheelchairs or other devices.
- Install access ramps to building and office areas.
- Widen doors and doorways to accommodate wheelchairs and other devices.
- Install raised letters and Braille on elevator controls.
- Provide visual and sound alarms.
- Install grab bars.
- Install raised toilet seats and wider stalls.
- Make paper towel dispensers accessible.
- Install paper cup dispensers at existing water fountains.
- Eliminate plush, low-density carpeting.

BOX 6-2 Sources of Information on the Americans with Disabilities Act

Office of the Americans with Disabilities Act
U.S. Department of Justice
P.O. Box 66118
Washington, D.C. 20035-6738
1-800-514-0301 (voice)
1-800-514-0383 (TDD)
Internet Web site (ADA home page): http://www.ada.gov
Architectural and Transportation Barriers Compliance Board
1111 18th Street NW, Suite 501
Washington, D.C. 20036
1-800-872-2253 (voice)
1-800-993-2822 (TDD)
Electronic bulletin board: 202-272-5448
Internet Web site: http://www.access-board.gov

Special attention should be directed to this act to ensure that the location of the massage business design complies with state and federal guidelines. The Justice Department issues accessibility specifications for offices, but some states have even stricter standards. Accessibility features must be incorporated into renovations of a building, and those features must be accessible from elsewhere in the building. For example, making a lobby bathroom accessible to a wheelchair client is not adequate if the client cannot get to the lobby. Box 6-1 lists recommendations for designing a barrier-free office.

The government estimates that the cost of incorporating accessibility features into new construction is less than 1% of construction costs. Because remodeling existing buildings usually is more costly, the requirements for them are less stringent. The law requires only "reasonable modifications" that are achievable with little effort; both are terms that may lead to litigation. Further information on any part of the Americans with Disabilities Act is available from the sources listed in Box 6-2 and the Web site (http://www.ada.gov or http://www.access-board.gov).

ADA & Massage

Design of the Reception Room

The *reception room* (the term *waiting room* has a negative connotation) is the gateway to the massage therapy environment and provides the client's first impression of the massage therapist. A warm atmosphere can be created in the reception room, furnishing a comfortable living room–type environment. The massage area should reflect the theme originating in the reception room (Fig. 6-1).

Clients should be able to check in with the massage therapist or receptionist at the desk as soon as they arrive. For privacy, clients should have access to a restroom off the reception room, and appropriate signs should direct them to this area.

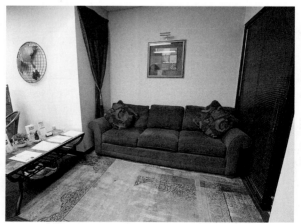

FIGURE 6-1. The reception room of a massage office reflects a theme. A reception room should have comfortable chairs and provide adequate seating space.

Seating in the reception room varies from office to office, depending on individual practice styles. A general rule is to provide two seats for each massage therapy treatment room in a general practice. Seating space is an important consideration. People usually do not like to have others sitting too close to them. When completing forms or other business activities, a person needs some privacy. Comfort should be the major concern when selecting furniture for this area. It needs to be sturdy but not too formal or too casual. Low, cushiony couches and armless chairs are sometimes difficult for even an agile person to get out of and even more difficult for an older adult or arthritic client. Figure 6-2 shows comfortable armchairs with a sturdy base.

Special amenities are a thoughtful gesture and include a desk-height table with an electrical outlet that makes it convenient for business people or students to bring laptop computers to use while waiting. A self-serve tea or juice bar is a considerate gesture for busy clients. These amenities send a message that the massage therapist respects the client's time and wants to make the office a friendly place to visit (Box 6-3). *Providing a wifi password*

Design of the Business Office

The business office workspace should provide a healthful, enjoyable environment that minimizes disruption and distraction. The factors involved in designing a business office work environment are motion economy, space planning, health issues, safety, and security. The following suggestions should be considered (Fig. 6-3):

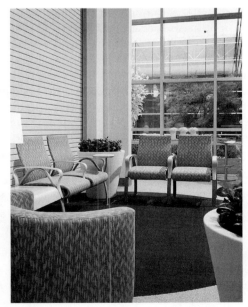

FIGURE 6-2. Open areas allow a client personal space and work areas. *(Courtesy of Dr. Neil Smith, Bridgman Massage, Bridgman, MI. In Finkbeiner BL, Finkbeiner CA: Practice Management for the Dental Team, ed 6, St. Louis, 2006, Mosby.)*

BOX 6-3	**Keys to Creating a Comfortable Reception Room**

1. A soft warning bell or chimes should announce the client's arrival in the reception area.
2. The client's arrival should be acknowledged immediately. A clear glass window affords privacy and allows the massage therapist or receptionist to see all the activity in the reception room. When a window is used, it commonly is 44 inches from the floor and at least 36 by 36 inches. A barrier-free environment can be created with the open concept. A desk area for physically challenged clients is positioned 27 to 29 inches from the floor (see 6-3).
3. Coat racks should be convenient for children and adults. A nearby bench benefits older adults, small children, and anyone putting on boots.
4. Magazine racks can be placed on a wall or table. They should be convenient for children and adults (see Fig. 6-4).
5. If appropriate to the massage practice, a small children's corner can be included.
6. The style and number of seats and tables depend on the clients' requirements. A combination of sofas and chairs provides a comfortable seating arrangement. Chairs should be of a height and depth that afford easy seating and exiting.
7. Cordial "no smoking" signs can be posted at the entrance and in the reception room.
8. An adjoining restroom eliminates trips to the inner office.
9. Warm, soft colors; wood paneling, fabric, and textured wallpaper; nature scenes or abstract artwork; a small, unobtrusive water feature; and mirrors add warmth to the reception room.
10. Signs directing clients to various rooms should be large and easy for all clients to read.
11. Full-spectrum lighting intensity and color should be adequate for easy reading of printed materials in any part of the room.
12. Soft, relaxing music of a general style (e.g., instrumentals) can be playing in the background.

1. If your office has a receptionist, the receptionist should be seated facing the reception room.
2. Two desk heights ensure comfort and efficiency. The keyboard level should be approximately 27 inches and the writing level about 29 inches. Twenty inches is an adequate depth for most working areas. A depth of more than 30 inches is excessive; it makes reaching inconvenient and reduces the amount of floor space in the office.
3. A counter approximately 44 inches high provides a writing area for clients and privacy for the assistant and for documents on the desk (Fig. 6-4).
4. The business office clock should be out of view of clients in the reception room.
5. Master controls for the music system, heating, cooling, and lighting also should be located in the business office.

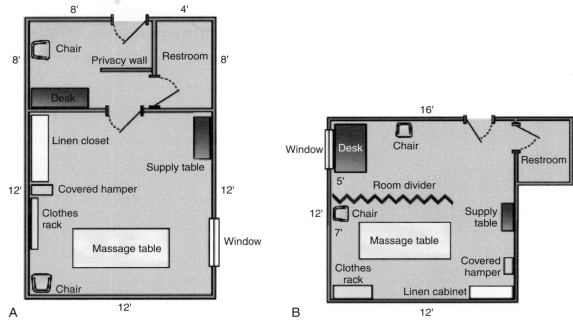

FIGURE 6-3. A, Example of the layout of a massage office with a separate business office and massage area. **B,** Example of the layout of a massage office with the business office and massage area in one room. *(From Fritz S:* Fundamentals of Therapeutic Massage, *ed 4, St. Louis, 2009, Mosby.)*

6. Lateral or open file cabinets (Fig. 6-5), at a depth of 18 inches, require less space than vertical file cabinets. These file cabinets are supplied in 30-, 36-, and 42-inch widths and with two to five drawers.

7. Cupboard space is necessary for storage of paper and supplies.

8. Small, compartmentalized areas above the desk provide easy access to items such as appointment cards and telephone message pads.

9. Telephones should be installed at each workstation and should be made hands free whenever possible.

10. Desk drawers should have full suspension for maximum use.

11. Inserts and dividers in drawers aid in organization of materials.

12. A small area adjacent to the business office set up for private calls and conversations with clients is convenient and can be used for completion of forms.

PRINCIPLES OF TIME AND MOTION

When determining the placement of office equipment and supplies, the principles of time and motion should be considered. *Time and motion* refer to the amount of time and degree of motion required to perform a given task.

In the early 1950s, researchers at the University of Alabama classified motions according to the amount of energy required to perform various tasks. These classifications (Box 6-4) apply to the business office tasks. Class I, II, and III motions require the least amount of energy and reduce stress.

To improve motion economy, it is often necessary to eliminate unnecessary steps or tasks, rearrange equipment and materials, organize procedures, simplify tasks, and evaluate the outcomes. The principles of motion economy (Box 6-5) can aid in accomplishing each of these goals, thereby reducing stress and increasing productivity in the practice.

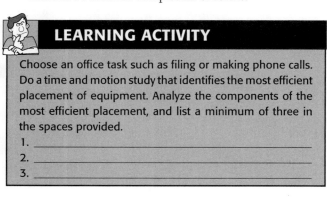

LEARNING ACTIVITY

Choose an office task such as filing or making phone calls. Do a time and motion study that identifies the most efficient placement of equipment. Analyze the components of the most efficient placement, and list a minimum of three in the spaces provided.

1. _____
2. _____
3. _____

SELF-REFLECTION

How do I support the environment in my personal and professional life? Do I recycle? Should I buy recycled products? Should I reduce paper waste and the use of hazardous chemicals? What can I do to improve conservation activities to the support the "green" philosophy? How to I think my life will change as newer forms of energy are better used and government regulations impose lifestyle changes?

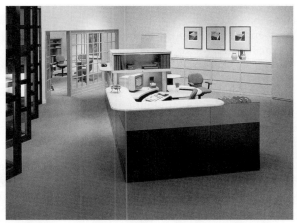

FIGURE 6-4. Counter space in the business office allows the client a comfortable position for business transactions. *(From Finkbeiner BL, Finkbeiner CA:* Practice Management for the Dental Team, *ed 6, St. Louis, 2006, Mosby.)*

BOX 6-5	**Applying the Principles of Motion Economy in the Business Office**

1. Position materials as close to the point of use as possible.
2. Use motions that require the least amount of movement.
3. Minimize the number of materials to be used for a given procedure.
4. Use smooth, continuous motions, not zigzag motions.
5. Organize materials in a logical sequence of use.
6. Position materials and equipment in advance whenever possible.
7. Use ergonomically designed stools or chairs to provide good posture and body support.
8. Use body motions that require the least amount of time.
9. Minimize the number of eye movements.
10. Provide lighting that eliminates shadows in work areas.
11. Avoid abrupt contrasts in room lighting to minimize eyestrain.
12. Position computer monitors to allow for line of sight to screen within 10 to 40 degrees of horizontal.
13. Provide work areas that are elbow level or 1 to 2 inches lower.

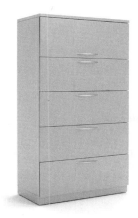

FIGURE 6-5. Lateral file. *(Courtesy of Steelcase, Grand Rapids, MI.)*

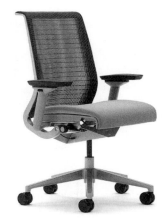

FIGURE 6-6. The Think Chair is an ergonomically designed office chair. *(Courtesy of Steelcase, Grand Rapids, MI.)*

BOX 6-4	**Classifications of Motion**

Class I: Fingers-only movement
Class II: Fingers and wrist movement
Class III: Fingers, wrist, and elbow movement
Class IV: Fingers, wrist, elbow, and shoulder movement
Class V: Arm extension and twisting of the torso

BODY POSITIONING

The massage therapist must consider proper seating arrangements during routine business activities. Just as body mechanics is a key issue in the practice of massage, the same occurs for the business functions. The following suggestions may be helpful.

When possible, all office activities should be performed in a seated position to avoid undue stress on the neck, back, and legs. A chair with a broad base, four or five casters, and a well-padded seat and back support is helpful (Fig. 6-6). Improper posture while standing or sitting can lead to fatigue, which affects productivity. The suggestions presented in Box 6-6 can help ensure the greatest comfort and efficiency. Much of the success of an office may be attributed to its efficiency and productivity without loss or waste. The goal in ergonomic body positioning should be to work smarter and not harder. Some suggestions follow:

- Top of monitor at or just below eye level
- Head and neck balanced and in-line with torso
- Shoulders relaxed
- Elbows close to the body and supported

- Lower back supported
- Wrist and hands in-line with the forearms
- Adequate room for keyboard and mouse
- Feet flat on the floor

Figure 6-7 illustrates proper seated posture while using a computer with a tabletop monitor.

BOX 6-6	Ergonomically Correct Body Positioning

1. When a person is seated, the thighs should be parallel to the floor, the lower legs vertical, and the feet firmly on the floor.
2. When a person is using a keyboard, the arms should be positioned so that the forearms and wrists are as horizontal as possible.
3. The distance from the eye to the computer screen should be 16 to 24 inches.
4. The keyboard should tilt 0 to 25 degrees.
5. The back and neck should be erect, and the upper arms should be perpendicular to the floor.
6. The buttocks should be well supported on the chair seat.
7. The feet should be flat on the floor.

HEALTH AND SAFETY ISSUES

A variety of factors can affect the health and safety of business office personnel. For example, spending hours each day looking at a computer screen can result in eyestrain and fatigue. Repetitive keyboarding can lead to wrist discomfort and possibly to carpal tunnel syndrome, although use of an ergonomically designed keyboard (Fig. 6-8) can help reduce this stress.

The following tips can help reduce fatigue and eyestrain when working at a computer:

- Make sure the screen is neither too dark nor too bright.
- If you are using the computer continuously, take a 10- to 15-minute break every hour or so.

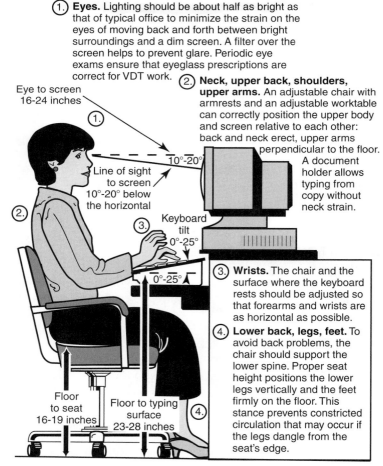

1. **Eyes.** Lighting should be about half as bright as that of typical office to minimize the strain on the eyes of moving back and forth between bright surroundings and a dim screen. A filter over the screen helps to prevent glare. Periodic eye exams ensure that eyeglass prescriptions are correct for VDT work.

2. **Neck, upper back, shoulders, upper arms.** An adjustable chair with armrests and an adjustable worktable can correctly position the upper body and screen relative to each other: back and neck erect, upper arms perpendicular to the floor. A document holder allows typing from copy without neck strain.

3. **Wrists.** The chair and the surface where the keyboard rests should be adjusted so that forearms and wrists are as horizontal as possible.

4. **Lower back, legs, feet.** To avoid back problems, the chair should support the lower spine. Proper seat height positions the lower legs vertically and the feet firmly on the floor. This stance prevents constricted circulation that may occur if the legs dangle from the seat's edge.

Eye to screen 16-24 inches

Line of sight to screen 10°-20° below the horizontal

10°-20°

Keyboard tilt 0°-25°

0°-25°

Floor to seat 16-19 inches

Floor to typing surface 23-28 inches

FIGURE 6-7. Good posture at a computer station. (*Courtesy of Nova Solutions. From Finkbeiner BL, Finkbeiner CA:* Practice Management for the Dental Team, *ed 6, St. Louis, 2006, Mosby.*)

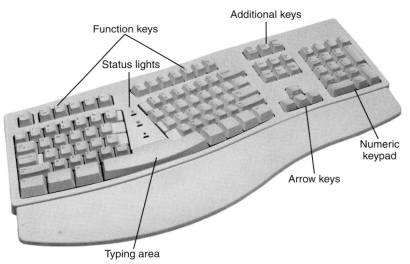

FIGURE 6-8. An ergonomic keyboard. *(Microsoft product reprinted with permission from Microsoft Corporation.)*

BOX 6-7	Potential Hazards

- Frayed or loose telephone cords or electrical wires
- Wires loosely secured to the floor
- Improperly grounded wall or floor switches
- Use of improper electric current to electronic equipment
- Spilled beverages or food on the floor
- Paper cutters, knives, or spindle files
- Loose floor covering on the stairs or floor
- Wearing of jewelry that can be caught in electronic equipment such as copiers
- Open files or drawers

- Use good posture.
- Stand up every half hour.
- Periodically look away from the screen for a few minutes.
- Use an ergonomically designed mouse, such as a trackball.
- Use an ergonomically designed chair.

Safety hazards can exist in the massage business office. In 1970, the Occupational Safety and Health Act was passed to ensure that workers in the United States have a safe working environment. The Occupational Safety and Health Administration (OSHA) requires employers to provide a hazard-free work environment, which is one without recognized dangers that can cause death, injury, or illness. Box 6-7 lists hazards that may be found in business offices. In massage offices, this list is compounded by the possibility of disease transmission (see Chapter 17). The lists in Boxes 6-7 and 6-8 can be used periodically to check for possible hazards.

Cleanliness and sanitation are essential. The business area needs to be cleaned at the end of each business day and checked periodically throughout the day. If beverages are offered, the area needs to be kept clean and sanitized, and the cups and other implements should be single use (e.g., paper cups) for sanitation purposes. Restrooms must be cleaned

BOX 6-8	Hazard Checklist

The following points should be evaluated routinely to ensure that safety measures have been observed:
- Floor coverings are durable and in good repair.
- Floor surfaces in clinical areas are hard and uncarpeted.
- Antislip protection is available on smooth floor surfaces.
- Electrical equipment and cords are in safe operating condition.
- Employees have been trained in proper operation of equipment.
- Only one drawer of a file cabinet is opened at a time.
- Office furniture has no sharp edges but does have stable arms and legs.
- First aid kits are well stocked and readily accessible.
- "No smoking" signs are posted in visible locations.
- All guidelines on infection control from the Occupational Safety and Health Administration (OSHA) are followed and are posted in visible locations.
- Hazard information (i.e., cleaning and disinfecting supplies) is posted and available for all employees.

and sanitized daily and checked often during the day. Whoever is responsible for cleaning needs to use standard precaution recommendations and be aware of the hazards of various cleaning materials. It is also important to be environmentally sensitive.

SELECTING OFFICE SUPPLIES

When first setting up a business office, determining what supplies will be needed may be an overwhelming task. Box 6-9 lists of the various forms and office supplies needed in a massage business office. Most office supply companies can assist you, and a variety of stationery suppliers can provide samples of stationery and forms. A walk through your favorite office

BOX 6-9	Basic Office Supplies

GENERAL SUPPLIES

Ballpoint pens
Calendar and calendar holder
Clear tape and tape dispenser
Erasers
Felt-tip markers
Hole puncher, three-hole puncher
Letter opener
Masking tape
Paper clips (small and large)
Pen holder
Pencil sharpener
Pencil tray
Pens and pencils
Rubber bands
Rubber stamps and pad
Scissors
Stapler, staples, staple remover
Utility tray (for paper clips, pens, pencils, and other small
    items)
Wastebasket

PAPER SUPPLIES

Adhesive notes
Assorted envelopes (e.g., coin mailers, large mailing
    envelopes)
Business cards
Copy paper (assorted sizes)
Drug reference
Fax paper
File folders
File folder labels
File guides
Index cards
Index tabs
Letterhead (second sheets)
Letterhead and envelopes
Medical and massage dictionaries and reference texts
Message reply forms
Note pads
Plain white paper
Preprinted office forms
Report covers
Ring binders
Ruled letter- and legal-size writing pads

Standard dictionary
Storage cartons
Telephone message pads

APPOINTMENT MANAGEMENT SUPPLIES

Appointment book (optional if computerized)
Appointment cards
Appointment schedule forms (optional if computerized)
Replacement sheets for appointment book (optional if
    computerized)
Work or school excuse forms

CLINICAL FORMS

Clinical charts
Colored filing labels
Consent forms
File guides
Health alert labels
Health questionnaire forms
Client file envelopes and folders
Referral forms
Registration forms
Update forms

FINANCIAL RECORD FORMS

Application for Employer Identification Number (SS-4)
Bank deposit slips
Bookkeeping forms (optional if not computerized)
Checkbook and replacement checks
Citizenship eligibility form (I-9)
Employee's withholding allowance certificate form (W-4)
Employer's quarterly tax return form (941)
Employer's annual federal unemployment tax return form
    (940)
Insurance claim forms
Ledger cards and forms (optional if not computerized)
Payroll forms
Statements
Transmittal of income and tax statements form (W-3)
Wage and tax statement form (W-2)

COMPUTER SUPPLIES*

Disks, CDs, DVDs
Cleaning materials
Cases, labels, mailers
Mouse pad
Printer ribbon
Toner cartridges

*When available, ergonomically designed supplies and materials should be purchased.

supply discount store can be fascinating, but buy only the supplies most needed, not one of everything available.

OFFICE ON THE GO

Many massage therapists work in multiple locations as independent contractors or travel to clients' homes or offices. In this case, it is necessary to have a portable office. Advances in technology, such as a small laptop computer and smartphones, make the portable office very efficient.

A miniaturized version of the content described in this chapter creates the business atmosphere. The atmosphere of the physical environment where you perform the massage can be created with soft, warm-colored linens, a table, carrying cases, and the professional appearance of your uniform.

A well-designed briefcase that has room for the computer acts as the business office. When choosing the briefcase, look for one that has multiple compartments for organizing business supplies and sleeves for file folders.

One of the most important activates is transporting the portable office and massage equipment to the location where services will be provided. Using roller bags and a rolling transport for the massage table is helpful. Be cautious when lifting the equipment from the vehicle. Avoid carrying equipment up and down stairs. When this is not possible, move equipment in stages. Do not attempt to carry multiple items at one time. Carry items on both sides of your body, switching often to avoid strain.

When setting up the massage area, be aware of health and safety issues. The massage table can slip on hard surface floors or mark plush carpet. A solution is to purchase large rubber coverings for the table legs or to have a separate rug

that does not slip (i.e., rubber backed) to place under the massage table. Soft music can be played on the computer or other portable device. A small fan works well to provide white noise and to improve air circulation. Make sure there are no slipping or tripping hazards. Massage lubricant on the bottoms of the feet can increase the tendency to slip.

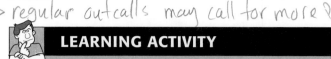

LEARNING ACTIVITY

Make a portable office, and share ideas with fellow students. The ability to work efficiently from the portable massage office increases your potential for servicing clients who desire this type of massage service.

Good Stuff from the Government

For your convenience, links to the information in this box are provided on the Evolve Web site. Log on to the Web sites of the Small Business Association (SBA), Occupational Health and Safety Association (OSHA), Centers for Disease Control and Prevention (CDC), and a division of the CDC, the National Institute for Occupational Safety and Health (NIOSH), for more information. On the SBA Web site, you can find information on these topics (http://www.sba.gov):

Commercial leasing: How to get the best commercial lease for your business.

Leasing checklist: Essential elements that should be on your lease agreement.

Zoning overview: Types of zones and their specific regulations.

Zoning problems: Sometimes, a lawyer can help you get around zoning regulations.

Signage tutorial: For help making the most of your commercial signage, visit SBA's signage tutorial.

Home-based business FAQs: If your business is home-based, look at the answers to these common questions.

Zip code locator: Find most zip codes in the country.

Home-based business and government regulations: Home-based businesses face daunting restrictions from the federal and local regulations described in this research report released by Advocacy.

For health and safety topics, visit the Centers for Disease Control Web site. Ergonomics research and recommendations can be found at the U.S. Department of Labor OSHA Web site. Their eTools are Web-based products that provide guidance information for developing a comprehensive safety and health program. Topics found on this Web site include good working positions, workstation components checklist, work process, workstation environment, monitors, keyboards, pointer or mouse, wrist and palm rests, document holders, desks, chairs, and telephones.

The mission of the National Institute for Occupational Safety and Health (NIOSH services) research program for the services sector is to eliminate occupational diseases, injuries, and fatalities among persons working in these industries through a focused program of research and prevention.

SUMMARY

The environment you create for your massage business is important. Efficiency is necessary for small business owners such as massage therapists because they often have to multitask. In the larger business offices with several massage therapists and others service providers, it is essential that the business office be

designed for function. Just like the body, structure (i.e., design) affects function (i.e., daily business activities). The importance of safety cannot be overemphasized. Each design element must be evaluated for safety. It is similar to pet- or child-proofing the home. Strive for a pleasant, warm atmosphere and neutral or generic design to best respect the tastes of most people.

Bibliography

Andress AA: *Saunders Textbook of Medical Office Management*, ed 2, St. Louis, 2003, Elsevier.

National Institute for Occupational Safety and Health: www.cdc.gov/NIOSH/

⊜ Evolve Annotated Web Links

http://evolve.elsevier.com/Fritz/business

U.S. Small Business Association:

Commercial leasing: http://www.sba.gov/smallbusinessplanner/start/pickalocation/SERV_BP_CLEASE.html

Leasing checklist: http://www.sba.gov/smallbusinessplanner/start/pickalocation/serv_bp_lclst.html

Zoning overview: http://www.sba.gov/smallbusinessplanner/start/pickalocation/SERV_BP_ZOVIEW.html

Zoning problems: http://www.sba.gov/smallbusinessplanner/start/pickalocation/SERV_BP_ZPROB.html

Signage tutorial: http://www.sba.gov/smallbusinessplanner/start/pickalocation/signage/index.html

Home-based business FAQs: http://www.sba.gov/smallbusinessplanner/start/pickalocation/SERV_BP_HOMEFAQ.html

Home-based business and government regulations: http://www.sba.gov/idc/groups/public/documents/sba_homepage/serv_sbp_rs35.pdf

Pick a location: http://www.sba.gov/smallbusinessplanner/start/pickalocation/index.html

Americans with Disabilities Act Home Page: http://www.ada.gov

Centers for Disease Control and Prevention: http://www.cdc.gov/

National Institute for Occupational Safety and Health (NIOSH services) Ergonomics: www.cdc.gov/NIOSH/

U.S. Department of Labor, Occupational Safety and Health Administration (OSHA), computer workstations: http://www.osha.gov/SLTC/etools/computerworkstations/index.html

United States Access Board: http://www.access-board.gov

Workbook

1. List eight suggestions for the design of a reception room.

   _____
   _____
   _____
   _____
   _____

2. Discuss 10 factors to consider when designing a business office.

   _____
   _____
   _____
   _____
   _____

3. Describe the impact of the Americans with Disabilities Act on a massage practice.

   _____
   _____
   _____
   _____
   _____

4. Describe the concept of time and motion as it applies to a massage business office.

   _____
   _____
   _____
   _____
   _____

5. On a separate piece of paper, use equipment suggested from the previous chapter and suggestions for office design from this chapter to develop an office design that could be used for a typical massage practice in your geographic area. Consider the latest electronic equipment, and include suggestions for color and texture of flooring, walls, and lighting.

7

DOCUMENTATION

KEY TERMS

Clinical abbreviations
Clinical record
Consent form
Health history
Health Insurance Portability and
  Accountability Act (HIPAA)

Important records
Information management
Records management
Statute of limitations
Unimportant
  records

Useful records
Vital records

LEARNING OUTCOMES

Mastery of the content in this chapter will enable the reader to:

- Define key terms
- Define HIPAA
- Describe how to implement HIPAA regulations in the massage office record management system
- Identify the types of records maintained in a massage office
- Categorize various types of records
- Distinguish between active and inactive records
- List the components of a clinical record
- Describe the function of the components of a clinical record

- Explain the rules for data entry on client records
- Explain the use of symbols and abbreviations in clinical records
- List the components of client financial records
- Identify the types of records required by the Occupational Safety and Health Administration (OSHA) to be maintained in a massage office
- Identify the types of employee records
- Explain the importance of maintaining accurate records
- Describe methods of records retention and transfer

ⓔ Guidelines for the Learning Activities and answers to the Workbook questions are located on Evolve at http://evolve.elsevier.com/Fritz/business.

Maintaining complete and accurate documents is an important part of the successful management of a massage practice. The massage therapist is required to maintain clinical, financial, employee, state, and federal records. Failure to perform any of these tasks can be a costly experience for the massage professional.

This chapter is a nuts and bolts chapter. This kind of information can be somewhat tedious to learn, but if business and client records are not attended to, the result can be frustrating and possibly illegal. Because the massage professional can work in multiple environments, from the very informal, single-person, part-time practice to a very formal, integrated, multidisciplinary health care practice, it is necessary to cover this topic in a comprehensive manner to prepare for multiple work environments. The implementation of a documentation system by the massage therapist depends on the focus of the massage business. It is better to do more documentation than less, because the various liability insurance programs for massage therapy can use the documentation to defend you in case of a lawsuit or insurance claim.

There are many aspects of the documentation and record keeping process. Various legislative actions influence how we keep records. One of the more comprehensive changes has been the implementation of the Health Insurance Portability and Accountability Act.

HEALTH INSURANCE PORTABILITY AND ACCOUNTABILITY ACT

The *Health Insurance Portability and Accountability Act* (HIPAA) of 1996, which became effective in April 2003, has affected the massage profession. It has generated much confusion about how massage therapists need to respond to the requirements of the act. Administrative simplification provisions of HIPAA have affected the massage profession whether the massage therapist is employed or works in the health care system. These provisions require national standards for electronic health care transactions. Massage therapists who transmit health information in an electronic transaction are required to use a standard format. The most affected area in the massage office is transmission of insurance claim forms, which are reviewed in Chapter 14. However, the impact of privacy in the management of client records is a primary concern, and in that regard, HIPAA reinforces the need for confidentiality in *records management* by the massage therapist even if they work in a non–health care environment, such as a day spa.

HIPAA laws may seem daunting at first. However, when you realize that the purpose is to protect and enhance clients' rights, it becomes a positive action because everyone is a client at one time or another. Protecting health information is the right thing to do, and it promotes safe practice for

everyone. It is also a good risk management, helping each massage professional to prevent potential litigation. Security regulations, which the Department of Health and Human Services released under HIPAA, were conceived to protect electronic client health information. Protected client health information is anything that ties a client's name or Social Security number to that person's health, health care, or payment for health care.

Each massage professional should become familiar with state and federal laws because these laws are often more stringent than federal laws. It would be necessary for the massage therapist working in an environment that is HIPAA compliant be trained to maintain HIPAA policies and procedures on the worksite. This would typically be the responsibility of the office manager in a health care environment, but it is still necessary for the massage therapist to understand the procedures and policies of the work environment (Fig. 7-1).

Specific HIPAA compliance training would include training on the forms used by the organization. The Notice of Privacy Practices policy presents information that the massage professional is required to give clients regarding the office's privacy practices. This form may need to be changed to reflect the massage practice's particular privacy policies or stricter state laws. The name of the practice should be on the notice, and it must be given to each client at the date of the first service. The notice should be posted in a clear and prominent location in the office that is visible to any client seeking service (Fig. 7-2).

Acknowledgement of Receipt of Notice of Privacy Practices (Fig. 7-3) is the form the client signs to acknowledge that he or she has received a copy of the Notice of Privacy Practices. If the client refuses to sign the form, it is indicated on the form that an attempt was made to have the client sign in the in-office section on the form. The client may also choose to sign a separate refusal form that may then be placed in the record.

Business Associate Contract Terms is a contract form that satisfies the obligation under the HIPAA and its implementing regulations issued by the U.S. Department of Health and Human Services. This form ensures the integrity and confidentiality of protected health information that a business associate may create or receive. To ensure that records are maintained for clients, a preprinted chart divider provides a permanent record of important HIPAA information for clients' files.

RECORDS MANAGEMENT

A massage office operates on information, which is created, processed, stored, printed, and distributed in many forms to various sites. The massage therapist must establish a logical, functional system for storing and retrieving information. This process is known as records management or

Who Should be Trained?

The HIPAA Privacy Rule stipulates that all members of the enterprise workforce receive training that is appropriate to their organizational roles. The "workforce" includes employees, volunteers, trainees, and other persons who work for a covered entity, whether or not they are paid by it. Some staff members will need to be trained in applying specific policies and procedures, such as provision of the notice of information practices or obtaining authorizations. Others, such as those who rarely have access to PHI, may require only an overview of HIPAA's background, objectives, principles, and general regulatory requirements.

New employees who join the organization must receive training within a reasonable period of time. It is often practical to include HIPAA privacy training in new employee orientation programs, particularly because privacy principles easily fit into discussions of the organization's mission and infrastructure. Workforce members who change jobs or receive new responsibilities must receive additional training if their new job duties include new patient privacy-related responsibilities. Further, the Privacy Rule requires retraining for each member of the covered entity's workforce whose functions are affected by a material change in the policies or procedures.

Covered entities also must document that privacy training has been provided. Though there is no requirement that members of the workforce sign a certificate following training, it is useful to document training completion by each worker, for future verification purposes.

What Should Your Training Program Cover?

The Privacy provisions do not prescribe the nature of the required training; HHS has left the design, approach, and specific content to the discretion of the covered entity. However, at the very least, it is recommended that the following topics be covered with all members of the workforce. In addition, more specialized training on detailed HIPAA requirements and internal procedural changes must be tailored for workforce groups that will be directly affected by them in the course of their work.

- Principles and objectives of HIPAA Privacy
- Background—What is protected health information (PHI)?
- Need for privacy of PHI
- Overview of HIPAA privacy regulations, including penalties
- Individual's rights regarding privacy
- Individual's rights regarding control of uses & disclosures of PHI
- Individual's right to request access, accounting, amendment
- New organizational privacy policies and procedures
- Sanction policy
- Notice of privacy practices
- Authorizations for use and disclosure
- Privacy Officer role and contact information
- Complaint policies and procedures
- Cooperating with investigations or audits
- How to report a violation and the whistleblower policy
- Organization's commitment to patient privacy integration with transactions standardization and security mandates

FIGURE 7-1. Health Insurance Portability and Accountability Act (HIPAA) document. *(Modified from D'Arcy GG: The first and last word in privacy compliance, Dallas, TX, Phoenix Health Systems, 2003. Available at http://www.hipaadvisory.com/regs/compliancecal.htm, (accessed June 2009). In Fritz S:* Mosby's Fundamentals of Therapeutic Massage, *ed 4, St. Louis, 2009, Mosby.)*

information management. Records begin with inception and end with disposition (Fig. 7-4):

Creation: This is the origination of the data. In the case of a client record, creation begins with the completion of a client registration form and health questionnaire. A permanent record usually is started on paper or the data entered into the computer. If the person is a transient client (comes in for just one massage), the form for recording the data may be different from the standard form, and the record may not be stored with the active clinical charts.

Distribution: In this stage, the information may be distributed manually or electronically. It includes sending the client's *clinical record* to the massage therapist if a receptionist is collecting the initial data or to a physician for diagnosis after the record has been completed and referral is indicated.

Notice of Privacy Practices (NPP) Policy

Effective date of policy: _____

Every client will receive a Notice of Privacy Practices. These practices may vary from business to business:

- It MUST be distributed to clients and you must get written documentation from the client that he/she received this notice.
- You must post an abbreviated notice prominently in the office.
- You may distribute it via e-mail with a return receipt.
- If you have a business Web site, it must be posted on the Web site.
- You must make a reasonable effort to assure that each client gets a Notice of Privacy Practice on his or her first date of service and document this effort in writing.

In the event that the client does not get a notice while in the office, you should mail the notice to him or her on the same day, and document why it was not given to the client at the time of service and that the notice was mailed.

This office will comply with all aspects as printed in our Notice of Privacy Practices and our privacy notice will be in compliance with all appropriate laws and regulations, federal, state, and local.

FIGURE 7-2. Client's privacy acknowledgement.

[Your Office Letterhead]

Sample HIPAA Acknowledgement Form

We are required to provide you with a copy of our Notice of Privacy Practices (NPP) policy, which states how we may use and/or disclose your health information. Please sign this form to acknowledge receipt of the Notice. You may refuse to sign this acknowledgement if you wish.

I acknowledge that I have received a copy of the office's Notice of Privacy Practices (NPP).

_____
Please print your name here.

_____
Signature

_____
Date

FIGURE 7-3. HIPAA acknowledgment form. *(From Fritz S: Mosby's Fundamentals of Therapeutic Massage, ed 4, St. Louis, 2009, Mosby.)* This form is available for use on Evolve at http://evolve.elsevier.com/Fritz/business.

Use: The massage therapist evaluates the data, develops the massage treatment or care plan, or refers the data to an appropriate location for maintenance.

Maintenance: This stage of the process involves determining whether the data or information should be retained. If it is to be retained, the massage therapist must decide the best way to store it for easy retrieval and how long it should

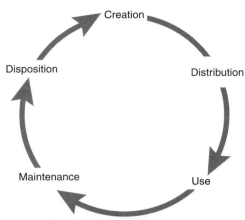

FIGURE 7-4. Life cycle of a record: creation, distribution, use, maintenance, and disposition. *(From Finkbeiner BL, Finkbeiner CA: Practice Management for the Dental Team, ed 6, St. Louis, 2006, Mosby.)*

be stored. If the client is to be seen again and become a client of record, the clinical record is filed alphabetically electronically or in a file folder and envelope in a protected file. Some components of the record, such as notes the massage therapist made during evaluation, can be destroyed. Only the pertinent data must be kept.

Disposition: At this stage, it must be determined whether the record should be destroyed because it no longer has value to the office or should be stored permanently as an important document. The clinical record is vital and must be retained for a period consistent with the state *statute of limitations.* Electronic data can be transferred to disks for storage. Paper records, which have no backup, must be kept in a safe, dry area.

SELF-REFLECTION

How organized are my closet, my kitchen, and my personal business records? Do I put off filing and picking up or putting away clutter? How long does the laundry pile up? After it is washed, do I put it away immediately? How long does it stay in the laundry basket? How many catch-all (junk) drawers do I have? Do I easily lose things? (*Note:* If most answers are yes, you need to regularly examine your documentation and record keeping. Put a note on your calendar to inspect records, or hire someone to assist you with this task.)

CATEGORIES OF RECORDS

The massage therapist must decide which records to keep, how to organize and store them, how long they legally must be retained, and when to dispose of them. In general, records can be categorized as vital, important, useful, or unimportant and as active or inactive.

Vital Records

Vital records are essential documents that cannot be replaced. They include client clinical and financial records and the practice records, such as rental agreement, insurance policies, and tax records. These records should be kept in a fireproof, theft-proof vault or safe, and copies often are kept in a protected, off-site location, such as a safe deposit box at a bank.

Important Records

Important records are extremely valuable to the operation of the office, but they are not vital. They include accounts payable and receivable, invoices, canceled checks, inventory and payroll records, and other federal regulatory records. Such records may be needed for a tax audit or if a question arises about a financial transaction. Important records should be retained for 5 to 7 years. Most offices keep them for about 7 years or in accordance with federal or state regulations.

Useful Records

Useful records include employment applications, expired insurance policies, petty cash vouchers, bank reconciliations, and general correspondence. This category is difficult to define, because one office may consider a document useful, whereas another may find it indispensable. These records usually are retained for 1 to 3 years.

Unimportant Records

Unimportant records are the documents that lie around, have little importance, and take up space. They include items such as notes to you, reminders of meetings, outdated announcements, and pamphlets. Common sense dictates when these materials may be discarded.

CLIENT RECORDS

Client records usually fall into two categories: clinical and financial. A recall system is another type of record that is retained separate from the clinical chart but which could be considered a type of clinical record. Clinical records are reviewed in this chapter; financial records are discussed in Chapter 15. The software packages typically have functions for these types of records. See the Evolve site for screen shot examples.

Clinical Record

The clinical record is a collection of all the information about the client's massage treatment. The client's clinical record is used during massage treatment, and updating and maintaining this record is the massage therapist's responsibility. Success in maintaining clinical records requires cooperation and efficiency from each member of the massage/health care team.

Accurate clinical records are vital for several reasons:

1. In treatment of the client, clinical records serve as a road map. They contain the client's history and outline future plans for massage intervention.
2. In a malpractice suit, the massage record is legally admissible as evidence. It can be used for or against the massage therapist.
3. In third-party payment plans, the consultants representing the carrier may review the clinical chart and other parts of the clinical record to determine whether services have been rendered adequately.
4. The record acts as verification of treatment rendered for Internal Revenue Service purposes.
5. If the client's health insurance covers massage treatment, the record should be recorded in a manner that is acceptable to the Insurance Company. To be on the safe side, use the subjective, objective, assessment, and plan (SOAP) format that is used in the medical field.

A client's clinical record commonly has the following components:

- Client file envelope or folder
- Registration form (e.g., name, address)
- Health questionnaire and update forms
- Medication history
- HIPAA acknowledgment form (if necessary)
- Clinical chart, including treatment record or progress notes (SOAP or other style)
- Consultation and referral reports (from other health care professionals or if you provide referral information)
- Massage treatment or session plan
- Consent forms
- Letters and postal receipts
- E-mail correspondence

With more massage practices moving toward computerized systems, client records and files are changing. More of the data will be stored in the computer, and the need for paper copies of these documents will decline. Purchased forms may need to be specifically adapted for massage therapy. As the profession grows, it is likely that more companies will produce forms specifically for massage. Major textbooks on massage education also have examples of forms.

CLIENT FILE ENVELOPE OR FOLDER

In most massage practices, use of an 8.5 by 11 inch file envelope or folder guards against misplacement of records. In practices in which clients do not return on a regular basis, a file may be created to hold a collection of these records. File envelopes may be plain or color-coded. They are supplied in a preprinted format with spaces for client information, including the client's name, address, and telephone number (Fig. 7-5). This type of envelope is widely used and satisfies the needs of many practices.

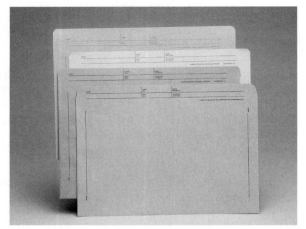

FIGURE 7-5. Envelopes for clients' files. *(Courtesy of Colwell, Division of Patterson Companies, Champaign, IL. In Finkbeiner BL, Finkbeiner CA: Practice Management for the Dental Team, ed 6, St. Louis, 2006, Mosby.)*

Another common type of storage for client records is an end-tab file folder with one or two two-hole fasteners (Fig. 7-6A and B). This type of folder requires the use of vertical-style records. The folders generally have a reinforced tab for easy label placement. They also are precut for quick insertion of a two-hole file fastener. Options include folders with pockets and diagonal cuts and expandable folders. Other auxiliary aids for these records include the hole punch, perm-clip fasteners, and polyvinyl pockets (Fig. 7-6C and D).

Whether folders or envelopes are used, some form of color-coding is necessary to make sorting, storing, and retrieval easier. Color-coding can be done as an alphabetical system or, in a group practice, can be categorized by practitioner.

CLIENT REGISTRATION FORM AND HEALTH HISTORY FORM

Although they are often combined, the client registration form and health history form contain two different types of data. They should be retained because they provide more detailed information about the client.

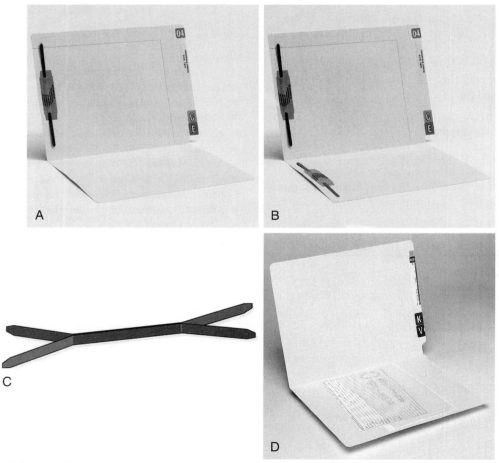

FIGURE 7-6. **A,** File folder with one two-hole fastener. **B,** File folder with two two-hole fasteners. **C,** Twin-prong fasteners for fastening pages to either side of a file folder. **D,** Polyvinyl pocket. *(A–D, Courtesy of Colwell, Division of Patterson Companies, Champaign, IL. In Finkbeiner BL, Finkbeiner CA: Practice Management for the Dental Team, ed 6, St. Louis, 2006, Mosby.)*

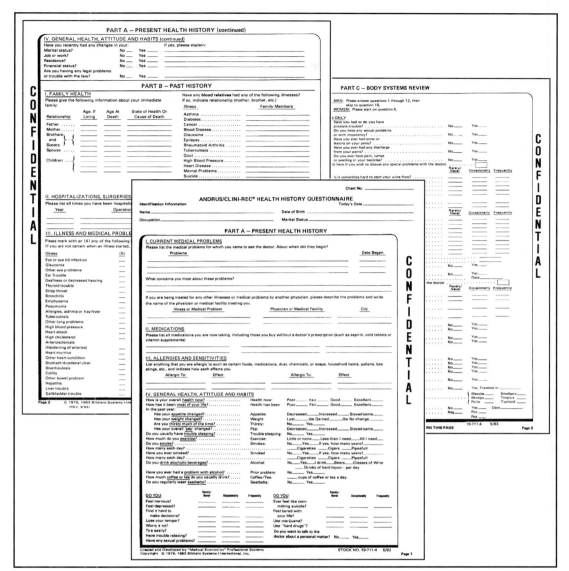

FIGURE 7-7. Examples of registration forms. *(Courtesy of Bibbaro Systems, Int'l.)*

The client registration form contains general information, such as addresses and telephone numbers, as well as employment and insurance information. Figure 7-7 shows common types of registration forms. Each client should fill out a *health history* form (Fig. 7-8) and date and sign it. If the massage therapist prefers to ask these questions in person, the client should verify the answers recorded and sign the form.

The health history form for children should be completed by a parent or guardian, not by the child or a babysitter. Make sure no nicknames are used and that all data are accurate, because this information is used later to complete insurance forms (Fig. 7-9; see Figs. 7-7 and 7-8).

The client's history should be reviewed when the person returns for treatment if several months have elapsed since the last visit. A health history update form should be completed periodically to keep the health history (Fig. 7-10A)

and the personal information (Fig. 7-10B) current. The client should sign and date this form.

Many types of client registration and health history forms are available. Figure 7-11 is an alternative registration and health history form for children. Regardless of the form used, it is important to remember that a current, accurate health history serves as a preventative measure in client treatment and as a defense in malpractice suits.

When collecting the data on these forms, consider the following points:

■ Give the client the form on a clipboard to which a black ballpoint pen (not a pencil) has been attached.
■ Do not ask the questions in the business office. Some answers may be embarrassing if overheard by other clients in the reception room. Clients often give more information if they do not have to respond orally.

CLIENT INTAKE INFORMATION FORM

Name: _____ Date: _____

Address: _____ City: _____ State: _____ Zip: _____

Phone: (day) _____ (eve) _____ Date of Birth: _____

Occupation: _____ Employer: _____

Referred by: _____ Physician: _____

Previous experience with massage:

_____

Primary reason for appointment/areas of pain or tension:

_____

Emergency contact—name and number: _____

**Please mark (X) for all conditions that apply now. Put a (P) for past conditions,
an (F) for family history of illness.**

Pain Scale: minor-1   2   3   4   5   6   7   8   9   severe-10

___ headaches, migraines	___ chronic pain	___ fatigue
___ vision problems, contact lenses	___ muscle or joint pain	___ tension, stress
___ hearing problems, deafness	___ muscle, bone injuries	___ depression
___ injuries to face or head	___ numbness or tingling	___ sleep difficulties
___ sinus problems	___ sprains, strains	___ allergies, sensitivities
___ dental bridges, braces	___ arthritis, tendonitis	___ rashes, athletes foot
___ jaw pain, TMJ problems	___ cancer, tumors	___ infectious diseases
___ asthma or lung conditions	___ spinal column disorders	___ blood clots
___ constipation, diarrhea	___ diabetes	___ varicose veins
___ hernia	___ pregnancy	___ high/low blood pressure
___ birth control, IUD	___ heart, circulatory problems	
___ abdominal or digestive problems	___ other medical conditions not listed	

Explain any areas noted above:

_____

_____

Current medications, including aspirin, ibuprofen, herbs, supplements, etc.:

_____

_____

Surgeries: _____

Accidents: _____

Please list all forms and frequency of stress reduction activities, hobbies, exercise, or
sports participation: _____

_____

FIGURE 7-8. Sample history form. This information is provided by the client. The key to completing the form is to ask questions. *(From Fritz S:* Mosby's Fundamentals of Therapeutic Massage, *ed 4, St. Louis, 2009, Mosby.)* ⊝ This form is available for use on Evolve at http://evolve.elsevier.com/Fritz/business.

- When making appointments for new clients, ask them to arrive 15 minutes early to allow time for completion of these forms.
- Make sure a parent or legal guardian completes the form for a child.
- Keep the information absolutely confidential. The client record is not for public review and should not become a feature of lunchtime gossip.

- Review the form to ensure that it has been completed and signed. Clients may avoid questions they do not understand or do not want to answer. If the client says, "I don't think this question has anything to do massage," explain how it relates to massage care. If the question cannot be justified, it should not be on the form.

Client ID number _____

Today's date _____

We strive to make each of your child's visits pleasant and comfortable.
Please fill out this form completely in ink.

Your child
Child's name _____ Sex _____ Age_____
Nickname _____Social security number_____Birthdate_____
School _____ Grade_____
Child's home address _____
City, State, Zip _____ Phone _____

Responsible party
Name _____ Relationship_____
Address _____
City, State, Zip _____ Phone _____
Social security number _____DL number _____
Who is responsible for making appointments?_____

Parent or guardian information   ☐ Mother   ☐ Stepmother   ☐ Guardian
Name_____
Home phone_____ Work phone_____
Employer_____ Occupation_____
Social security number_____ DL number_____
Marital status ☐ Single   ☐ Married   ☐ Divorced   ☐ Separated   ☐ Widowed

Parent or guardian information   ☐ Father   ☐ Stepfather   ☐ Guardian
Name_____
Home phone_____ Work phone_____
Employer_____ Occupation_____
Social security number_____ DL number_____
Marital status ☐ Single   ☐ Married   ☐ Divorced   ☐ Separated   ☐ Widowed

Primary insurance
Insured's name _____ Relationship_____
Birthdate _____Social security number_____
Employer _____ Date employed_____ Occupation_____
Insurance company_____ Group number_____ Employee number_____
Insurance company address _____City_____State _____ Zip _____
Deductible _____ Copay _____ Amount already used_____Maximum annual benefit _____

Additional insurance
Insured's name _____ Relationship_____
Birthdate _____ Social security number_____
Employer_____ Date employed_____ Occupation_____
Insurance company _____ Group number_____ Employee number_____
Insurance company address _____City_____State _____ Zip _____
Deductible _____Copay_____Amount already used _____Maximum annual benefit _____

FIGURE 7-9. Registration and health history form for children used in health care. (*Courtesy of SYCOM, Madison, WI. In Finkbeiner BL, Finkbeiner CA:* Practice Management for the Dental Team, *ed 6, St. Louis, 2006, Mosby.*)

LEARNING ACTIVITY

Create a client registration and health history form. Pair with a series of partners, and complete the client registration and health history forms created after reading the guidelines in this section. Remember that a person's privacy is protected by law. Some questions shown as examples may be considered discriminatory or in violation of a client's rights. Consequently, the massage therapist must be aware of the state laws that protect a person's rights and change the form to accommodate these rights.

CLINICAL CHART

A wide selection of massage charts is available for use in the massage office. The massage therapist may purchase a standard form or may design one specifically suited for the needs of the practice.

Most charts are 8.5 by 11 inches, made of heavy paper stock, and printed on both sides. Many of these charts are die-punched to fit into a file folder. One side of the record contains a massage chart, a review of the client's health history, and general client information. The reverse side provides space for entering the treatment plan and recording services rendered. Some charts have space for entering the fee, but this should not become the client's financial ledger

HEALTH HISTORY UPDATE

Client: ______________________________ Date: ______________

1. Have there been any changes in your health since your last visit?

   ____

   ____

2. Have you recently required other health services? ______________

   If yes, nature of care ______________________________

3. Physician's name: ______________________________

4. Have you been hospitalized since your last visit? ______________

   If yes, nature of problem ______________________________

5. Any new illnesses? ______________________________

   ____

6. Are you taking any medication(s) now? ______________________

   To treat: ______________________________

   Name & dosage: ______________________________

7. Do you have any new allergies or reactions to any medications or drugs?

   ____

8. Women only: Are you pregnant? ________ If yes, due date: __________

9. Any other new diseases, conditions, or problems you think we should know about? ______________________________

   ____

Client Signature: ______________________________

Massage Therapist Signature: ______________________________

Form 4051 • 12/93 **SYCOM®** 1-800-356-8141

A

FIGURE 7-10. **A,** Health history update form. **B,** Personal information update form. *(Courtesy of SYCOM, Madison, WI. Modified from Finkbeiner BL, Finkbeiner CA:* Practice Management for the Dental Team, *ed 6, St. Louis, 2006, Mosby.)*

■■■■■■ PERSONAL INFORMATION UPDATE ■■■■■

Name_____ Date _____

1. Has your name changed since your last visit here? _____ yes   _____ no
   If yes, what was the old name? _____
   What name do you use for insurance if different than above? _____
   _____

2. If you have a new or different address since your initial visit here, please
   indicate below:

                        _____
                        _____
                        _____

   Please indicate if any apartment # or P.O. Box # _____

3. Has your marital status changed? _____ yes   _____no

4. Has your telephone number changed? _____ yes   _____no
   Please indicate your correct telephone number _____

5. Has your employment changed? _____yes   _____no
   Please indicate your new employer name and address:

                        _____
                        _____
                        _____

   New employer telephone #: _____

6. Have you changed insurance companies? _____yes   _____no
   If yes, please indicate your new insurance carrier and address.

   Primary _____   Secondary _____
           _____   _____
           _____   _____
   Group Nos. _____   Group Nos._____
   Subscriber Nos. _____   Subscriber Nos. _____

7. Who is responsible for this bill? _____

8. Signature _____

Thank you for your assistance.

Item 4595 • 08/94 • SYCOM® 1-800-356-8141

B

FIGURE 7-10, cont'd

CHILD REGISTRATION ████████████████████

Child's name _____ Date _____

Birth date _____ Age _____

Nickname _____ Hobbies _____

Parent's name_____

Residence-street_____

City _____ State _____ Zip _____

School_____

Telephone: Residence _____ School_____

Father employed by _____

Present position _____ How long held _____

Mother employed by _____

Present position _____ How long held _____

Referred by _____

Who will pay this account _____

Purpose of call _____

Name of father's insurance co._____

Policy number _____

Name of mother's insurance co. _____

Policy number _____

Parents' Social Security numbers: Father _____

                                   Mother _____

Parent's birth dates: Father _____

                                   Mother _____

Item 539 • 12/93 **SYCOM**● 1-800-356-8141

A

FIGURE 7-11. Alternative registration (**A**) and health history (**B**) form for children. *(Courtesy of SYCOM, Madison, WI. In Finkbeiner BL, Finkbeiner CA:* Practice Management for the Dental Team, *ed 6, St. Louis, 2006, Mosby.)*

Information For Emergency Treatment

Date of last medical examination _____

Does child have or has child ever had: Yes   No

    Anemia ....   _____   _____

    Diabetes...   _____   _____

    Hepatitis..   _____   _____

    Allergies ....   _____   _____

        To penicillin ....   _____   _____

        To local anesthetic..   _____   _____

    Abnormal heart condition..   _____   _____

    Abnormal bleeding from a cut..   _____   _____

    Rheumatic fever..   _____   _____

    Heart murmur...   _____   _____

    Is your child under the care of a physician now......................   _____   _____

    Is any medication being taken now...   _____   _____

    If so, what _____

    _____

    Other physical conditions_____

    _____

    _____

    Name of physician _____

    Telephone number_____

    Information given by (signature) _____

Date	Service Rendered	Charge	Credit	Balance

B

FIGURE 7-11, cont'd

Birthdate _____ Age _____

Date of last medical examination _____

Do you have or have you ever had: Yes   No

REGISTRATION/HEALTH HISTORY

Client's name _____

If a child, parent's name _____

Single _____ Married _____ Widowed _____ Divorced _____ Separated _____

Address _____

City _____ State _____ Zip _____

Business address _____

Telephone: Residence _____ Business _____

Patient employed by _____

Present position _____

In case of emergency, who should be notified _____

Phone _____

Referred by _____

Who will pay this account _____

Purpose of call _____

Spouse's name _____

Spouse's birthdate _____

Spouse employed by _____

Do you have insurance that may cover any part of our services   ☐ Yes   ☐ No

If so, name of primary company _____

Is policy connected with your union   ☐ Yes   ☐ No

If yes, name of union _____

Policy no. _____ Group no. _____

Local no. _____

Social Security no. of person covered _____

Any secondary insurance _____

Name of company _____

Social Security no. of person covered _____

Your signature _____ Date _____

Item 119 - 12/89 SYCOMe Madison, WI Printed in U.S.A.

	Charge	Credit	Balance

FIGURE 7-12. Short-form registration and health history form applicable to a health care practice. *(Courtesy of SYCOM, Madison, WI. In Finkbeiner BL, Finkbeiner CA: Practice Management for the Dental Team, ed 6, St. Louis, 2006, Mosby.)*

card, and it need not include a record of payments and balances. Several of the illustrations can help to familiarize you with some of the different types of clinical charts (Figs. 7-12 to 7-14; see Figs. 7-10 and 7-11).

MASSAGE ASSESSMENT AND TREATMENT FORM

The massage assessment and treatment form includes the massage therapist's assessment of the client and the recommended treatment plan (see Figs. 7-13 and 7-14). In many cases, the client can select options in the treatment plan, such as the addition of essential oils or hydrotherapy methods, if the massage therapist is trained to provide them. After the assessment has been completed and treatment has been

accepted by the client, the form is signed by the client (parent or guardian in the case of a minor).

CONSULTATION AND REFERRAL REPORT

In some cases, the massage therapist refers a client to another health care professional or different type of bodywork practitioner for examination, evaluation, treatment, and diagnosis. The form shown in Figure 7-15 includes information about the client, the reason for the referral, and an anticipated treatment plan. This form is sent to the referring professional, and a copy is given to the client. The consultant enters an evaluation and recommendation on the form and returns it to the massage therapist.

MASSAGE ASSESSMENT/PHYSICAL OBSERVATION/PALPATION AND GAIT

Client Name: _____ Date: _____

PRE
POST

OBSERVATION & PALPATION				
ALIGNMENT	**RIBS**		**SCAPULA**	
Chin in line with nose, sternal notch, navel	Even		Even	
	Springy		Move freely	
Other:	Other:		Other:	
HEAD	**ABDOMEN**		**CLAVICLES**	
Tilted (L)	Firm and pliable		Level	
Tilted (R)	Hard areas		Other:	
Rotated (L)	Other:		**ARMS**	
Rotated (R)	**WAIST**		Hang evenly (internal) (external)	
EYES	Level		(L) rotated ☐ medial ☐ lateral	
Level	Other:		(R) rotated ☐ medial ☐ lateral	
Equally set in socket	**SPINE CURVES**		**ELBOWS**	
Other:	Normal		Even	
EARS	Other:		Other:	
Level	**GLUTEAL MUSCLE MASS**		**WRISTS**	
Other:	Even		Even	
SHOULDERS	Other:		Other:	
Level	**ILIAC CREST**		**FINGERTIPS**	
(R) high / (L) low	Level		Even	
(L) high / (R) low	Other:		Other:	
(L) rounded forward	**KNEES**		**PATELLA**	
(R) rounded forward	Even/symmetrical		(L) ☐ movable ☐ rigid	
Muscle development even	Other:		(R) ☐ movable ☐ rigid	
Other:				

FIGURE 7-13. Sample physical assessment form. This information is obtained by observing (looking and feeling) and by measuring. The key to completing the form is to identify what is the same on the two sides of the body and what is different. *(From Fritz S: Mosby's Fundamentals of Therapeutic Massage, ed 4, St. Louis, Mosby, 2009.)* ⊖ This form is available for use on Evolve at http://evolve.elsevier.com/Fritz/business.

(Continued)

ANKLES		TRUNK		LEGS	
Even		Remains vertical		Swing freely at hip	
Other:		Other:		Other:	
FEET		**SHOULDERS**		**KNEES**	
Mobile		Remain level		Flex and extend freely through stance and swing phase	
Other:		Rotate during walking		Other:	
ARCHES		Other:		**FEET**	
Even		**ARMS**		Heel strikes first at start of stance	
Other:		Motion is opposite leg swing		Plantar flexed at push-off	
TOES		Motion is even (L) and (R)		Foot clears floor during swing phase	
Straight		Other:		Other:	
Other:		(L) swings freely		**STEP**	
SKIN		(R) swings freely		Length is even	
Moves freely and resilient		Other:		Timing is even	
Pulls/restricted		**HIPS**		Other:	
Puffy/baggy		Remain level		**OVERALL**	
Other:		Other:		Rhythmic	
HEAD		Rotate during walking		Other:	
Remains steady/eyes forward		Other:			
Other:					

FIGURE 7-13, cont'd

CONSENT FORM

A *consent form* (Fig. 7-16) is commonly used in massage as a preventive measure against malpractice suits. It is impossible to have a consent form for every circumstance that may occur, and it is unrealistic to believe that a general consent form covering every possible procedure would be upheld in court. A written summary of the treatment plan, as agreed on by the client and massage therapist, dated, and signed by both parties, is a more acceptable format for such consent.

LETTERS

Copies of all written communications sent to or concerning a client should become part of the client's clinical record. The fact that these documents may become evidence in a malpractice suit warrants caution in writing and retaining them.

Entering Data on a Clinical Chart

Several types of data are entered in the various components of a client's record, such as charting of existing conditions, recording of treatment procedures on progress notes (written in clear, concise detail), treatment plans, and discussions with the client about recommended treatment. Some clinical charts provide space for data entry on the back of the form. As entries are made and the form becomes complete or as a separate form, many massage therapists choose to use a progress sheet to enter clinical data. All data entered in a client's clinical chart or progress note should be dated,

accurate, complete, and initialed by the treating massage therapist (see Fig. 7-13). One of the major concerns in legal action is the incompleteness of data on a client's record. All action should be recorded in the clinical record. If a client declines referral, this notation should be entered on the record, dated, and signed. Failure to document any activity completely and accurately may prove costly in a lawsuit. Box 7-1 lists several rules for entering data, beginning with creation of the record.

Clinical abbreviations are short versions of or initials for common clinical terminology. Table 7-1 is a detailed list of abbreviations commonly used for data entry on massage records. The massage therapist should be cautious about using any abbreviations that are not universally used or not represented by a key someplace in the client record. When in doubt, it is prudent to write out the word.

Records Retention

The question often is asked, "How long should a client's records be retained?" The answer is awkward. The record should be retained for the period of time consistent with the statute of limitations within the state. The statute of limitations, the period within which a civil suit for alleged wrongdoing may be legally filed, varies from state to state. The average minimum for retention of a client's records is approximately 6 years after performance of the last treatment, but it is better to retain the records longer than that. Chapter 8 offers suggestions for longer-term storage.

TREATMENT PLAN

Client Name: _____

Choose One: ☐ Original plan   ☐ Reassessment date _____

Short-term client goals:
Quantitative: _____
Qualitative: _____

Long-term client goals:
_____
_____

Therapist objectives:
_____
_____

(1) Frequency, (2) length, and (3) duration of visits:
(1) _____ (2) _____ (3) _____

Progress measurements to be used: (e.g., pain scale, range of motion, increased ability to perform function) _____
_____

Dates of reassessment:
_____

Categories of massage methods to be used: (e.g., general constitutional, stress reduction, circulatory, lymphatic, neuromuscular, connective tissue, neurochemical)
_____
_____

Additional notes:
_____
_____
_____

Client Signature: _____   Date: _____

Therapist Signature: _____   Date: _____

FIGURE 7-14. A sample form for a care or treatment plan specific to message therapy. *(From Fritz S:* Mosby's Fundamentals of Therapeutic Massage, *ed 4, St. Louis, 2009, Mosby.)* ⊜ This form is available for use on Evolve at http://evolve.elsevier.com/Fritz/business.

Records Transfer

Requests for transfer of records are made for many reasons. The client may want to change massage therapists; the client is moving out of the area; the massage therapist wants to consult with another massage therapist; or the client is being referred to another massage therapist or health care practitioner.

Care must be taken in completing a request for transfer of a client's records. By law, any information regarding a client's care and treatment is confidential and privileged. This privilege belongs to the client, not to the massage therapist. For the massage therapist's protection, it is prudent to obtain a written consent signed by the client or the client's legal representative before transferring records to anyone other than the client. Certain exceptions exist to this privilege prohibiting disclosure, such as legal action or court orders involving the massage therapist. In general, if the following suggestions

are followed, record transfer can be handled efficiently and confidentially:

- Provide accurate and complete massage records.
- Never change massage records without maintaining the readability of the original entry. Date any changes, and record the reason for the change.
- Obtain a signed consent form from the client or the advice of legal counsel before providing copies of or allowing access to a client's massage records to anyone other than the client.
- Retain records in accordance with the state statute.
- Keep original records.
- Charge a reasonable clerical fee for furnishing records in accordance with local standards.
- Charge a reasonable professional fee for preparing and furnishing a narrative report for the client.

CONSULTATION/REFERRAL REPORT ▬▬▬▬▬▬▬▬▬▬▬▬▬▬▬

Luke Fritz, MT, NCTMB
2050 Leisure Lane
Lapeer, MI 48446
123-456-7890

Date:

Referral to:

Client:

Age: _____ Sex: _____

Family physician:

Client history:

Planned massage treatment:

Reason for referral:

Appointment scheduled for: _____ AM / PM

_____
Signature of Massage Therapist

Consultant's reply: _____

_____

_____

_____

_____

_____

_____

_____

_____

_____

_____

_____

_____

_____

_____

_____

_____   _____
Date   Signature of Massage Therapist

White - To recipient of referral - return to referral source   *Yellow* - To recipient of referral for retained copy   *Pink* - Retain as file copy until white is returned

Form 4052 • 8/88 SYCOM® Madison, WI Printed in U.S.A.

FIGURE 7-15. Consultation and referral report form. *(Modified from SYCOM, Madison, WI. In Finkbeiner BL, Finkbeiner CA:* Practice Management for the Dental Team, *ed 6, St. Louis, 2006, Mosby.)*

Informed Consent Process

A new client arrives for a massage.

The massage professional shows the client an informational brochure explaining massage, why it works, the procedures and process of massage, the benefits of massage, and the general contraindications. The client is asked to read the information. The massage professional then discusses the information with the client. In general terms, the massage professional explains alternatives to massage, such as exercise and self-hypnosis, that provide benefits similar to massage.

The massage professional then tells the client about his or her professional background: that he or she graduated from a state-licensed massage therapy school 2 years ago after a training program of 1000 hours, that he or she has been nationally certified by the National Certification Board for Therapeutic Massage, that he or she has been in professional practice part time for 2 years and averages eight massages a week, and that he or she has taken additional training in myofascial approaches and massage for elderly persons (approximately 100 hours for each). The client also is given information on methods of reporting misconduct of the massage therapist to state agencies, national professional organizations, and the police.

The client is given the policy and procedures booklet or statement and asked to read it. After he or she has done so, the massage professional goes over the booklet with the client, point by point, so that he or she understands the rules and requirements of the massage therapist. The massage professional makes sure that the requirements to report abuse and threat of deadly harm, as well as the release of files by court order, are discussed.

The massage professional hands the client a form that states the following:

I, (client's name) _____, have received a copy of the rules and regulations for Massage Works operated by Sue and John Grey. I have read the rules and regulations and I understand them. The massage procedures, information about massage in general, general benefits of massage, contraindications for massage, and possible alternatives have been explained to me. The qualifications of the massage professional and reporting measures for misconduct have been disclosed to me.

I understand that the massage I receive is for the purpose of stress reduction; relief from muscular tension, spasm, or pain; and to increase circulation. If I experience any pain or discomfort, I will immediately inform the massage practitioner so that the pressure or methods can be adjusted to my comfort level. I understand that massage professionals do not diagnose illness or disease or perform any spinal manipulations, nor do they prescribe any medical treatments, and nothing said or done during the session should be construed as such. I acknowledge that massage is not a substitute for medical examination or diagnosis and that I should see a health care provider for those services. Because massage should not be performed under certain circumstances, I agree to keep the massage practitioner updated as to any changes in my health profile, and I release the massage professional from any liability if I fail to do so.

Client's Signature _____ Date _____

Therapist's Signature _____ Date _____

Consent to Treat a Minor

By my signature, I authorize_____ to provide therapeutic massage to my child or dependent.

Signature of Parent or Guardian _____ Date _____

For clients who will have several sessions, the next step is completion of the needs assessment and initial treatment plan.

FIGURE 7-16. Informed consent process and consent forms. *(From Fritz S:* Mosby's Fundamentals of Therapeutic Massage, *ed 4, St. Louis, 2009, Mosby.)* ⊜ This form is available for use on Evolve at http://evolve.elsevier.com/Fritz/business.

(Continued)

Informed Consent Process—cont'd

Modified Informed Consent Form for Single Session
For clients who will be seen only once (such as might occur if the professional is working on a cruise ship, doing sports massage at an event, or doing promotional chair massage at a health fair), the following modification in informed consent can be made.

I, (client's name) _____ , have received a copy of the rules and regulations for (name of business) _____ ,operated by (owner) _____ .
I have read the rules and regulations and I understand them. The general benefits of massage and contraindications for massage have been explained to me. I have disclosed to the therapist any condition I have that would contraindicate massage. Other than to determine contraindications, I understand that no specific needs assessment has been performed. The qualifications of the massage professional and reporting measures for misconduct have been disclosed to me.
I understand that the massage I receive is for the purpose of stress reduction; relief from muscular tension, spasm, or pain; and to increase circulation. If I experience any pain or discomfort, I will immediately inform the massage practitioner so that the pressure or methods can be adjusted to my comfort level. I understand that massage professionals do not diagnose illness or disease or perform any spinal manipulations, nor do they prescribe any medical treatments. I acknowledge that massage is not a substitute for medical examination or diagnosis and that I should see a health care provider for those services.
I understand that a single massage session or massage used on a random basis is limited to providing a general, nonspecific massage approach using standard massage methods and does not include any methods to address soft tissue structure or function specifically.

Client's Signature _____ Date _____

Therapist's Signature _____ Date _____

Consent to Treat a Minor

By my signature, I authorize_____ to provide massage work to my child or dependent.

Signature of Parent or Guardian_____ Date _____

FIGURE 7-16, cont'd

BOX 7-1 | Rules for Entering Data on a Clinical Record

- Transfer the information from the registration and health history form to the physical assessment form completely and accurately.
- Enter general information about the client neatly. The clinical record must be completed in ink, or it may be keyboarded.
- Underline in red any notation about a serious illness or allergies. Small, brightly colored labels may also be used to draw attention to special notations.
- The massage therapist may make the entries for services rendered in the clinical record. Data can be entered on a keyboard in the massage room or on a keyboard outside the massage treatment room. Both methods provide a neater record.
- Check information to ensure that it has been transferred or entered correctly.
- Place the record in the file envelope or folder with the client's name visible on the record.
- After each client has been seen, check each record carefully to determine if it has been completed for the day.
- Verify that the record has been initialed.
- Ensure that all codes and charting techniques are consistent with the system used in the office. A list of these codes and symbols should be posted in each massage treatment room and available to all staff members.
- Never make a derogatory remark about a client in the record that could prove damaging in a lawsuit.

TABLE 7-1	Clinical Abbreviations		
ABBREVIATION	**TERM**	**ABBREVIATION**	**TERM**
@	at	Lt	left
Ad	to, up to	MDR	minimum daily requirement
AIDS	acquired immune deficiency syndrome	Med	medicine, medical
Amt	amount	mg	milligram
Anat	anatomy	Micro	microscopic
Ant	anterior	ML	midline
Approx	approximate	MM	mucous membrane
BP	blood pressure	mm	millimeter
CC	chief complaint	MS	multiple sclerosis
Cond	condition	Narc	narcotic
CV	cardiovascular	Nc, NC	no change, no charge
CVA	cerebrovascular accident	NCP	not clinically present
D	distal	Neg	negative
Dbl	double	Norm	normal
Dg or Dx	diagnosis	Opp	opposite
DOB	date of birth	P	pulse
DR	doctor	Path	pathology
Emerg	emergency	PDR	Physicians' Desk Reference
EMT	emergency medical treatment	Ped	pediatrics
ENT	ears, nose, and throat	PO, postop	postoperative
Epith	epithelial	Preop	preoperative
Est	estimate, estimation	Prep	preparation, prepare for treatment
Et	and	PRN	as needed
et al	and others	Prog	prognosis
Etc	and so on, and so forth	Pt	client
Eval	evaluate, evaluation	q	every
Ext	extract, external	qd	every day
F	Fahrenheit, female, field, formula	qh	every hour
FB	foreign body	q2h	every 2 hours
FH	family history	qid	four times daily
FR or frac	fracture	qn	every night
Frag	fragment	R	respiration
Freq	frequent, frequency	Rx, RX	prescribed
GP	general practitioner	Rad	radiograph
HBP	high blood pressure	Reg	regular
Hosp	hospital	Req	requisition
Hr	hour	Resp	respiration
Hs	hour of sleep	RHD	rheumatic heart disease
Ht	height	ROA	received on account
Hx	history	Sig	write on label
IH	infectious hepatitis	Sol	solution
IM	intramuscular	Stat	immediately
Inf	infected, inferior, infusion	Stim	stimulate, stimulator
Inj	injection, injury	Strep	*Streptococcus pyogenes*
IV	intravenous	Surg	surgery, surgeon
L	lingual	Sx	symptom
Lab	laboratory	T	temperature
Lac	laceration	Tab	tablet
Lat	lateral	TB	tuberculosis
Lig	ligament	Temp	temperature
Liq	liquid	tid	three times a day
LLQ	lower left quadrant	TLC	tender loving care
LN	lymph node	TMJ	temporomandibular joint
LRQ	lower right quadrant	TPR	temperature, pulse, respiration

(Continued)

TABLE 7-1	Clinical Abbreviations—cont'd		
ABBREVIATION	TERM	ABBREVIATION	TERM
Tr.P	treatment plan	URQ	upper right quadrant
U, u	unit	Wnd	wound
Unk	unknown	X, x	times (e.g., 4×), x-ray
ULQ	upper left quadrant	YOB	year of birth
URI	upper respiratory infection	yr	year

From Finkbeiner BL, Finkbeiner CA: Practice Management for the Dental Team, ed 6, St. Louis, Mosby, 2006.

- Require advance payment for clerical and preparation service in accordance with local standards.
- If records are mailed, send them by certified mail with a return receipt requested. The receipt will verify that the materials were received.

BUSINESS RECORDS

Financial records are as important as clinical records but must be maintained separately. A financial record protects the client and the massage therapist, provides information for tax purposes, and verifies data for a business analysis. Inadequate or incomplete financial records can result in poor public relations and can create unnecessary legal problems with state and federal governments and third-party payers. Chapter 15 details the step-by-step procedure for creating and managing various financial records.

Several employee records must be maintained in the office. These must be accurate and must be maintained with strict confidentiality. The massage therapist who employs others is responsible for periodically updating these records. Many of the records relate to payroll, and they are discussed in Chapter 16.

Employee records are classified in various ways. Employment forms:

- Applications for employment (see Chapter 18)
- Employment agreements (see Chapter 18)
- Merit evaluation forms (see Chapter 18)
- Health and medical records form (Fig. 7-17)
- Federal employment eligibility verification forms (Form I-9) (Fig. 7-18)

Employment tax information forms (see Chapter 16):

- Employer identification number
- Amounts and dates of all wage, annuity, and pension payments
- Names, addresses, Social Security numbers, and documents of employees and recipients
- Periods for which employees and recipients are paid while absent due to sickness or injury and the amount and weekly rate of payments made by the massage therapist or third-party payers
- Copies of employees' and recipients' income tax withholding allowance certificates
- Employee copies of federal form W-2 that were returned as undeliverable
- Dates and copies of tax deposits made
- Copies of returns filed

Confidential employee medical record

Employee medical record
Employee name _____
Employee address _____
_____
_____
_____

Employee social security number _____
Employee starting date _____
Employee termination date (if any) _____
History of HBV vaccination _____
_____
(date received, or, if not received, a brief explanation of why not)
History of other immunizations _____
_____

History of exposure incident(s) (dates, brief explanation, attachments)
_____
_____
_____
_____
_____

Results of medical exams and follow-up procedures regarding exposure
incident or hepatitis B immunity, including written opinion of healthcare
professional (dates, brief explanation, attachments)
_____
_____
_____
_____

Information provided to the health care professional regarding hepatitis B
vaccination and/or exposure incident(s) (dates, brief explanation, attachments)
_____
_____
_____
_____
_____
_____

Attach pre-employment health records to this document.
Note: maintain the record for duration of employment plus 30 years

FIGURE 7-17. Employee health and medical records form. *(Courtesy of SYCOM, Madison, WI. In Finkbeiner BL, Finkbeiner CA:* Practice Management for the Dental Team, *ed 6, St. Louis, 2006, Mosby.)*

U.S. Department of Justice
Immigration and Naturalization Service

OMB No. 1115-0136
Employment Eligibility Verification

Please read instructions carefully before completing this form. The instructions must be available during completion of this form. **ANTI-DISCRIMINATION NOTICE.** It is illegal to discriminate against work eligible individuals. Employers **CANNOT** specify which document(s) they will accept from an employee. The refusal to hire an individual because of a future expiration date may also constitute illegal discrimination.

Section 1. Employee Information and Verification. To be completed and signed by employee at the time employment begins

Print Name: Last	First	Middle Initial	Maiden Name

Address (Street Name and Number)	Apt. #	Date of Birth (month/day/year)

City	State	Zip Code	Social Security #

I am aware that federal law provides for imprisonment and/or fines for false statements or use of false documents in connection with the completion of this form.

I attest, under penalty of perjury, that I am (check one of the following):
☐ A citizen or national of the United States
☐ A Lawful Permanent Resident (Alien # A_____
☐ An alien authorized to work until_____/_____/_____
(Alien # or Admission #_____

Employee's Signature

Date (month/day/year)

Preparer and/or Translator Certification. (To be completed and signed if Section 1 is prepared by a person other than the employee.) I attest, under penalty of perjury, that I have assisted in the completion of this form and that to the best of my knowledge the information is true and correct.

Preparer's/Translator's Signature	Print Name

Address (Street Name and Number, City, State, Zip Code)	Date (month/day/year)

Section 2. Employer Review and Verification. To be completed and signed by employer. **Examine one document from List A OR examine one document from List B and one from List C** as listed on the reverse of this form and record the title, number and expiration date, if any, of the document(s)

List A	OR	List B	AND	List C

Document title: _____ _____ _____

Issuing authority: _____ _____ _____

Document #: _____ _____ _____

Expiration Date (if any): ___/___/___ ___/___/___ ___/___/___

Document #: _____

Expiration Date (if any): ___/___/___

CERTIFICATION - I attest, under penalty of perjury, that I have examined the document(s) presented by the above-named employee, that the above-listed document(s) appear to be genuine and to relate to the employee named, that the employee began employment on (month/day/year)____/____/____ and that to the best of my knowledge the employee is eligible to work in the United States. (State employment agencies may omit the date the employee began employment).

Signature of Employer or Authorized Representative	Print Name	Title

Business or Organization Name	Address (Street Name and Number, City, State, Zip Code)	Date (month/day/year)

Section 3. Updating and Reverification. To be completed and signed by employer

A. New Name (if applicable)	B. Date of rehire (month/day/year) (if applicable)

C. If employee's previous grant of work authorization has expired, provide the information below for the document that establishes current employment eligibility.

Document Title:_____ Document #:_____ Expiration Date (if any): ___/___/___

I attest, under penalty of perjury, that to the best of my knowledge, this employee is eligible to work in the United States, and if the employee presented document(s), the document(s) I have examined appear to be genuine and to relate to the individual.

Signature of Employer or Authorized Representative	Date (month/day/year)

Form I-9 (Rev. 11-21-91) N

FIGURE 7-18. Federal employment eligibility verification form (Form I-9). *(From the U.S. Citizenship and Immigration Services.)*

LISTS OF ACCEPTABLE DOCUMENTS

LIST A		LIST B		LIST C
Documents that Establish Both Identity and Employment Eligibility	**OR**	**Documents that Establish Identity**	**AND**	**Documents that Establish Employment Eligibility**

LIST A — Documents that Establish Both Identity and Employment Eligibility

1. U.S. Passport (unexpired or expired)

2. Certificate of U.S. Citizenship *(INS Form N-560 or N-561)*

3. Certificate of Naturalization *(INS Form N-550 or N-570)*

4. Unexpired foreign passport, with *I-551 stamp or* attached *INS Form I-94* indicating unexpired employment authorization

5. Alien Registration Receipt Card with photograph *(INS Form I-151 or I-551)*

6. Unexpired Temporary Resident Card *(INS Form I-688)*

7. Unexpired Employment Authorization Card *(INS Form I-688A)*

8. Unexpired Reentry Permit *(INS Form I-327)*

9. Unexpired Refugee Travel Document *(INS Form I-571)*

10. Unexpired Employment Authorization Document issued by the INS which contains a photograph *(INS Form I-688B)*

OR

LIST B — Documents that Establish Identity

1. Driver's license or ID card issued by a state or outlying possession of the United States provided it contains a photograph or information such as name, date of birth, sex, height, eye color, and address

2. ID card issued by federal, state, or local government agencies or entities provided it contains a photograph or information such as name, date of birth, sex, height, eye color, and address

3. School ID card with a photograph

4. Voter's registration card

5. U.S. Military card or draft record

6. Military dependent's ID card

7. U.S. Coast Guard Merchant Mariner Card

8. Native American tribal document

9. Driver's license issued by a Canadian government authority

For persons under age 18 who are unable to present a document listed above:

10. School record or report card

11. Clinic, doctor, or hospital record

12. Day-care or nursery school record

AND

LIST C — Documents that Establish Employment Eligibility

1. U.S. social security card issued by the Social Security Administration *(other than a card stating it is not valid for employment)*

2. Certification of Birth Abroad issued by the Department of State *(Form FS-545 or Form DS-1350)*

3. Original or certified copy of a birth certificate issued by a state, county, municipal authority or outlying possession of the United States bearing an official seal

4. Native American tribal document

5. U.S. Citizen ID Card *(INS Form I-197)*

6. ID Card for use of Resident Citizen in the United States *(INS Form I-179)*

7. Unexpired employment authorization document issued by the INS *(other than those listed under List A)*

Illustrations of many of these documents appear in Part 8 of the Handbook for Employers (M-274)

Form I-9 (Rev. 11-21-91) N

FIGURE 7-18, cont'd

Good Stuff from the Government

www.business.gov: This site has a business forms catalog with more than 500 forms used in small business operations. U.S. Environmental Protection Agency (EPA, http://www.epa. gov/p2/pubs/assist/sbg.htm): Going green by reducing the use of paper in the business setting.

EPA history: In July 1970, the White House and Congress worked together to establish the EPA in response to the growing public demand for cleaner water, air, and land. Before the establishment of the EPA, the federal government was not structured to make a coordinated attack on the pollutants that harm human health and degrade the environment. The EPA was assigned the daunting task of repairing the damage already done to the natural environment and of establishing new criteria to guide Americans in making a cleaner environment a reality.

SUMMARY

Record keeping is probably one of the most time-consuming tasks for a massage therapist, and it is important to follow the same procedures for each record. HIPAA is related to clients' records because it was conceived to protect their health information, which relates to following the same procedures for each record created and keeping the clients' records in a safe place and out of the hands of others. The procedures you follow for the SOAP note should always be the same, especially if submitting to an insurance company.

The client's record can contain numerous forms, including the client registration form, health history form, signed HIPAA form, medication history, massage assessment and treatment forms, SOAP notes, referral forms, signed informed consent, and letters. Each record should remain consistent, and if you are using symbols or abbreviations, make sure a key is used so others in the massage practice can decipher the chart. Manage your active and inactive files appropriately. Many store inactive files (those that have not been used in some time) in a different location to save room for the active files. Remember: organization, management, and consistency.

Bibliography

Fulton PJ: *General Office Procedures for Colleges*, ed 12, Cincinnati, OH, 2003, South-Western.

Mosley DC et al: *Supervisory Management*, ed 6, Cincinnati, OH, 2004, South-Western.

Evolve Annotated Web Links

http://evolve.elsevier.com/Fritz/business

Business.gov: http://www.business.gov/forms/

HIPAAcomply, HIPAA FAQs: http://www.hipaacomply.com/hipaafaq.htm

Phoenix Health Systems, HIPAA Advisory: http://www.phoenixhealth.com/hipaadvisory/

U.S. Department of Health and Human Services, Health Information Privacy: http://www.hhs.gov/ocr/hipaa

U.S. Environmental Protection Agency, Preserving Resources, Preventing Waste: http://www.epa.gov/epaoswer/non-hw/reduce/wstewise/targeted/rcc.htm#paper

U.S. Environmental Protection Agency: http://www.epa.gov/epahome/aboutepa.htm

1. Describe the impact of HIPAA on a massage practice. Why is this important to you as a client and health care professional?

_____

_____

_____

_____

_____

_____

2. List the various categories of records, and give examples of massage office documents that fit each category.

_____

_____

_____

_____

_____

_____

3. Explain why the clinical record is a vital record in the massage office.

_____

_____

_____

_____

_____

_____

4. Describe the parts of a clinical record.

_____

_____

_____

_____

_____

_____

5. Describe the retention and transfer of clinical records in the massage office.

_____

_____

_____

_____

_____

_____

6. Using a clinical chart obtained from the massage practice of an employer or instructor, transfer the information from a completed health questionnaire. This questionnaire may be completed in a classroom or obtained from a client record in an office of employment.

STORAGE OF BUSINESS RECORDS

KEY TERMS

Alphabetical filing system

Card file

Chronologic filing system

Cross-referencing

Geographic filing system

Lateral file

Numeric filing system

Open-shelf filing

Retrieval

Subject filing system

Tickler file

Vertical file

LEARNING OUTCOMES

Mastery of the content in this chapter will enable the reader to:

- Define key terms
- Identify and distinguish among the different storage systems
- Apply basic alphabetical indexing rules
- Determine the most efficient storage methods for various documents in a massage office
- Select supplies for the storage of records

Guidelines for the Learning Activities and answers to the Workbook questions are located on Evolve at http://evolve.elsevier.com/Fritz/business.

Disposition by destruction or storage is the final stage of a massage record (see Chapter 7). This chapter discusses records storage. A massage practice produces many kinds of information, including clinical and financial records, correspondence, employee records, tax and insurance records, accounts receivable and payable records, and possibly Occupational Safety and Health Administration (OSHA) records. Inability to find a document quickly is frustrating. Although computer storage is becoming the method of choice, many forms of information are still on paper and need to be filed manually. To many massage therapists, filing is one of those dreaded, procrastinated, routine jobs done when you can "get around to it" or "have the time."

Anyone with office experience knows that records must be readily available. Wise planning can save a tremendous amount of time and effort. The heart of any professional office is its filing system. Business office files should not be a place to *put* materials, but rather a place to *find* materials. A systematic plan for storage, retrieval, transferring, protection, and retention must be established. When planning for the office files, consider ease in retrieval, confidentiality, and safety. The needs of the office, the size of the massage practice, and the space available for equipment are determining factors in establishing an efficient filing system.

PREPARING RECORDS FOR FILING

Filing

Certain routines should be followed in preparing materials for filing:

1. Set aside some time each day or every few days for filing paper records.
2. Keep papers or records to be filed in a basket marked *To Be Filed.*
3. File electronic records immediately, and make backup copies of all electronic files as you complete them.

Before mastering the different filing systems, it is necessary to understand some basic steps, which usually are done in the order of inspecting, indexing, coding, sorting, and storing:

Inspecting: Review each record to determine if it is something that must be filed. If you are certain it can be disposed of, dispose of it. If it is to be retained, continue to the next step.

Indexing: Determine under which caption or name an item is to be filed. Indexing is a mental process that requires you to make a decision. For instance, if the record is a receipt for a payment that was just made from the massage therapist's checking account, you must decide into which file to place the receipt. If files are organized by subject, you may file the receipt under the subject to which it pertains (e.g., a receipt for an electric bill may be filed under "utilities" or "electricity"). For a client's clinical record, you

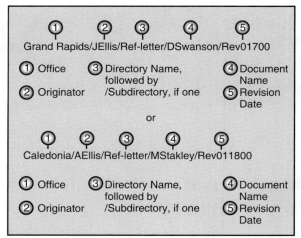

FIGURE 8-1. This figure provides an example of how documents are cross referenced in the computer so that they can be pulled up with multiple search terms. Electronic coding at the bottom of a document refers to the originator of the document, the directory name, the subdirectory (if used), and the document name. *(From Finkbeiner BL, Finkbeiner CA:* Practice Management for the Dental Team, *ed 6, St. Louis, 2006, Mosby.)*

commonly use an alphabetical system and break down the name into first, second, and third units to consider for filing. Electronic records are indexed by determining on what disk and in what directory the file should be located and by following a uniform procedure for naming the files. Do not name electronic files with characters or words that do not identify the subject of the record.

Coding: After you have determined the caption or title of the record, you must assign a code by highlighting, typing, or writing a caption on a paper record or by giving the electronic file a name. If an electronic file also exists in paper form, the file name on the document allows quick, easy retrieval. Examples of coding are shown in Figure 8-1. The clinical record is coded with the client's name, and the electronic document is coded with the name of the originator and other important information about the document.

Sorting: The records are arranged in the order in which they are to be placed in the file (e.g., if the file is alphabetical, put the records in alphabetical order). Electronic files are sorted as you save the files in the correct directory or on the correct disk. The system then sorts the files for you alphabetically by file name, date, or any other designation you make.

Storing: Put documents in folders and bulkier records in file drawers. Check and double-check that you are filing a document correctly.

Two other aspects of document storage, cross-referencing and retrieval, deserve special consideration:

Cross-referencing alerts staff members that a record normally kept in a specific location has been stored elsewhere. A cross-reference can be provided by making a copy of the record and filing it in the referenced file with a note that it is a copy, or a cross-reference sheet can be put in the file. A cross-reference sheet contains the name of the document, the date it was filed, a brief description of the subject of the record, and the places where the record could be found.

Retrieval is the removal of records from files using proper "charge-out" methods. When an entire file folder is removed, an out-folder is put in the place of the removed folder. The out-folder has the name of the individual or department that removed the folder and the date it was removed. Out-guides or substitution cards may be used instead of an out-folder. Although it does not commonly happen with clinical charts during routine massage session, a record may need to be removed from a file and used in another location for consultation or study. In such cases, the out-folder should denote the area to which the record has been taken.

SELF-REFLECTION

What do my personal files look like? What can be improved? Do I have a filing system, or is it a piling system? Are my records organized or thrown in a box? How will my management of personal records influence my business?

Retention of Records

It is not cost-effective to maintain unnecessary records and filing cabinets. Records are retained in accordance with state statutes. The National Archives and Records Service, a federal agency, has produced a helpful reference, *Guide to Record Retention Requirements*. It is available from the Superintendent of Documents, U.S. Government Printing Office, Washington, D.C. 20402.

Retention and destruction of files have taken on additional importance since the federal Revised Rule 26 of the Rules of Civil Procedure was approved in December 1993. This rule requires organizations to make available all relevant records that must be kept in compliance with prevailing statutes and regulations. Delay or failure to find information makes an office vulnerable to financial loss and adverse legal judgments (Box 8-1).

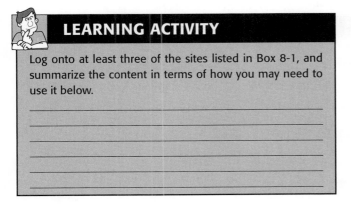

LEARNING ACTIVITY

Log onto at least three of the sites listed in Box 8-1, and summarize the content in terms of how you may need to use it below.

_____

_____

_____

_____

_____

_____

FILING SYSTEMS

Classification of Filing Systems

The five basic classification systems of filing are the alphabetical system, the geographic system, the numeric system, the subject system, and the chronologic system. All these methods except the chronologic system apply alphabetical procedures.

Selecting the Appropriate Filing System

ALPHABETICAL SYSTEM

In an *alphabetical filing system*, the arrangement of names appears in sequence from A to Z. This is the most common method used by massage therapist that are self-employed. The alphabetical filing system accounts for about 90% of the filing a person is likely to perform and can be applied to various captions. Standard rules exist for alphabetizing correctly. Box 8-2 illustrates alphabetical indexing rules applied to a variety of situations.

GEOGRAPHIC SYSTEM

In a *geographic filing system*, location is the important factor of reference. The principle of geographic filing is essentially the same as alphabetical filing, except that geographic filing is done by a territorial division (e.g., state, city, or street) rather than by name. Coding should be done in a manner similar to that of the alphabetical system by marking the caption under which the item will be filed (see Fig. 8-1).

NUMERIC SYSTEM

The *numeric filing system* uses a method of assigning numbers to each new client. Numbers assigned are then recorded on an alphabetical card index or computer file for future reference. Additional papers relating to the same person or account are subsequently filed according to the number originally allocated. In large clinics with access to computer centers, a numeric system can be used to great advantage because computers handle numeric data faster than alphabetical characters.

SUBJECT SYSTEM

The *subject filing system* is the alphabetical arrangement of papers according to the subject or topic of the papers. This system is used when it is more desirable to assemble information by topic than by name. For example, a subject file may be preferred if the massage therapist is involved in research or writing for publications. If a subject area is very broad, it can be broken down into smaller divisions by the use of secondary guides.

CHRONOLOGIC SYSTEMS

The *chronologic filing system* is a method of filing by date. It can be used within an alphabetical, geographic, subject, or numeric system by filing the most recent correspondence

---

BOX 8-1 Recordkeeping: Guidelines and Resources

The following information is useful in knowing what records to keep, and what records to shred, when running your own business. Use this as a resource as you start a new small business.

GUIDELINES FROM THE INTERNAL REVENUE SERVICE (IRS) ON RECORDKEEPING

(Information below from http://www.irs.gov/businesses/small/article/0,,id=98513,00.html)

The length of time you should keep a document depends on the action, expense, or event the document records. Generally, you must keep your records that support an item of income or deductions on a tax return until the period of limitations for that return runs out.

The period of limitations is the period of time in which you can amend your tax return to claim a credit or refund, or that the IRS can assess additional tax. The following information contains the periods of limitations that apply to income tax returns. Unless otherwise stated, the years refer to the period after the return was filed. Returns filed before the due date are treated as filed on the due date.

Note: Keep copies of your filed tax returns. They help in preparing future tax returns and in making computations if you file an amended return.

1. You owe additional tax and situations (2), (3), and (4), below, do not apply to you; keep records for 3 years.
2. You do not report income that you should report, and it is more than 25% of the gross income shown on your return; keep records for 6 years.
3. You file a fraudulent return; keep records indefinitely.
4. You do not file a return; keep records indefinitely.
5. You file a claim for credit or refund after you file your return; keep records for 3 years from the date you filed your original return or 2 years from the date you paid the tax, whichever is later.
6. You file a claim for a loss from worthless securities or bad debt deduction; keep records for 7 years.
7. Keep all employment tax records for at least 4 years after the date that the tax becomes due or is paid, whichever is later.
   The following questions should be applied to each record as you decide whether to keep a document or throw it away.

ARE THE RECORDS CONNECTED TO ASSETS?

Keep records relating to property until the period of limitations expires for the year in which you dispose of the property in a taxable disposition. You must keep these records to figure any depreciation, amortization, or depletion deduction and to figure the gain or loss when you sell or otherwise dispose of the property.

Generally, if you received property in a nontaxable exchange, your basis in that property is the same as the bases of the property you gave up, increased by any money you paid. You must keep the records on the old property, as well as on the new property, until the period of limitations expires for the year in which you dispose of the new property in a taxable disposition.

WHAT SHOULD I DO WITH MY RECORDS FOR NONTAX PURPOSES?

When your records are no longer needed for tax purposes, do not discard them until you check to see if you have to keep them longer for other purposes. For example, your insurance company or creditors may require you to keep them longer than the IRS does.

ADDITIONAL GOVERNMENT RESOURCES

IRS Documentation Maintenance: (http://www.irs.gov/businesses/small/article/0,,id=98575,00.html)

Keeping records: (http://www.irs.gov/businesses/small/article/0,,id=98862,00.html#6)

OSHA record keeping guide: (http://www.osha.gov/recordkeeping)

Fair Labor Standards Act (FLSA) Recordkeeping Requirements: (http://www.dol.gov/esa/regs/compliance)

Audit Information related to Recordkeeping: (http://www.sec.gov/rules/final/33-8180.htm)

Department of Transportation (DOT) Recordkeeping Requirements: (http://www.nhtsa.dot.gov/cars/rules/rulings/NAFTA/recordkeeping.htm)

SMALL BUSINESS ASSOCIATION RESOURCES

General Recordkeeping Guidelines: (http://www.sba.gov/library/pubs/fm-10.txt)

Small Business Association's YouTube video: (http://www.youtube.com/sba)

Small Business Television: On SBTV.com you'll find: technical information on how to run your business; inspirational success stories from entrepreneurs across the country; information about small business conferences and associations; and resources that can provide you with the right solutions for your business. http://www.sbtv.com

BOX 8-2	Indexing Rules for the Alphabetical System

Names of individuals are indexed by units. The last name (surname) is the key unit, followed by the first name (given name), which is the second unit, and then by the middle name or initial, the third unit. Alphabetize names by comparing the first units of the names, letter by letter. Consider second units only when the first units are identical. Consider third units only if the first and second units are identical, and so on.

NAME	1	2	3
Alice J. Gooding	Gooding	Alice	J.
Alice Marie Goodman	Goodman	Alice	Marie
William Grafton	Grafton	William	

If the last names are the same, consider the second indexing unit.

NAME	1	2	3
Frank Martin	Martin	Frank	
George Martin	Martin	George	
George C. Martin	Martin	George	C.

If the last names are the same but vary in spelling, consider each letter.

NAME	1	2	3
Joy Read	Read	Joy	
Janice Reed	Reed	Janice	
Phyllis J. Reid	Reid	Phyllis	J.

Initials are considered the same as a whole word and are filed before names beginning with the same initial. Names with no initial are filed before those with an initial (i.e., nothing before something).

NAME	1	2	3
Arthur Stone	Stone	Arthur	
C. Stone	Stone	C.	
Charles Stone	Stone	Charles	

If two people have the same name, they are indexed according to the alphabetical order of the city of residence, then by state. If two people have the same name and live in the same city, they are indexed according to street name.

NAME	1	2	3
Richard Murphey (Grand Rapids)	Murphey	Richard	Grand Rapids
Richard Murphey (Grandville)	Murphey	Richard	Grandville

Surname prefixes are considered part of the last name, not separate words. A hyphenated surname (e.g., Meyer-Schafer) is considered a single indexing unit. A compound personal name that is not hyphenated (e.g., Catherine Myers Schafer) is treated as separate indexing units.

NAME	1	2	3
Connie MacDonald	MacDonald	Connie	
Connie McDonald	McDonald	Connie	
Alice Meyer-Schafer	Meyer-Schafer	Alice	
Martin O'Connor	O'Connor	Martin	
Frank M. O'Dell	O'Dell	Frank	M.
Catherine Myers Schafer	Schafer	Catherine	Myers

If the first word in a compound surname is one of the standard prefixes (e.g., St. in St. James), the surname is indexed as a single unit.

NAME	1	2	3
Edward St. James	Saint James	Edward	
William St. Johns	Saint Johns	William	
James E. Sutton	Sutton	James	E.

(Continued)

BOX 8-2	Indexing Rules for the Alphabetical System—cont'd

Titles and degrees are disregarded but may be placed in parentheses after the names.

NAME	1	2	3
Professor Joseph C. Kline	Kline	Joseph	C. (Prof.)
Father Patrick O'Reilly	O'Reilly	Patrick (Fr.)	
Capt. C. J. Walters	Walters	C.	J. (Capt.)

A seniority designation is not considered an indexing unit but is used as an identifying element to distinguish between identical names.

NAME	1	2	3
Charles D. Flynn Jr.	Flynn	Charles	D. (Junior)
Charles D. Flynn Sr.	Flynn	Charles	D. (Senior)

Titles used without a complete name should be considered as the key indexing unit.

NAME	1	2	3
Father Patrick	Father	Patrick	
Sister Mary Martha	Sister	Mary	Martha

Articles, conjunctions, and prepositions are disregarded in indexing.

NAME	1	2	3
The Litton Massage Clinic	Litton	Massage	Clinic (The)

A firm or business name is indexed in the order written unless it contains an individual's name.

NAME	1	2	3	4	5
The Harvey F. Andrews Massage Practice	Andrews	Harvey	F.	Massage	Practice (The)
Grand Rapids Massage Practice	Grand	Rapids	Massage Practice		
Fritz Sports Massage	Fritz	Massage Practice			

Agencies of the federal government are indexed under United States Government and then according to department, division, subdivision, and location for adequate differentiation.

NAME	1	2	3	4	5	6
Federal Bureau of Investigation	United	States (Dept. of)	Govt. (Bur. of)	Justice	Federal	Investigation
Bureau of Labor	United	States (Dept. of)	Govt. (Bur. of)	Labor	Labor	Statistics

State, county, and city governments are indexed according to location and then by department, division, or subdivision.

NAME	1	2	3
Park Department, Kent	Kent	County	Park (Dept.) County
Michigan State	Michigan	State	Education (Dept. of) Department of Education
Grandville Department	Grandville	City	Health (Dept.) of Health

Numbers spelled as words in business names are filed alphabetically. Numbers written in digit form are filed before letters or words.

NAME	1	2	3	4
5-Cent Copy Center	5	Cent	Copy	Center
Four Seasons Health Spa	Four	Seasons	Health	Spa
Seventh Street Photo Center	Seventh	Street	Photo	Center

Names of schools are first indexed by the name of the city in which the school is located and then by the name of the school.

Local banking or other institutions with branch offices are indexed as the name is written. However, if banks from several cities are involved, the first indexing unit is the city where the bank is located, and the name of the bank follows.

Numbers, including Roman numerals, are filed before alphabetical information. However, all Arabic numerals come before Roman numerals.

Acronyms, abbreviations, and television and radio call letters are treated as one unit, and company names are filed as you see them. Hyphenated last names are indexed by the second last name.

Modified from Finkbeiner BL, Finkbeiner CA: *Practice Management for the Dental Team,* ed 6, St. Louis, 2006, Mosby.

in the front of the file folder. This system can also be used for treatment records in a client's clinical chart. The most current treatment data sheet appears first, followed by past treatment records.

Another type of chronologic classification system is a *tickler file,* or follow-up file. The most common type of tickler file contains the days of the month and the months of the year. The captions on a tickler file are most commonly the days of the month, from 1 to 31. Items to be completed are filed in the slot of the day you plan to complete the task. Take time each day to review the tickler file. Perform the task to be done on that day, or move the notation to the appropriate day if the activity has been rescheduled. Care should be taken to ensure that an activity is not placed on a weekend day or holiday on which you may not be able to complete the task. The files for these days should be carefully checked in advance to ensure that the task is done before the weekend or holiday or that the task is placed in the slot of a later day.

ELECTRONIC FILES

Storage of electronic records requires a knowledge of computer systems and the storage of word processing, database, or spreadsheet files, as well as knowledge of tasks that require you to sort, search, retrieve, and print reports. In a massage practice, you probably will most often use a manual filing system, but you may also use at least one type of electronic storage system. Special attention must be paid to the storage of electronic storage systems to prevent damage and loss of data. Each manufacturer may recommend specific care for its products, but in general, they should be protected from dust, magnetic fields, extreme temperatures, liquids, and vapors. Box 8-3 presents several suggestions for ensuring safe storage of data.

STORAGE EQUIPMENT

After an appropriate filing system has been chosen, the massage therapist must determine what types of supplies and equipment are necessary to maintain the system. The equipment should be practical for day-to-day use and for storage.

The term *filing equipment* refers to the structures that store files or records. Most manufacturers supply a variety of models in different colors with assorted features. Many practices still use vertical file cabinets, but open-shelf and lateral file cabinets have become very popular, especially if space is limited. A *vertical file* cabinet stores records in drawers; file folders are placed on the folder's edge and arranged according to the filing method selected. Vertical file cabinets are available with one to five or more drawers and may accommodate an 8.5 by 11 inch (letter size) or 8.5 by 14 inch (legal

| **BOX 8-3** | Diskette Care |

- Never touch the internal disk; handle disks only by the protective outer cover.
- Do not expose disks to magnetic fields, such as those produced by telephones, radio speakers, or computer screens.
- Keep disks at temperatures of 50 to 140°F (10 to 60°C); avoid extreme temperatures.
- Protect disks from dust and foreign particles.
- Do not expose disks to water or other liquids.
- If disks contain permanent information, use the *write protect* system to prevent data loss. Write protect is a feature on a disk or tape that prevents writing over existing data.

From Finkbeiner BL, Finkbeiner CA: *Practice Management for the Dental Team,* ed 6, St. Louis, 2006, Mosby.

size) file. These are not the best file cabinets to use for saving space. You must allow room for the cabinet and for the pull-out drawer space. This means you need approximately double the space of the vertical cabinet.

A *lateral file* (Fig. 8-2) cabinet is similar to a vertical file cabinet, except that the longest side opens, and the files are stored as if they were placed on a bookshelf. Lateral file cabinets have the added advantage of providing a countertop for reviewing files removed from the cabinet or for displaying books and other materials. Like their vertical counterparts, lateral file cabinets are designed to accommodate letter- or legal-size files. These cabinets can store more files and require less floor and pull-out drawer space.

Open-shelf filing saves space and speeds filing and retrieval. The visibility and accessibility of open-shelf filing have proved to be two of the many advantages of this arrangement (Fig. 8-3). Compared with a closed drawer filing system, open-shelf units hold twice as many files on one half of the floor space. The files give a visible sense of location and allow the users to take full advantage of index guides and color-coding techniques. Misfiled information becomes less of a problem. However, because the files are open, dirt and dust may accumulate if covers are not used.

A *card file* can be used to store small cards (i.e., 3 by 5 inch, 4 by 6 inch, or larger) that are used for specialized systems. Such a system can also be used for a recall system. A card with the client's name, telephone numbers, and other pertinent information may be set up in a metal or wooden box and used as a quick reference. Another example of the card system that allows for quick reference to clients' names, addresses, telephone numbers, and special notations about the family is the rotary or Rolodex file (Fig. 8-4). A second rotary file can be useful for addresses, e-mail addresses, and telephone numbers related to business activities such as maintenance and suppliers.

When selecting filing equipment, you should consider a fire-protection file. As a precaution against fire destruction,

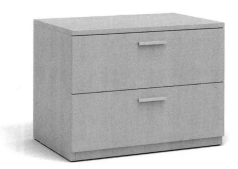

FIGURE 8-2. Lateral file cabinet. *(Courtesy of Steelcase, Grand Rapids, MI.)*

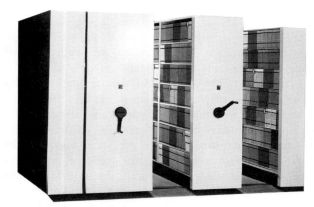

FIGURE 8-3. Open-shelf filing system. *(Courtesy of Kardex Systems, Marietta, OH. In Finkbeiner BL, Finkbeiner CA: Practice Management for the Dental Team, ed 6, St. Louis, 2006, Mosby.)*

the clients' ledger cards, the appointment book, disk copies, and other vital records should be placed in the file at the end of each workday.

STORAGE SUPPLIES

Filing supplies for paper storage include file guides, file folders, folder labels (in a variety of colors for color-coding), cross-reference sheets, and out-guides.

File guides, usually heavy cardboard, divide the file drawer into separate sections. The division is indicated by a tab that extends above the guide. The guides divide the alphabet into sections, or they may show a division in a numeric sequence. The file drawer is marked on the outside to correspond with the division of the filing arrangement.

File folders are usually made of manila paper or another heavy type of material. Folders may be obtained in a variety of cuts. Using a variety of cuts allows the tabs to be arranged

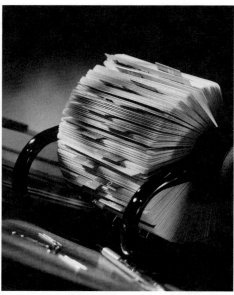

FIGURE 8-4. Rolodex file. *(From Finkbeiner BL, Finkbeiner CA: Practice Management for the Dental Team, ed 6, St. Louis, 2006, Mosby.)*

in a staggered fashion. The tabs may be on the far-left side, or they may be center cut, one-third cut, or one-fifth cut.

Most massage practices prefer to use client file folders or envelopes with labels that come in a variety of colors. This type of file and label guards against misplaced records and provides space for the client's name, address, and telephone number. Most file folders can be labeled with gummed labels, available in a variety of styles (i.e., rolls of labels, peel-off labels, and continuous folded strips) and colors that make the folders easier to locate and refile (Fig. 8-5). In a group practice, a different color may be used to designate the clients of each massage therapist or other practitioner.

Several points should be remembered when making the labels. The labels should be keyed, not handwritten; keying should begin two or three spaces from the left edge of the label and at a uniform distance (usually one line space) from the top edge of the label; the name may be keyed in all capital letters, or the first letter of each important word may be capitalized; and the established format should be followed consistently.

Color-coding of file folders aids in fast retrieval and refiling. Figure 8-6 shows a typical open-shelf, end-tab filing system that uses colored filing labels on each file folder to translate the alphabetical rules discussed earlier into a color code. The assignment of color to each alphabetical character has long been recognized by efficiency experts as a time and energy saver. When clients' charts are filed alphabetically and when each letter in the alphabet has a different file label color, color block patterns begin to form

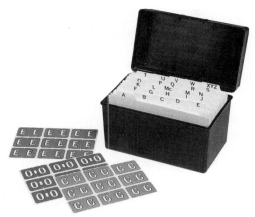

FIGURE 8-5. Label kit with assorted labels. *(Courtesy of SYCOM, Madison, WI. In Finkbeiner BL, Finkbeiner CA:* Practice Management for the Dental Team, *ed 6, St. Louis, 2006, Mosby.)*

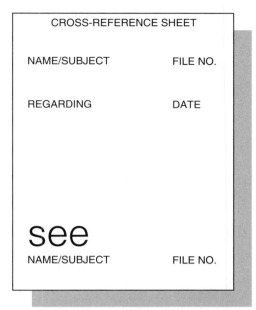

FIGURE 8-7. Cross-reference sheet. *(From Finkbeiner BL, Finkbeiner CA:* Practice Management for the Dental Team, *ed 6, St. Louis, 2006, Mosby.)*

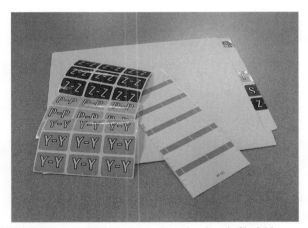

FIGURE 8-6. Filing labels are used on the client's file folder. *(From Finkbeiner BL, Finkbeiner CA:* Practice Management for the Dental Team, *ed 6, St. Louis, 2006, Mosby.)*

in the open-shelf system—block patterns that immediately direct the eye toward the proper filing areas. This virtually eliminates the misfiling common in non-color-coded systems.

Sometimes, cross-referencing is necessary within the filing system. Cross-referencing helps locate or file the information in its proper location. For example, if a letter is to be filed by the business name rather than by the name of the individual who has written the letter, you may look under the individual's name and find the cross-reference sheet that directs you to the name of the business (Fig. 8-7).

The electronic supplies necessary for records management include specially designed storage units for disks or tapes. These may be small plastic or fabric units that hold one to five disks, plastic or wooden desktop boxes, rotary files, or ring binders with vinyl pages that have pockets. Similar boxes are available for compact disks. A tape backup system is necessary when large amounts of data stored on hard disks must be recorded. Some of these systems store the entire contents of a hard disk on a single minicassette.

MANAGING WORKSTATION RECORDS EFFECTIVELY

Regardless of the types of records or systems used, organization of the workstation is an absolute necessity for successful records management. Almost all massage therapists spend some of their workday filing records of some type. Even if your filing duties are limited to organizing your own files, you need to develop and follow a simple system. The goal should be to establish a system that allows for easy retrieval. Successful retrieval means you will be able to find a record or document when needed in a minimal amount of time. This type of efficiency eliminates time and motion and ultimately financial loss. Box 8-4 presents tips for successful records management.

SUMMARY

Massage therapists must prepare records for filing, set up filing systems, and maintain current and archived records. There are different types of filing systems, and an important business management function is selecting the appropriate filing system to best serve the business. The business office is becoming paperless, and knowledge of electronic

BOX 8-4	Tips for Successful Records Management

PAPER RECORDS

1. Organize incoming and outgoing papers in an In/Out box. Use a stackable style that has two or three trays. Label each tray In, Out, or Hold. The Hold tray is for papers that do not have to be acted on immediately.
2. Use desk drawer files for personal records, forms, stationery, procedural handbooks, and other routinely used items.
3. Use logbooks to record recurring events or data, such as long distance telephone calls, petty cash, and appointment call lists.
4. Keep correspondence in a loose-leaf binder called a *correspondence* or *chronological file*, and date each folder for the year. This provides a fingertip reference of all correspondence pertaining to any client or given activity.
5. Plan a work schedule that includes filing as a daily routine.
6. When placing records in a folder, remove the folder from the file far enough so that the material can be placed completely in the folder and does not extend over the top edge of the folder or tab.
7. Be careful to place materials *in* a folder, not behind or in front of another folder.
8. Do not use paper clips on filed material. It is easy for other materials to attach themselves to the clips. Staples are better if materials must be held together, but remove the first staple before adding another.
9. To avoid filing errors, designate as few people as possible to file and retrieve records.
10. When searching for lost records, check transposition and alternate spellings of names.
11. Replace folders as they become worn out.
12. Avoid overuse of the *Miscellaneous* file.

ELECTRONIC RECORDS

1. Store disks in a file box specifically designed for the disk style.
2. Label each disk with a general classification.
3. Print an index of the documents on disk each time a new document is added. The index can be folded and placed in the jacket or kept in a reference notebook.
4. When a disk becomes full and you want to use the same label for a new disk, number the disks in consecutive order (e.g., "Letters 1," "Letters 2"). Mark each new disk with the date it was first used.
5. Store documents in electronic folders named to represent the activity (e.g., "Correspondence," "Recall," "Client charts").

From Finkbeiner BL, Finkbeiner CA: *Practice Management for the Dental Team,* ed 6, St. Louis, 2006, Mosby.

Good Stuff from the Government

All of the links for this chapter are on the Evolve Web site.

INTERNAL REVENUE SERVICE: RECORDKEEPING (http://www.irs.gov)

Why should I keep records? Good records will help you to monitor the progress of your business, prepare your financial statements, identify source of receipts, keep track of deductible expenses, prepare your tax returns, and support items reported on tax returns (http://www.irs.gov/businesses/).

What kinds of records should I keep? You may choose any recordkeeping system suited to your business that clearly shows your income and expenses. Except in a few cases, the law does not require any special kind of records. However, the business you are in affects the type of records you need to keep for federal tax purposes (http://www.irs.gov/businesses/).

How long should I keep records? The length of time you should keep a document depends on the action, expense, or event the document records. You must keep your records as long as they may be needed to prove the income or deductions on a tax return (http://www.irs.gov/businesses/).

How long should I keep employment tax records? You must keep all of your records as long as they may be needed; however, keep all records of employment taxes for at least 4 years (http://www.irs.gov/businesses/).

How should I record my business transactions? Purchases, sales, payroll, and other transactions you have in your business generate supporting documents. These documents contain information you need to record in your books (http://www.irs.gov/businesses/).

What is the burden of proof? The responsibility to prove entries, deductions, and statements made on your tax returns is known as the burden of proof. You must be able to prove (substantiate) certain elements of expenses to deduct them (http://www.irs.gov/businesses/).

RELATED TOPICS

Publication 583, Starting a Business and Keeping Records (http://www.irs.gov/publications/p583/index.html).

Online Classroom, Lesson 1: What you need to know about federal taxes and your new business (http://www.irs.gov/businesses/small/article/0,,id=97726,00.html).

Business with Employees (http://www.irs.gov/businesses/).

Operating a Business (http://www.irs.gov/businesses/).

files processes and procedures and of storage equipment is important. The various types of storage equipment and supplies must be considered. The way in which records and procedures are maintained provides a platform for organization of the business. As always, there are good things from the government to add to or expand the information in this chapter.

Bibliography

Fulton PJ: *General office procedures for colleges*, ed 12, Cincinnati, OH, 2003, South-Western.

Mosley DC et al: *Supervisory management*, ed 6, Cincinnati, OH, 2004, South-Western.

Evolve Annotated Web Links

http://evolve.elsevier.com/Fritz/business

Internal Revenue Service: http://www.irs.gov/publications/p583/ar02.html#d0e2170

Workbook

1. List four steps for preparing materials to be filed.

2. Define the five basic methods of filing.

3. Describe the use of the following filing equipment:

   a. Vertical file

   b. Open-shelf file

   c. Card file

   d. Rolodex™ file

   e. Tickler file

   f. Electronic file

4. Explain how color-coding can be used in the massage office files.

5. List five helpful hints for more efficient filing.

6. Assume that the following list of names with addresses represents the accounts payable for the massage practice.

   a. Index each name by keying the name in proper indexing form.

   b. Using a manual system, arrange the cards in alphabetical order, and prepare a list of alphabetical names.

Apex Business Supplies
1816 S. Riverfront
Elgin, IL 26582

T. S. Davis
26058 S. State
Chicago, IL 26528

Quality Massage Supplies
P.O. Box D-1
Minneapolis, MN 48807

J. P. T. Uniforms
22803 Third Avenue
Benton Harbor, MI 23062

Davis & Davis Office Supplies
4800 N. Baseline
Grand Rapids, MI 27501

M & M Creative Systems
11015 Orange Avenue
Los Angeles, CA 90025

Tasha D. Apple
3668 N.W. Territorial
Buffalo, NY 32506

Quick Copy
1108 Third Street
Des Moines, IA 42106

QT Physical Therapy Supplies
1556 Eighth Street SW
Dubuque, IA 42013

Roberta S. Davis, C.P.A.
90724 S. Hubbard
Gary, IN 30682

Mark C. Sylvester
2601 Beck Boulevard
Albany, NY 30582

Telcom Credit Bureau
914 E. Michigan
Madison, WI 78034

C. V. Talbot
2247 Hamilton
Charleston, WV 82506

Batch & Associates
839 Frederick
Hampton, VA 26809

B B Waste Paper Co.
1308 Cadillac
Charlotte, NC 89045

Brian Baumgartner
6262 Shield
Jamestown, ND 45902

Consumer Counseling
590 Bridge Street
Charleston, SC 78032

E. S. Comstock
1255 Harbour Cove
Los Altos, CA 91256

Community Coop
2236 Stadium Drive
Kansas City, MO 64119

Krauss & Krauss Accounting
152 Barkber Boulevard
Kansas City, KS 78566

9

WRITTEN COMMUNICATION

KEY TERMS

Attention line
Body
Complimentary close
Date line

Electronic mail (e-mail)
Interoffice memorandum
Keyboarded signature
Mixed punctuation

Open punctuation
Reference initials
Salutation
Subject line

LEARNING OUTCOMES

Mastery of the content in this chapter will enable the reader to:

- Describe the various types of written communication in a massage office
- Select stationery supplies
- Identify the characteristics of effective correspondence
- Identify the parts of a letter

- Review rules of punctuation and capitalization
- Describe the basic steps for preparing written communication
- Apply various formatting styles to written communication
- Describe standard procedures for preparing outgoing mail

Guidelines for the Learning Activities and answers to the Workbook questions are located on Evolve at http://evolve.elsevier.com/Fritz/business.

LEARNING OUTCOMES—Cont'd

- Observe ethical and legal obligations in written communication
- Explain the use of e-mail in the massage office
- Apply common business etiquette to the use of e-mail

- Identify the classifications of mail
- Identify special mail services
- Explain the function of a postage meter
- Explain the procedure for sorting incoming mail

You will be surprised how often you will communicate in written form in the business setting. This chapter may seem to be a reminder of high school English. We thought the information we had to learn in high school was useless, but as adults, we need to be reminded of how to complete a task, such as writing a business letter.

Good business and professional writing should sound like a person talking to another person. Unfortunately, some of the writing produced in our professional lives does not seem to be written by caring people. Using an easy-to-read style makes the reader respond more positively to your ideas. You can make your writing easier to read in two ways. First, you can make individual sentences and paragraphs easy to read so the reader can easily skim the first paragraph or read the entire document in as short a time as possible. Second, you can make the document visually pleasant and structured.

Good business and professional writing is closer to a conversation and less formal than the style of writing that has traditionally earned high marks on college essays and term papers. Most people have several styles of talking that they vary instinctively depending on the audience; the same is true of your writing in the massage practice. A letter to a massage therapist regarding a professional technique or a letter to a massage supplier demanding better service may be formal, whereas an e-mail to a colleague probably is informal and perhaps even chatty.

In Chapter 7, we examined the various types of documents generated in the massage office. It is time to review other types of written communication in a massage practice, specifically the use of letters, forms, and newsletters. These documents are created for a variety of reasons. This chapter discusses the creation and production of written communication and how it is distributed and describes how incoming communication in manually written and electronic forms are processed.

LETTERS

Many types of written documents are generated in the massage office, but none is as important as the letters that seek to enhance public relations with clients and professional colleagues. These letters should be original and create a professional image. The letter should be one that you are proud to mail from the office.

With the increased use of word processing in the massage office, the dreaded task of creating an original letter each time

one is needed can be eliminated. You can have a supply of sample letters stored as templates in an electronic file. When necessary, you can transform the sample into an original letter that is professional and that can be personalized within minutes.

The types of written communication most commonly sent from a massage office include thank you notes for referral of clients, letters of appreciation, birthday or holiday greetings, congratulatory letters, sympathy messages, client transfer letters or letters of consultation, collection letters, order letters, and newsletters.

Thank You for Referral Letter

The massage therapist should be appreciative of the confidence expressed by a client who refers a new client to the office and should acknowledge such a referral with a personally signed letter. Although this letter should mention the name of the referred client, it should not divulge any confidential information about the treatment. An example of this type of thank you letter is shown in Figure 9-1. You will note that the content varies according to the situation.

Letter of Appreciation

A massage therapist should acknowledge a client who is prompt for appointments, maintains a regular payment plan, and cooperates with suggested self-plans. This is an opportunity to give sincere compliments. When the opportunity presents itself, try writing a letter as in Figure 9-2 and see how appreciative your clients are. A letter of appreciation should be sincere, state the purpose briefly, and be written as though you were conversing with the client in person.

Birthday Letter and Holiday Greetings

People, especially children and older adults, like to be recognized on their birthdays. These letters should be cheerful. Figure 9-3 shows a letter that could be sent to an older adult on a special birthday. Another method of handling this form of public relations is to send a birthday card (Fig. 9-4).

Congratulatory Letter

Through conversations with clients and by reading the daily newspaper, you can learn about the outstanding achievements of clients. These accomplishments should not go

Leisure Massage/Luke Fritz, MT, NCTMB
222 Relaxation Drive, Your Town, State 00000
(123) 456-7890 leisuremassage@massage.com

September 15, 20__

Mr. Bob Smith
333 Comfort Zone Drive
Lapeer, MI 48446

Dear Mr. Smith:

It was so good to meet your friend, Randy Jones, last week. My staff and I are always glad to offer our massage services to you and your friends whenever possible. Thank you so much for the referral.

You, as well as your family and friends, have been very valuable clients to my practice, and we appreciate the opportunity to serve you. I am confident we can offer Randy the same quality massage treatment that you, your family, and friends have enjoyed over the years.

Our best to you,

Luke Fritz, MT, NCTMB

ah

FIGURE 9-1. Letter thanking a client for a referral. ⊜ This letter template is posted on Evolve at http://evolve.elsevier.com/Fritz/business.

unnoticed by the massage office staff. A letter sent to congratulate a client must be sent promptly. Include how you learned of the event and a sincere expression of congratulations (Fig. 9-5). Congratulations can also be sent for the birth of a child, a wedding, or a graduation. A greeting card or brief letter is appropriate.

Referral

When appropriate, the massage therapist can refer the client to other professionals. A different massage therapist may better serve the client, another form of bodywork may be indicated, or the client's condition may need to be evaluated by a physician. Alternatively, someone may refer a client to you. When this is the case, written communication as an aspect of the referral and thank you letters to those who have referred to you are advisable (Fig. 9-6).

Sympathy Message

Many people find it difficult to express sympathy in a letter. One of the best ways to handle this difficult situation is to send a sympathy card. It is the unexpected message that often means a great deal to family members in their time of grief.

Miscellaneous Letters

Many letters are not public relations letters and are not included in this chapter. Specific examples of recall, broken appointment, and collection letters are discussed in the chapters that specifically address each of these topics (Fig. 9-7).

LEARNING ACTIVITY

Choose one of the letter types discussed in this chapter, and write a fictitious letter that meets the recommendations.

NEWSLETTERS AS MARKETING DEVICES

As massage therapists seek to address the consumer market, marketing becomes part of the business of massage therapy. If done ethically and with concern for the values of the community and the education of the public, marketing can be a valuable tool.

Automated systems in the massage office have made it easier to incorporate marketing procedures into the massage business. One of the products of automated systems is a client newsletter. A newsletter can educate your clients about

Leisure Massage/Luke Fritz, MT, NCTMB
222 Relaxation Drive, Your Town, State 00000
(123) 456-7890 leisuremassage@massage.com

September 15, 20__

Mr. Bob Jones
333 Comfort Zone Drive
Lapeer, MI 48446

Dear Mr. Jones:

Our philosophy at Leisure Massage includes a partnership in well-being with each client. I wanted to take an opportunity to thank you for being a good partner in your care. My staff and I are grateful for the courtesy that you show us regarding your appointments, prompt payment of your account, and your diligence on your self-help plan.

We always look forward to your appointments and feel you bring a positive attitude when calling on our office. We hope you continue to enjoy the investment you are putting into your life. We promise to continue providing our very best massage services and any assistance you need to help you benefit the most from your massage.

Thank you again for your continued loyalty.

Sincerely,

Luke Fritz, MT, NCTMB

ah

FIGURE 9-2. Letter of appreciation to a cooperative client. ⊜ This letter template is posted on Evolve at http://evolve.elsevier.com/Fritz/business.

Leisure Massage/Luke Fritz, MT, NCTMB
222 Relaxation Drive, Your Town, State 00000
(123) 456-7890 leisuremassage@massage.com

September 15, 20__

Mr. Bob Smith
333 Comfort Zone Drive
Lapeer, MI 48446

Dear Mr. Smith:

Happy birthday! My staff and I wish to send you our very best wishes for a wonderful day. We hope you will enjoy your special day and take time out to reflect on your accomplishments over the past year.

Birthdays are a time for celebration and a renewed dedication to your goodness and health. We hope your day finds you marking the event with loved ones.

Again, best wishes on your birthday and continued health in the future. We look forward to seeing you in 2 weeks.

Sincerely,

Luke Fritz, MT, NCTMB

ah

FIGURE 9-3. Letter acknowledging the birthday of an older adult. ⊜ This letter template is posted on Evolve at http://evolve.elsevier.com/Fritz/business.

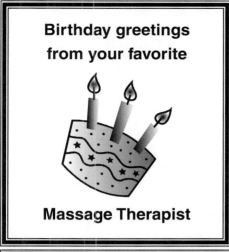

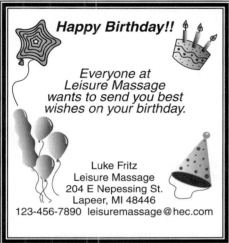

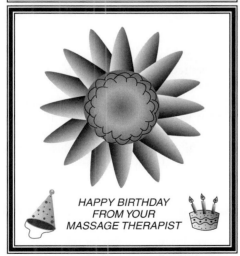

FIGURE 9-4. Birthday postcards. *(Modified from Colwell, Division of Patterson Companies, Champaign, IL.)*

new ideas and research in massage therapy, basic massage related health concepts, community trends, and ideas your business is promoting, such as a Mother's Day special.

Newsletters may be a single page or many pages (Fig. 9-8) and should be mailed regularly—quarterly or biannually.

Software packages can be used to generate the original copy, which then can be duplicated at a discount printer. Others have the entire newsletter generated and produced outside the office.

Newsletters can be sent by e-mail. If this is your choice for correspondence including newsletters, it will be necessary to collect e-mail addresses during the intake process. Regardless of the method of production, it is important that the content originate from the massage therapist and the staff, with their own philosophy and image influencing the final product.

SELECTING STATIONERY SUPPLIES

If you begin working in an established massage practice, stationery supplies will be available. However, in a new business, you must choose business supplies as part of the start-up process. Many of these supplies are described in Chapter 6.

The business stationery (letterhead) is usually selected on the basis of simplicity, neatness, and quality. Bond paper, because of its quality, is often used. It can be made from all-cotton fiber (sometimes called rag), from all sulfite (a wood pulp), or from any proportion of the two. High-cotton fiber bond indicates quality and prestige, and it ages without deterioration or chemical breakdown.

The following information may be used as a guide for future stationery needs:

Letterhead for standard office use: business size 8.5 by 11 inches, usually 16- or 20-pound bond, 25% cotton fiber (rag)

Letterhead for executive use: standard and Monarch size (7.25 by 10 inches), usually 24-pound bond, 100% cotton fiber

Matching envelopes for standard office use: no. 10 (4.125 by 9.5 inches), same weight and fiber content as letterhead

Matching envelopes for executive use: no. 10 and no. 7 (3.875 by 7.5 inches), same weight and fiber content as letterhead

A color theme may be used for stationery items, such as letterheads, envelopes, appointment cards, and notepads. Color coordinates such as light and dark mauve or blue or contrasting tones of gray with black print are attractive combinations. Most stationery supply houses have samples of stationery stock and logo designs from which you may select.

A popular alternative to purchasing stationery is to create the letterhead using appropriate computer software. A fine bond paper can be purchased. When a new letter is to be keyboarded, the letterhead is removed from the file where it is stored, the letter is prepared, and it is printed on bond paper. This method is less expensive and allows for more frequent changes and creativity. Clip art makes it easy to create

Leisure Massage/Luke Fritz, MT, NCTMB
222 Relaxation Drive, Your Town, State 00000
(123) 456-7890 leisuremassage@massage.com

September 15, 20__

Mr. Bob Smith
333 Comfort Zone Drive
Lapeer, MI 48446

Dear Mr. Smith:

It was great to hear the news about your promotion at work!

It is always such a pleasure to learn about the accomplishments of our clients, and we send our very best wishes for success in your new position.

Again, best wishes on your awesome achievement.

Sincerely,

Luke Fritz, MT, NCTMB

ah

FIGURE 9-5. Congratulatory letter. ⊖ This letter template is posted on Evolve at http://evolve.elsevier.com/Fritz/business.

a professional letterhead that provides you many options. Labels with the same clip art and office information can also be created in this manner. The labels that are selected must be compatible with the office printer.

CHARACTERISTICS OF AN EFFECTIVE LETTER

Effective letters (including e-mails) that generate good public relations have certain common elements. Direct, simple writing is easier to read. The best word depends on the context, including the situation, the purpose, the audience, and the words you have already used. Use words that are accurate, appropriate, and familiar. Accurate words mean what you want to say. Appropriate words convey the attitudes you want to create and fit well with the other words in your document. Familiar words are easy to read and understand.

Use technical terminology sparingly. The exception to this rule is communication with another professional, when you need to describe a condition or treatment in technical terms. However, when communicating with clients or laypersons, it is wise to use a plain English equivalent instead of a technical term.

Use active verbs most of the time. This is common in writing for a job application or referring a client. If the verb describes something that the subject is doing, the verb is active. If the verb describes something that is being done to the grammatical subject, the verb is passive:

> Active: I recommend that the client's knee be assessed for joint damage.
> Passive: It was recommended by me for the client to have his knee assessed for joint damage.

Tighten your writing. Eliminate words that say nothing, and combine sentences to eliminate unnecessary words. Put the meaning of the sentence into the subject and verb. Cut words if the idea is already clear from other words in the sentence. Substitute single words for wordy phrases.

> Wordy: Keep this information in the client's file for future reference.
> Tighter: Keep this information for reference.
> Tighter: File this information.

Phrases beginning with *of*, *which*, and *that* can often be shortened:

> Wordy: The issue of most importance
> Tighter: The most important issue

Leisure Massage/Luke Fritz, MT, NCTMB
222 Relaxation Drive, Your Town, State 00000
(123) 456-7890 leisuremassage@massage.com

September 15, 20__

Gerald L. Jones, D.O.
555 Main Street
Lapeer, MI 48446

Dear Dr. Jones:

Please accept this letter as a referral of my client, Jolanda Randall, age 25, to your office for a physical and evaluation. Ms. Randall will be calling your office for an appointment.

On September 2, 20--, Ms. Randall indicated during her regular massage treatment that she was experiencing unexplained breathing difficulties that do not have a logical cause such as an upper respiratory infection.

Enclosed you will find copies of the release of information form, initial intake data, assessment notes, and other relevant information.

I appreciate your assistance with this client. Please let my office know if we can provide any further information.

Sincerely,

Luke Fritz, MT, NCTMB

ah

FIGURE 9-6. Referral of a client to a chiropractor. ⊖ This letter template is posted on Evolve at http://evolve.elsevier.com/Fritz/business.

Wordy: It is the case that certified massage therapists are more qualified to practice in our office.

Tighter: Certified massage therapists are more qualified for in our office.

Combine sentences to eliminate unnecessary words. In addition to saving words, combining sentences focuses the reader's attention on key points, makes your writing sound more sophisticated, and sharpens the relationship between ideas, making your writing more coherent.

Wordy: I conducted a survey by telephone on Monday April 17th. I questioned 18 massage practitioners, some massage technicians without certification, and some certified massage therapists, who according to the state directory were all currently working. The purpose of this survey was to find out how many of them were working in health care. I also wanted to find out if there were any differences between their salaries.

Tighter: On Monday, April 17th, I phoned certified and noncertified working massage professionals to determine (1) if they were working in health care and (2) whether there was a distinction between salaries for these two credentials.

Vary sentence length and sentence structure. A readable letter mixes sentence lengths and varies sentence structure. A short sentence is less than 10 words and can add punch to your letter. Long sentences of 30 to 40 words can raise a danger flag.

A simple sentence has one main clause:

We will open a new office this month.

A compound sentence has two main clauses joined with *and*, *but*, *or*, or another conjunction. Compound sentences are

Leisure Massage/Luke Fritz, MT, NCTMB
222 Relaxation Drive, Your Town, State 00000
(123) 456-7890 leisuremassage@massage.com

<<Today's date in words>>

<<Client's name>>
<<Client's street address>>
<<Client's city, state zip code>>

Dear <<Client's name>>:

Welcome to Leisure Massage! Our staff looks forward to meeting you on <<appointment date>> at <<appointment time>>. It is always our goal to ensure that the time you spend with us is pleasant and worthwhile.

Please bring with you the completed client information sheet (enclosed), as well as any applicable insurance forms if your health insurance covers massage therapy.

During your first visit we will complete an assessment and customize a treatment plan that meets your specific needs. If you have any quesitons, please don't hesitate to contact our office.

Looking forward to meeting you,

Luke Fritz, MT, NCTMB

ah

FIGURE 9-7. Form letter from a massage therapist to welcome a new client. ⊖ This letter template is posted on Evolve at http://evolve.elsevier.com/Fritz/business.

used best when the ideas in the two clauses are closely related:

We have hired three new massage therapists, and they will complete their orientation next week.
We hired a new massage therapist, but he will be unable to begin work until the end of the month.

Complex sentences have one main and one subordinate clause. They are good for showing logical relationships:

When the new office opens, we will have an open house for potential clients and offer refreshments and door prizes.
Because we already have a strong client base in Livingston County, we expect the new office will be as successful as the Ann Arbor office.

Use parallel structure. Parallel structure puts words, phrases, or clauses in the same grammatical and logical form. Clarity eliminates long, meaningless words and uses language that the reader will understand. You can be certain each statement will not be misinterpreted:

Nonparallel: The position is prestigious, challenging, and also offers good money.
Parallel: The position offers prestige, challenge, and money.
Nonparallel: The steps in the planning process include the following: determining the objectives, an idea of who the reader is, and a list of the facts.
Parallel: Determine the objective, consider the reader, and gather the facts.

Put your readers in your sentences. Use second person pronouns (you) rather than third person (he, she, one) or first person (I, we) to give your writing a greater team approach. The "you" approach to letter writing requires the

Getting the most out of your massage

Volume 1, Issue 2	Newsletter Date

Special points of interest:

- Nutrition
- Water
- Rest
- Sleep Schedule
- Disease
- Essential Oils
- Memory

Sandy Fritz

204 Nepessing

Lapeer, MI 48446

123-456-7890

Diet, Water, Rest

This probably isn't the first time you've heard this. Drink more water, eat a nutritious diet, get enough sleep. Well, you're going to hear it again. Why, because I believe everyone out there is trying to live a perfect life. Let's be honest with ourselves. Really think about the answer to this scenario: To live the perfect life probably means feeling a whole lot better than you are feeling at the present moment. Do you have an ailment, little or big? It could be as little as getting a cold sore or as big as diabetes or high blood pressure. So let's help ourselves by taking a small step and giving up just one bad food in our diet—whether it is a food with high fructose corn syrup, a drink such as "pop" or "soda." Or cut out the French fries when going out to eat and replace with a vegetable or salad. It's not as hard as you think. What it takes is perseverance and the desire to live a better life than you did yesterday. Adjusting your pure clean water intake, if you don't drink enough already, would help tremendously. The amount needed is still in debate, but the general rule is your body weight divided in half equals the amount of water in ounces you should drink a day. For some that's true, but others need to drink more. For instance, my assistant had some substantial tests done; she doesn't hold her water so she needs to drink a liter of water a day, and she is a tiny person. Remember—after a massage you need to drink more than usual because the massage is getting things moving so toxins are probably wanting to come out. So drink your water to let those toxins out. Last but not least—Rest. If you are tired during the day, you're probably overworked. So get to bed before 10 pm and if that isn't doable then try 11 pm and after awhile try 10:30 pm and so on. This is to let your circadian rhythm do its job. The melatonin in your body depends on darkness and 12 hours to

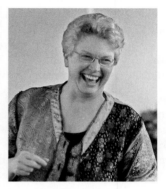

work its magic. Again, let it do its job. If you want more research on it, go on the internet and search for the importance of darkness while sleeping. For those who work nights, get some really good black-out shades and hopefully that'll do the trick. All this will help you get the best results from your massage.

Essential Oils

One of the passions that I have developed after becoming a massage therapist is making essential oils. Yes, I actually make my own. Sure, I buy them too, but making your very own is very rewarding. Essential oils is really a secret that many don't know about even though they have been used for a long time. Essential oils have been used throughout history for healing purposes. I use them for the same reason and also for relaxation. They can also bring about a calming effect. For instance, have you ever walked into someone's house and thought, "I know that smell; it reminds me of my mom or grandma"? Many smells trigger those memories we had as a child or even as adults. Smell and memory are closely linked because the olfactory bulb is part of the brain's limbic system. If this intrigues you, go into a natural food store and ask for some essential oils—you'll be amazed at what memories they may trigger.

FIGURE 9-8. Newsletter from a massage office to a client. ⊜ This newsletter template is posted on Evolve at http://evolve.elsevier.com/Fritz/business.

writer to place the reader at the center of the message. When writing the letter, put yourself in place of the reader.

> Third person: Referrals for clients in this office are made by our office manager, and the client will be contacted as soon as the appointment has been confirmed with the specialist.
> Second person: After you are referred to a specialist, you will receive a confirmation of your appointment from our office manager.

In addition to the ideas previously discussed, you should review the basic characteristics of effective correspondence. These factors should be used in a review of the letter before it is sent. Remember that the letter sent from the massage office is representative of the quality of work or treatment produced in that practice. Reading the correspondence out loud can help detect areas that are unclear or that may read in a clumsy manner.

Review your letter for the following:

Completeness: Include all of the data the reader needs to make a decision or take action.
Conciseness: Be brief.
Confidentiality: Release information only about the case that is relative to the contents of the letter and only after the client has given consent to release specific information.
Courtesy: Use good manners for good public relations. Do not make derogatory statements.
Accuracy: All of the data must be correct. Check details carefully, and use correct spelling and grammar.
Neatness: Avoid smudges, tears, or wrinkles.
Attitude: Use positive words that indicate you are helpful and caring (Box 9-1).
Orientation: Use second person style when writing the letter. Pronouns should be "you oriented."

Parts of a Business Letter

A review of the parts of a business letter and the proper placement and purpose for each part is appropriate before you select a letter style or begin to create the letter. Most business letters contain the following parts:

- Date line
- Inside address (letter address)
- Salutation
- Body
- Complimentary close
- Keyboarded signature
- Reference initials
- Special notations, such as an attention line, a subject line, or enclosures

When using most word processing software, many preformatted letter styles are available. Dates are automatic,

BOX 9-1	Positive and Negative Words

POSITIVE WORDS
I will
Congratulations
Concern
Pleasure
Thank you
Satisfactory
I can
Welcome
NEGATIVE WORDS
I'm sorry
Complaint
Difficult
Unpleasant
No
Can't
Careless
Error
Inconvenient
Disappointed

and in most systems, alignment and letter parts are already defined.

DATE LINE

The *date line* contains the date the letter is keyboarded. When using printed letterhead stationery, the date usually begins a double line space below the lowest line of the letterhead. The letterhead usually takes up about 2 inches, but this depends on the style and design of the letterhead. Window envelopes require the date line to be placed on a line 2 inches below the top of the page.

The length of the letter often determines whether the heading should be started lower on the paper; use good judgment. When keyboarding a personal business letter, the individual's return address is placed as the first two lines directly above the date line. The position of the date line can be affected by the length of the letter. When using the computer, you may go to Print Preview to check the appearance of the letter, and necessary changes can be made before printing. General guidelines that relate to letter length are shown in Table 9-1.

INSIDE ADDRESS

The inside address provides all of the information for mailing the letter. The letter address should match the envelope address. When using word processing, the envelope often is addressed from the letter address by a minor key function on the computer. The address information includes the recipient's name, the name of company (if appropriate), street number and name, city, state, and zip code. Three lines of space are left between the date and the first line of the letter address.

TABLE 9-1	Placement of a Date Line	
LETTER LENGTH	SIDE MARGINS	TOP AND BOTTOM MARGINS
Short (less than 100 words)	2 inches	3 inches
Average (101 to 200 words)	1.5 inches	2 inches
Long (201 to 300 words)	1 inch	1 inch

Use titles preceding the individual's name (Mr., Mrs., Ms., or Dr.). Do not use a double title, such as Dr. L. B. Bildice Ph.D.; this is redundant. An official title, such as President, may follow the name, such as Ms. M. P. Coleman, President. The person's official title is often placed on the second line if it helps to balance the inside address lines. The city, state, and zip code are placed on the last line. The appropriate two-letter state abbreviation should be set in capital letters without a period. Leave two spaces after the abbreviation before entering the zip code.

SALUTATION

The *salutation* formally greets the reader. If the writer wishes the letter to be directed to an individual within a firm, it is acceptable to use an attention line. The salutation line should begin one double line space below the letter address and should be even with the left margin. If you are writing to an individual, the most appropriate salutation is the individual's name. For example, if the letter is addressed to Mr. Ted Monroe, the salutation is "Dear Mr. Monroe." The salutation can be altered to "Dear Ted" if you are a close friend of the recipient. This change in formality should be recognized before keyboarding the letter. Special situations occur when the letter is to be sent to unknown individuals or to more than one person. Suggestions for salutations to be used in common situations are shown in Box 9-2, as are addresses and salutations used for governmental and academic officials.

BODY OF THE LETTER

The *body* of the letter contains the message. It begins a double line space after the salutation. The paragraphs within the body are single spaced with double spacing between paragraphs. Paragraphs may or may not be indented, depending on the format selected (see Figs. 9-1 to 9-3 and 9-10). Many illustrations in this chapter demonstrate variations in format styles.

COMPLIMENTARY CLOSE

The *complimentary close* provides a courteous ending to the letter. It is keyboarded a double space after the last line of the body of the letter. The complimentary close is entered at the same point as the date line position if using the modified block style or aligned with the left margin if using the block style. Only the first word of the complimentary close should be capitalized. The most common complimentary closes are "Very truly yours" and "Sincerely." Other acceptable closures are "Yours very truly" and "Sincerely yours."

KEYBOARDED SIGNATURE

The *keyboarded signature* appears four line spaces below the complimentary close. If the name and title of the individual are short, they may be placed on the same line and separated by a comma. If the name and title are relatively long, the name is keyboarded on the first line, and the title is placed on the second line. The comma is not placed after the name. You should attempt to make the lines as even as possible.

REFERENCE INITIALS

If someone else has typed the letter for you, *reference initials* are the initials of the person who keyboards the letter. They should appear in lowercase one double line space after the keyboarded signature, even with the left margin.

ATTENTION LINE

You may wish to direct a letter to a particular individual or department within an organization. This can be done by using an attention line. The following example illustrates how an attention line is used if the letter has been addressed to a firm:

Apex Massage Supplies
Attention Ms. W. W. Thomas, President
1616 W. Riverfront Street
Any Town, Any State 00000-0000

The *attention line* indicates that the letter writer prefers that the letter be directed to a particular individual. The salutation should agree with the inside address, not the attention line.

SUBJECT LINE

The *subject line* clearly states what the letter is about. For example, if writing to a client regarding the office policy on broken appointments, the subject line is written as follows—Subject: Missed Appointments. The subject line is entered a double line space after the salutation and is followed by a double line space before continuing with the body of the letter. The subject line may be centered, begun at paragraph point, or aligned with the left margin when using block style. The style of letter often determines the best position for the subject line. The word subject or abbreviation RE may be entered in all capital letters or in capitals and lowercase, or it may be underlined. Acceptable methods using the subject line are illustrated as follows:

Dear Mrs. Calloway:
SUBJECT: Missed Appointments
or

BOX 9-2	Salutations

APPROPRIATE SALUTATIONS FOR VARIOUS SITUATIONS

One person, sex unknown: Dear M.R. Rieger
One person, name unknown, title known: Dear Director of Surgical Technology
One woman, title unknown: Dear Ms. Hartwig
Two or more women, titles known: Dear Ms. Martin, Mrs. Leverett, and Ms. Grey
If all women are married: Dear Mrs. Franks, Mrs. Johnson, and Mrs. Sullens, or Dear Mesdames Franks, Johnson, and Sullens
If all women are unmarried: Dear Miss Franks, Miss Johnson, and Miss Sullens, or Dear Misses Franks, Johnson, and Sullens
If all recipients are women: Dear Ms. Franks, Johnson, and Sullens, or Dear Mses. or Mss. Franks, Johnson, and Sullens
A woman and a man: Dear Ms. Johnson and Mr. Ladley
A group or organization composed entirely of women: Ladies or Mesdames
A group or organization composed entirely of men: Gentlemen
A group composed of women and men: Ladies and Gentlemen

ADDRESSES AND SALUTATIONS FOR GOVERNMENT AND ACADEMIC OFFICIALS

The following addresses and salutations are recommended in correspondence with governmental or academic officials. In each case, the proper ways to address letters are illustrated. On the left are addresses, and on the right are salutations. When additional examples are given, they are arranged in order of decreasing formality.

Correspondence with Government Officials

The President

The President	Sir, Madam
The White House	Mr. (Mrs. or Ms.) President
Washington, DC 20500	Dear Mr. (Mrs. or Ms.) President

or
The President of the United States
The White House
Washington, DC 20500

Chief Justice of the Supreme Court

| The Chief Justice of the United States | Sir, Madam |
| Washington, DC 20543 | Mr. or Madam Chief Justice |

or
The Honorable (full name)
United States Supreme Court
Washington, DC 20543

Associate Justice of the Supreme Court

The Honorable (full name)	Sir, Madam
Associate Justice of the Supreme Court	Mr. or Madam Justice
Washington, DC 20543	My dear Justice (surname) Dear Justice (surname)

Cabinet member

The Honorable (full name)	Sir, Madam
Secretary of State	Dear Sir, Madam
Washington, DC 20520	My dear Mr. or Madam Secretary

or
Dear Mr. or Madam Secretary

The Secretary of State
Washington, DC 20520

Senator

The Honorable (full name)	Sir, Madam
The United States Senate	Dear Sir, Madam
Washington, DC 20510	My dear Mr. or Madam Senator

or

| My dear Senator (surname) | Senator (full name) |
| | Dear Senator (surname) |

The United States Senate
Washington, DC 20510

Representative

The Honorable (full name)	Sir, Madam
The House of Representatives	Dear Sir, Madam
Washington, DC 20515	My dear Representative (surname)

or
Dear Representative (surname)
Representative (full name)
The House of Representatives
Washington, DC 20515

Chief, Director, or Commissioner of a Government Bureau

Mr., Ms., Mrs., or Miss (full name)	Sir, Madam
Director of Public Information	Dear Sir, Madam
Department of Justice	My dear Mr., Ms., Mrs., or Miss (surname)
Washington, DC 20530	Dear Mr., Ms., Mrs., or Miss

or
Director of Public Information
Department of Justice
Washington, DC 20530

Governor

The Honorable (full name)	Sir, Madam
Governor of Ohio	Dear Sir, Madam
Columbus, OH 43215	My dear Governor (surname)

or

| Dear Governor (surname) | The Governor of Ohio |
| | Dear Governor |

Columbus, OH 43215

State Senator

The Honorable (full name)	Sir, Madam
The State Senate	Dear Sir, Madam
Columbus, OH 43215	My dear Senator

or
My dear Senator (surname)

Senator (full name)	Dear Senator (surname)
The State Senate	My dear Mr., Ms., Mrs., or Miss (surname)
Columbus, OH 43215	Dear Mr., Ms., Mrs., or Miss

State Representative

The Honorable (full name)	Sir, Madam
House of Representatives	Dear Sir, Madam
Columbus, OH 43215	My dear Representative (surname)

or

BOX 9-2	Salutations—cont'd

Dear Representative (surname)		**Dean of a college**	
Representative (full name)	My dear Mr., Ms., Mrs., or Miss (surname)	Dean (full name)	My dear Sir, Madam
		College of Business Administration	Dear Sir, Madam
House of Representatives	Dear Mr., Ms., Mrs., or Miss	University of Cincinnati	My dear Dean (surname)
Columbus, OH 43215	(surname)	Cincinnati, OH 45221	Dear Dean (surname)
Mayor of a city		*or*	
The Honorable (full name)	Sir, Madam	Dr. (full name)	
Mayor of the City of Ann Arbor	My dear Sir or Madam	Dean of the College of Business Administration	
City Hall	Dear Sir or Madam	University of Cincinnati	
Ann Arbor, MI 48105	Dear Mr. or Madam Mayor	Cincinnati, OH 45221	
	My dear Mayor (surname)	(If the individual has a doctorate degree, the salutation may be	
	Dear Mayor (surname)	Dear Dr. Wilson instead of Dear Dean Wilson.)	
Correspondence with Educators		**Professor (college or university)**	
President (college or university)		(full name), Ph.D.	My dear Sir, Madam
Dr. (full name)	My dear Sir, Madam	Dr. (full name)	Dear Sir, Madam
or		Vanderbilt University	My dear Professor (surname)
Dear Sir, Madam		Nashville, TN 37203	Dear Dr. (surname)
(full name), Ph.D.	My dear President (surname)		Dear Mrs. Mr. Ms., or Miss (surname)
President	Dear President (surname)		
Ohio University			
Athens, OH 45701			

Dear Mrs. Calloway:
RE: Missed APPOINTMENTS
or
Dear Mrs. Calloway:
RE: Missed Appointments

ENCLOSURES

Papers, pictures, or other materials sometimes are enclosed with the letter. When the letter mentions that an item is enclosed or attached, an enclosure notation should be made. This notation is keyboarded a double line space below the reference initials or in that area if reference initials are not used, even with the left margin. Two acceptable methods are as follows:

Enclosure
or
Enclosures 2

COPY NOTATION

When additional copies of the letter are made for distribution to various persons, reference to each recipient is commonly made in the copy notation. This informs the recipient to whom copies were sent. Several types of notations are possible, including mail, copy, blind copy, postscript, and second-page headings.

Special Mailing Notations

Notations such as REGISTERED MAIL, SPECIAL DELIVERY, or CERTIFIED are keyboarded in all capital letters between the date and inside address, and they are aligned with the left margin. Other special notations, such as CONFIDENTIAL or PERSONAL, are entered in the same location.

Types of Copy Notations

With the use of word processing software, copies of correspondence are stored electronically; however, paper copies of all business correspondence should be available in the office. When additional copies are made for distribution, it is necessary for the addressee to know this. A notation is keyboarded a double line space below the enclosure, if used, or below the reference initials if there is no enclosure. When more than one person is to receive a copy, list each person on a succeeding line, indenting three spaces from the left margin. Because not all copies are photocopies or computer copies, variations may be used as they apply to the various copy styles. The notation may be keyboarded as follows:

Copy to O.J. Fox
or
c O.J. Fox (copy)
or
cc O.J. Fox (courtesy copy)
or
cc O.J. Fox (courtesy copies to multiple parties)
R.C. Campbell
M.A. Reynolds

Blind Copy

If the person who receives the original letter does not need to know that a copy is being sent to a particular person, a blind copy notation can be made. To do this, the original copy is removed from the computer or machine, and the

Very truly yours,

Jana Larke, MT, NCTMB

ah

PS. Thank you so much for suggesting a lighting dimmer for the massage room. The dimmer lets me adjust the lighting as needed and also provide a relaxing ambiance for our clients.

FIGURE 9-9. Example of a postscript.

notation is keyboarded on the copy 1 inch from the top at the left margin, as in the following example:

bc Barbara Rice

Postscript

A postscript is often used to highlight a particular point. It is not necessarily an item that has been omitted in the body of the letter. If a postscript is used, it is the last line entered. It is not necessary to precede the postscript with P.S.; however, the postscript paragraph should be blocked or indented, depending on the style of letter used (Fig. 9-9).

Second-Page Heading

When writing a client referral letter, it is sometimes necessary to send a lengthy letter to provide adequate information about the client. If a second page is necessary, the continuation is made on plain paper that is the same size, color, and quality as the letterhead. Leave a 1-inch bottom margin on the first page. Include at least two lines of a paragraph at the bottom of the first page, and continue with at least two lines of the same paragraph on the succeeding page. A heading consisting of the addressee, page number, and date is single spaced, 1 inch (line six) from the top of the sheet. The following are two acceptable arrangements for beginning the second page. Block form is used when the letter is in block style:

Ms. Margaret Thompson
Page 2
October 27, 0000

Horizontal form is used when the letter is in modified block style:

Ms. Margaret Thompson 2 October 27, 0000
(triple space)

Punctuation Styles In Business Letters

Two common styles of punctuation are used in business letters: open punctuation and mixed or standard punctuation. *Open punctuation* omits all punctuation (except periods after abbreviations) in the salutation and complimentary close lines. *Mixed* or *standard punctuation* requires a colon after the salutation and a comma after the complimentary close. Either style of punctuation may be used with any of the basic letter styles.

If you use titles and academic degrees in writing, the traditional rule is to never omit the period after the element of an academic degree or religious order and never include internal spaces: B.S., Ph.D., or Ed.D. This rule may need to be altered, however, in contemporary use when addressing envelopes or completing specialized federal, state, or insurance forms that limit space for computerization or scanning. Addressing envelopes is discussed in greater detail later in this chapter.

Correct punctuation is based on certain accepted rules and principles rather than on the whim of the writer. Punctuation enables the reader to correctly interpret the writer's thoughts. The summary of rules given in this chapter will be helpful in using correct punctuation. The common use of periods, commas, colons, and other types of punctuation is illustrated in Boxes 9-3 to 9-13.

CAPITALIZATION

In addition to understanding the rules for punctuation, it is necessary to review the rules for capitalizing various initials and words. A summary of the rules for capitalization is convenient for reference purposes and is listed in Box 9-14.

TELEPHONE NUMBERS

There are several ways of entering telephone numbers in a letter. The parentheses method—(734) 956-9800—is frequently used, but it does not work well in text material when the telephone number as a whole has to be enclosed in parentheses. Parentheses are also avoided because of the growing use of the mandatory area code where there is a shortage of numbers. In these areas, the use of the parentheses with the telephone number may suggest you would not need to use the area code. Three other methods of entering telephone numbers are 707-555-3998, 707 555 3998, and 707.555.3998. The latter system, which uses periods to separate the elements, seems to be gaining popularity. The periods resemble the dots in e-mail addresses.

BOX 9-3	The Period

1. The period indicates a full stop and is used at the end of a complete declarative or imperative sentence.
2. It is also used after an abbreviation and after a single or double initial that represents a word (does not apply to addressing envelopes).

    acct.   etc.   Ph.D.

    U.S.   viz.   p.m.

    N.E.   i.e.   pp.
3. Some abbreviations that are made up of several initial letters do not require periods.

    FDIC (Federal Deposit Insurance Corporation)

    AMA (American Massage Association)

    AAA (American Automobile Association)

    YWCA (Young Women's Christian Association)
4. Insert a period between dollars and cents (period and cipher are not required when an amount in even dollars is expressed in numerals).

    $42.65 $1.47 $25
5. Insert a period to indicate a decimal.

    3.5 bushels   12.65%   6.25 feet

BOX 9-4	The Comma

The comma indicates a partial stop and is used in the following instances:

1. To separate coordinate clauses that are connected by conjunctions, such as *and, but, or, for, neither,* or *nor,* unless the clauses are short and closely connected:

    We have a supply on hand, but I think we should order an additional quantity.

    She had to work late, because the auditors were examining the books.
2. To set off a subordinate clause that precedes the main clause:

    Assuming that there will be no changes, I suggest that you proceed with your instructions.
3. After an introductory phrase containing a verb form:

    To finish his work, he remained at the office after hours.

    After planning the program, she proceeded to put it into effect.
4. Introductory phrases are set off by commas to make sentences easier to read and to avoid confusion:

    After much deliberation the plan was revoked. Because of the vacation period we have been extremely busy.
5. To set off a nonrestrictive clause:

    Our group, which had never lost a debate, won the grand prize.
6. To set off a nonrestrictive phrase:

    The beacon, rising proudly toward the sky, guided the pilots safely home.
7. To separate from the rest of the sentence a word or a group of words that breaks the continuity of a sentence:

    The business manager, even though his work was completed, was always willing to help others.
8. To separate parenthetical expressions from the rest of the sentence.

    We have, as you know, two persons who can handle the reorganization.
9. To set off names used in direct address or to set off explanatory phrases or clauses:

    I think you, Mr. Bennett, will agree with the statement.

    Ms. Linda Tom, our vice-president, will be in your city soon.
10. To separate from the rest of the sentence expressions that may be interpreted incorrectly without punctuation:

    Misleading: Ever since we have filed our reports monthly.

    Better: Ever since, we have filed our reports monthly.
11. To separate words or groups of words when they are used in a series of three or more:

    Most executives agree that dependability, trustworthiness, ambition, and judgment are required of their office workers.

    I emphasize that factory organization, correlation of sales and production, and good office organization are all necessary for maximum results.
12. To set off short quotations from the rest of the sentence:

    He said, "I shall be there."

    "The committees have agreed," he said, "to work together on the project."
13. To separate the name of a city from the name of a state:

    Our southern branch is located in Atlanta, Georgia.
14. To separate abbreviations of titles from the name:

    William R. Warner, Jr.

    Ramona Sanchez, Ph.D.

BOX 9-5 | The Semicolon

The semicolon is used in the following instances:
1. Between independent groups or clauses that are long or that contain parts that are separated by commas:
   He was outstanding in his knowledge of word processing, databases, spreadsheets, and related software applications; however, he was lacking in many desirable personal qualities.
2. Between the members of a compound sentence when the conjunction is omitted:
   Many executives would rather dictate to a machine than to a secretary; the machine will not talk back.
3. In a series of well-defined units when special emphasis is desired:
   Emphatic: The prudent secretary considers the future; he or she ensures that all requirements are obtained, and he or she uses his or her talents to attain the desired goal successfully.
   Less emphatic: The prudent secretary considers the future, ensures that all requirements are obtained, and uses his or her talents to attain the desired goal successfully.

BOX 9-6 | The Colon

The colon is used in the following instances:
1. After the salutation in a business letter, except when open punctuation is used:
   Ladies and Gentlemen:
   Dear Ms. Carroll:
2. After introductory expressions, such as *the following*, *as follows*, and other expressions that precede enumerations:
   Please send the following by parcel post:
   Officers were elected as follows: president, vice-president, and secretary-treasurer.
3. To separate hours and minutes when indicating time:
   2:10 PM   4:45 PM   12:15 AM
4. To introduce a long quotation:
   The agreement read: "We the undersigned hereby agree …"
5. To separate two independent groups having no connecting words between them and in which the second group explains or expands the statement in the first group:
   We selected the machine for one reason: in competitive tests, it surpassed all other machines.
   There are several reasons for changing the routine of handling mail: to reduce postage, to conserve time, and to place responsibility.

BOX 9-7 | The Question Mark

The question mark (interrogation point) is used in the following instances:
1. After each direct question:
   When do you expect to arrive in Philadelphia?
2. An exception to the foregoing rule is a sentence that is phrased in the form of a question as a matter of courtesy, although it is a request:
   Will you please send us an up-to-date statement of our account.
3. After each question in a series of questions within one sentence:
   What is your opinion of the IBM word processor? The Xerox? The CPT?

BOX 9-8 | The Exclamation Point

The exclamation point is used ordinarily after words or groups of words that express a command, a strong feeling, an emotion, or an exclamation:
Don't waste office supplies!
It can't be done!
Stop!

BOX 9-9   The Dash

The dash is used in the following instances:
1. To indicate an omission of letters or figures:
   Dear Mr.—   Date the letter July 16, 20—
2. Sometimes a dash is used in letters, especially sales letters, to cause a definite stop in reading the letter. The dash typically is used in such cases for increased emphasis, but be careful not to overuse the dash:
   This book is not a revision of an old book—it is a brand new book.
3. To separate parenthetical-type expressions when unusual emphasis is desired on the parenthetical expression:
   These sales arguments—and every one of them is important—should result in getting the order.

BOX 9-10   The Apostrophe

The apostrophe should be used in the following instances:
1. To indicate possession:
   the client's record
   the massage therapist's coat
   the assistants' responsibilities
   the massage therapists' records.
2. To form the possessive singular, add 's to the noun:
   man's work
   bird's wing
   hostess's plans
3. An exception to this rule is made when the word following the possessive begins with an s sound:
   for goodness' sake
   for conscience' sake
4. To form the possessive of a plural noun ending in an s or z sound, add only the apostrophe to the plural noun:
   workers' rights
   hostesses' duties
5. If the plural noun does not end in an s or z sound, add 's to the plural noun:
   women's clothes
   alumni's donations

6. Proper names that end in an s sound form the possessive singular by adding 's:
   Williams's house
   Fox's automobile
7. Proper names ending in s form the possessive plural by adding the apostrophe only:
   The Walters' property faces the Jones' swimming pool.
8. To indicate the omission of a letter or letters in a contraction.
   it's (it is)
   you're (you are)
   we'll (we shall)
9. To indicate the plurals of letters, figures, words, and abbreviations.
   Don't forget to dot your i's and cross your t's.
   I can add easily by 2's and 4's, but I have difficulty with 6's and 8's.
   More direct letters can be written by using shorter sentences and by omitting and's and but's.
   Two of the speakers were Ph.D.'s.

BOX 9-11   Quotation Marks

The following rules should be followed when using quotation marks:
1. When a quotation mark is used with a comma or a period, the comma or period should be placed inside the quotation mark:
   She said, "I plan to complete my program in college before seeking a position."
2. When a quotation mark is used with a semicolon or a colon, the semicolon or colon should be placed outside the quotation mark.
   The treasurer said, "I plan to go by train"; others in the group stated that they would go by plane.
3. When more than one paragraph of quoted material is used, quotation marks should appear at the beginning of each paragraph and at the end of the last paragraph.
   "_____
   _____.
   "_____
   _____."

Quotation marks are used in the following instances:
1. Before and after direct quotations:
   The author states, "Too frequent use of certain words weakens the appeal."
2. To indicate a quotation within a quotation, use single quotation marks:
   The author states, "Too frequent use of 'very' and 'most' weakens the appeal."
3. To indicate the title of a published article.
   Have you read the article, "Automation in the Office?"
   He asked, "Have you read 'Automation in the Office'?"

BOX 9-12 | Omission Marks or Ellipses

Ellipses marks (… or ***) are frequently used to denote the omission of letters or words in quoted material. If the material omitted ends in a period, four omission marks are used (….). If the material omitted is elsewhere in the quoted material, three omission marks are used (…).

He quoted the proverb, "A soft answer turneth away wrath: but … ."

She quoted Plato, "Nothing is more unworthy of a wise man … than to have allowed more time for trifling and useless things than they deserved."

From Fulton PJ: General Office Procedures for Colleges, ed 11, Cincinnati, OH, South-Western, 1998.

BOX 9-13 | Parentheses

Although parentheses are frequently used as a catch-all in writing, they are correctly used in the following instances:

1. When amounts expressed in words are followed by figures:.
   He agreed to pay twenty-five dollars ($25) as soon as possible.
2. Around words that are used as parenthetical expressions:
   Our letter costs (excluding paper and postage) are much too high for this type of business.
3. To indicate technical references:
   Sodium chloride (NaCl) is the chemical name for common table salt.
4. When enumerations are included in narrative form.
   The reasons for his resignation were three: (1) advanced age, (2) failing health, and (3) a desire to travel.

BOX 9-14 | Rules for Capitalization

Apply capitalization in the following instances:

1. The first word of every sentence should be capitalized.
2. The first word of a complete direct quotation should be capitalized.
3. The first word of a salutation and all nouns used in the salutation should be capitalized.
4. The first word in a complimentary close should be capitalized.
5. Capitalize the first word in each section of an outline form.
6. Capitalize the first word after a colon only when the colon introduces a complete passage or sentence having independent meaning.
   In conclusion I wish to say: "The survey shows that …"
7. If the material following a colon depends on the preceding clause, the first word after the colon is not capitalized:
   I present the following three reasons for changing: the volume of business does not justify the expense; we are short of people; and the product is decreasing in popularity.

NAMES

1. Capitalize the names of associations, buildings, churches, hotels, streets, organizations, and clubs:
   The American Massage Association, Merchandise Mart, Central District Massage Society, Peabody Hotel, Seventh Avenue, Administrative Management Society, Chicago Chamber of Commerce
2. Capitalize all proper names:
   Great Britain, John G. Hammitt, Mexico
3. Capitalize names that are derived from proper names:
   American, Chinese
4. Do not capitalize words that are derived from proper nouns and that have developed a special meaning:
   pasteurized milk, china dishes
5. Capitalize special names for regions and localities:
   North Central states, the Far East, the East Side, the Hoosier State
6. Do not capitalize adjectives derived from such names or localities that are used as directional parts of states and countries:
   far eastern lands, the southern United States, southern Illinois
7. Capitalize names of government boards, agencies, bureaus, departments, and commissions:
   Civil Service Commission, Social Security Board, Bureau of Navigation
8. Capitalize names of the deity (deities), the Bible, holy days, and religious denominations:
   God, Easter, Yom Kippur, Genesis, Church of Christ

BOX 9-14	Rules for Capitalization—cont'd

9. Capitalize the names of holidays:
   Memorial Day, Labor Day
10. Capitalize words used before numbers and numerals, with the exception of the common word, such as page, line, and verse:
    The reservation is Lower 6, Car 27.
    He found the material in Part 3 of Chapter X.

TITLES USED IN BUSINESS AND PROFESSIONS

1. Any title that signifies rank, honor, and respect, and that immediately precedes an individual's name should be capitalized:
   She asked President Harry G. Sanders to preside.
   He was attended by Dr. Howard Richards.
2. Academic degrees should be capitalized when they precede or follow an individual name:
   Constance R. Collins, Ph.D., was invited to direct the program.
   Fred R. Bowling, Master of Arts
3. Capitalize titles of high-ranking government officers when the title is used in place of the proper name in referring to a specific person:
   Our Senator invited us to visit him in Washington.
   The President will return to Washington soon.
4. Capitalize military titles signifying rank:
   Captain Meyers, Lieutenant White, Lieutenant Commander Murphy

PREPARING AN EFFECTIVE LETTER

To prepare an effective letter, it is necessary to follow several basic steps:

1. Collect the information
2. Make an outline
3. Develop the letter
4. Select a format style
5. Review and revise the letter
6. Produce the letter
7. Proofread the letter
8. Distribute the letter
9. Store the document

Before beginning each step of letter writing, it is necessary to determine who will receive the letter and what the person knows about the subject you are writing. If a letter is to be written to another massage therapist or to a physician about a client, it will require using technical language. If a client is to receive a letter about an unknown subject, the educational level of the person needs to be determined so the letter can be written in understandable language.

Collecting Information

Before you begin to write the letter, you need to gather the important facts to be included in the letter. You should gather the following information: to whom the letter is being sent, by whom the letter is being written, and the subject of the letter. If it is a letter of referral, you will need the name of the client and any necessary personal information for which consent has been given, the nature of the problem or reason for referral, enclosures (if any), anticipated response, deadline dates, and how the client will make contact. If it is a letter of inquiry, the nature of the inquiry, product names if available, quantity or specifications of the product or service, and date of needed reply are required.

Making an Outline

You may wonder why it is necessary to make an outline. After writing several letters, you may find that it is natural for you to be organized. If you are a beginner or someone who dislikes letter writing, making an outline can provide organization and a framework that forces you to get your thoughts on paper, and in the process, you may discover that you do not have all the facts you need. An outline helps you to see relationships between topics and determine if your letter is written in a logical sequence.

Developing the Letter

It is often said that after the outline is completed, you are nearly finished with the letter. This is partially true, but you do need to give special attention to how each part of the letter is developed and determine its format. A variety of format styles are illustrated in this chapter.

As you begin to develop the letter, remember that the first paragraph is the most important paragraph of any letter. It should get the reader's attention and set the tone for the letter. This paragraph places the emphasis on the reader and uses the second person approach. Review each paragraph in the letter to determine if it gets the reader's attention and clearly states the purpose of the letter. Make a natural transition from one paragraph to the next. Special consideration should be given to factors such as data and confidentiality that are included in various types of letters. Box 9-15 includes suggestions for writing several types of letters.

BOX 9-15 | Special Considerations for Letter Content

ORDER LETTER
- Indicate quantity.
- Provide a description of the material or product.
- List the price.
- Define the method of payment.
- Indicate your shipping preference.

REFERRAL LETTER
- Provide the complete and proper name of the client.
- State the condition and expected type of consultation or examination.
- Refer to enclosures.
- Indicate timeliness if necessary.
- Maintain confidentiality and provide only information for which consent is given.
- Extend courteous expression of appreciation.

INQUIRY LETTER
- State the objective.
- Give all the necessary facts.
- Close with good will.

THANK YOU LETTER
- State the purpose.
- Explain your appreciation.
- Maintain confidentiality.
- Close with a sincere expression of good will.

Selecting the Format

You may select a template from the word processing software in the office, but the letter still requires decisions about punctuation styles. Most word processing software provides several templates for a variety of letter styles, which can be modified to meet the massage therapist's preference and saved in the letter file as a specialized template. The block style with mixed punctuation is shown in Figure 9-10. Other styles include the block style with open punctuation, modified block style with mixed punctuation, block style with attention line and enclosure, and the Administrative Management Society (AMS) simplified style. The AMS simplified style can be put to good use when informing all clients about a policy change or announcing that an associate will be joining the practice. The style has two basic rules.

1. The letter must have a subject line. The word *subject* is omitted, and the subject line is keyboarded in all capital letters with a triple line space before and after the subject line.
2. The writer's name and title are keyboarded in all capital letters at least four lines below the last line of the letter.

Reviewing the Letter

After the letter has been written, you need to determine if the letter meets all of the criteria of an effective letter, as described in Box 9-15. If the letter does not meet most of

these criteria, take time to modify it. If you are unsure about a letter, ask another person to review and evaluate it. Make the necessary changes until all criteria are met.

Producing the Final Letter

Before the final printing of the letter, use spell-check and grammar-check functions, if available. Whether the letter is created on a typewriter or electronically using word processing software, the letter needs to be produced on quality stationery that creates a professional image of the office.

Proofreading the Letter

You cannot rely completely on an electronic system to proofread your letter. Although software packages provide spell-check programs, many massage terms are not in the dictionary, unless you have inserted them. Likewise, English words are often misused, such as *there* and *their*. Both of these words are read by the computer as correct, but you might have misused them. Not all word processing systems can be relied on for complete grammar accuracy. Make a final review of the letter to be certain the grammar, spelling, and punctuation are correct. Proofreading a letter is much like the final check of the margins on an amalgam restoration. It is your creation, and you want it to be perfect. Reading the letter out loud is a good strategy. The letter should sound smooth and be easy to read.

Distributing the Letter

There are several methods of distributing the letter: E-mail, traditional postal services, fax, or some form of specialized mail service. Each of these is explained in detail later in this chapter. Before creating the letter, you should be aware of the method of distribution to determine the type of envelope or mailing label necessary for production.

Storing the Document

If the letter is to be stored electronically, the procedure discussed in Chapter 8 should be followed. If not, a hard copy should be made and filed in the client record or other location that is appropriate for the document. If you are striving for the paperless office, you need to maximize the use of the electronic filing system.

Preparing the Envelope

It is possible to prepare the envelope as part of the word processing procedure, or the envelope may be keyboarded on a typewriter. Larger mailing envelopes may require special labeling. In either case, it is necessary to prepare the envelope or package with a standardized delivery address. Most postal services use automatic sorting equipment, which begins an

Leisure Massage/Luke Fritz, MT, NCTMB
222 Relaxation Drive, Your Town, State 00000
(123) 456-7890 leisuremassage@massage.com

September 15, 20__

Gerald L. Jones, D.O.
555 Main Street
Lapeer, MI 48446

Dear Dr. Jones:

I appreciated your assistance with my client on September 14th. The time you spent with my client discussing her breathing disorder was very generous, and our practice thanks you!

If you ever find a need for my assistance, please don't hesitate to contact me. I look forward to working with you in the future.

Sincerely,

Luke Fritz, MT, NCTMB

ah

FIGURE 9-10. Block-style letter with mixed punctuation.

automatic sorting process with an optical character reader (OCR). A standardized address, readable by an OCR, contains the correct city name, state, and zip code. To obtain zip codes for any address, visit the U.S. Postal Service Web site at www.usps.com, and select the zip code navigation bar. The address on the envelope should agree with the inside address of the letter, although the inside address may contain punctuation not recommended by the postal service for the envelope.

The address is should be single spaced, even if the address is only two lines. In this case, the name of the individual or firm is on the first line, and the city, state, and zip code are on the second line. The two-letter state abbreviations, approved and recommended by the U.S. Postal Service, should be used. These abbreviations appear in Box 9-16. For further information, request Publication 28, Postal Addressing Standards, from your local Postal Business Center or by calling the National Address Information Center in Memphis, Tennessee, at 800-238-3150. Figure 9-11 shows how an address should be keyboarded on various business envelopes.

Other important elements of the address are suffixes, directional designations, apartment or suite numbers, post office box numbers, and complete rural or highway contract route addresses with box numbers. All of these elements must be spelled correctly and clearly written. If the address is not electronically readable, the letter or package will be delayed for manual handling.

ADDRESS FORMAT

Using the universal format for addresses expedites the processing capability of automated equipment at the post office. The format requires that you use a uniform left margin. Type the address in uppercase letters as follows:

MS MARY BALL
3347 MAPLE RD
ANY TOWN, MI 00000-0000

A secondary address unit, such as an apartment (APT) or suite (STE) number, should be printed as part of the address. Always use APT or STE rather than the pound sign (#).

BOX 9-16	Two-Letter Abbreviations for States		
Alabama	AL	Montana	MT
Alaska	AK	Nebraska	NE
Arizona	AZ	Nevada	NV
Arkansas	AR	New Hampshire	NH
California	CA	New Jersey	NJ
Colorado	CO	New Mexico	NM
Connecticut	CT	New York	NY
Delaware	DE	North Carolina	NC
District of Columbia	DC	North Dakota	ND
Florida	FL	Ohio	OH
Georgia	GA	Oklahoma	OK
Hawaii	HI	Oregon	OR
Idaho	ID	Pennsylvania	PA
Illinois	IL	Rhode Island	RI
Indiana	IN	South Carolina	SC
Iowa	IA	South Dakota	SD
Kansas	KS	Tennessee	TN
Kentucky	KY	Texas	TX
Louisiana	LA	Utah	UT
Maine	ME	Vermont	VT
Maryland	MD	Virginia	VA
Massachusetts	MA	Washington	WA
Michigan	MI	West Virginia	WV
Minnesota	MN	Wisconsin	WI
Mississippi	MS	Wyoming	WY
Missouri	MO		

Common designations are APT, BLDG FLOOR (FL), STE, UNIT, ROOM (RM), and DEPARTMENT (DEPT). Using this format, the address line may appear as follows:

1334 RIVERSIDE APT 201
or
3745 KINSEY DR STE 301
or
845 KELSAY BLVD BLDG 5
or
1234 KELLOGG PL RM 136

If your letter or package is sent to the attention of an individual, that information precedes the line of the name of the firm or building. The attention line varies from the traditional format that many people have used:

ATTN: MS MARY CLINE
ACME MASSAGE COMPANY
134 FLETCHER
ANYTOWN, OH 00000-0000

Avoid using dual addresses, even though you may have a box number and street address available. Place the delivery address on the line immediately above the city, state, and zip code (ZIP4).

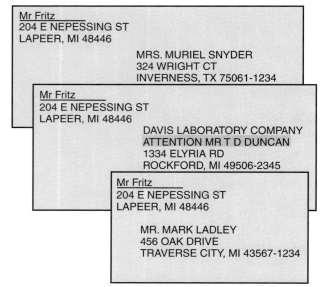

FIGURE 9-11. Address styles for different sizes of envelopes. Notice placement of the attention line.

PUNCTUATION ON ADDRESS LABELS

The U.S. Postal Service prefers that you do not use punctuation, special characters, or multiple blanks in the address, with the exception of a hyphen in the ZIP4 code or a hyphen that appears in the primary number of the delivery address, such as 51-234 HANCOCK ST. Spell out city names completely. If an abbreviation must be used because of labeling or space constraints, use existing abbreviations first for suffix or directional words, as in these examples:

EAST MARKET becomes E MARKET
JEFFERSON MOUNTAIN becomes JEFFERSON MT

The eight standard directional designations can be abbreviated by one or two characters, as in the following example:

255 NW WASHINGTON ST
or
133 CHERRY DR S

If the first word in a street name is a directional word and no other directional designation is to the left of it, abbreviate it, as in these examples:

NORTH CHERRY ST becomes N CHERRY ST
or

LAKE DRIVE WEST becomes LAKE DRIVE W

When two directional words appear before the street name, the first one is abbreviated:

NORTH EAST SUGAR ST becomes N EAST SUGAR ST

Folding and Inserting the Letter

After all enclosures have been checked to be certain they correspond to the letter and that the items are correct, the letters must be signed, and you must be sure that the right letter gets in the right envelope (letters get in the wrong envelopes surprisingly often). The letter is placed in the envelope so that the date and inside address are visible on opening the letter. The reader should not be forced to turn the paper around to begin reading the letter. Figure 9-12 shows a step-by-step procedure for folding and inserting the letter in the proper size of envelope.

ELECTRONIC MAIL

Use of E-mail

With the wide use of computers today, *electronic mail* (e-mail) has opened the doors to sending mail between computers within networked locations. E-mail within a large clinic has

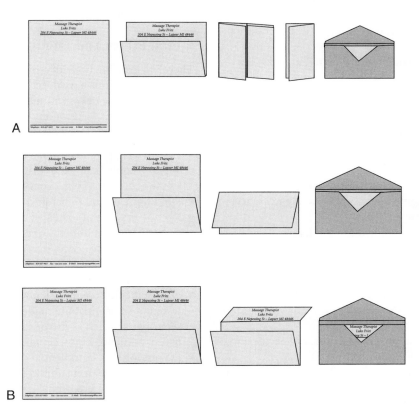

FIGURE 9-12. Folding and inserting a letter. **A,** Small envelope. **B,** Large envelope. *(Modified from Finkbeiner BL, Finkbeiner CA: Practice Management for the Dental Team, ed 6, St. Louis, 2006, Mosby.)*

become the choice for sending memoranda to the staff. With more clients having e-mail, this becomes another source of communication between the staff and clients. Consideration should be given to include this on the personal questionnaire on admission. The client's e-mail can be integrated into various software programs and may even be used to confirm appointments or act as a reminder for routine recalls. E-mail has many advantages as a communication tool:

- E-mail reaches its destination in a matter of seconds after it is sent, even if its destination is across the world.
- Multiple individuals may be sent the same message, with all the recipients receiving the message instantly.
- Paper is saved. It is not necessary to make a hard copy of e-mail.
- E-mail may be filed electronically for later reference.
- E-mail may be forwarded to another party.
- E-mail may be destroyed immediately after it is read.
- E-mail takes less time to write than a paper letter. Only the receiver's name, the sender's name, and the body of the letter need to be entered. The date and time is entered automatically, and the letter or envelope does not need to be printed.
- Other documents and graphic images may be transferred as attachments through e-mail.
- The recipient is notified of the arrival of an e-mail by a message that appears at the bottom of the computer screen or by an audio signal that is emitted through the computer.
- A hard copy of the e-mail may be printed if necessary for retention in a manual file.
- Notations such as "confidential" and "urgent" can be made on the e-mail message.

As with any new system, a person often overlooks the need to follow basic protocol. E-mail should not become a quick system for communication with no concern given to punctuation or formatting. Consider the following guidelines when using e-mail:

- Be certain you have thought about the purpose of the e-mail before you begin writing; know what you are trying to achieve with your e-mail message.
- Be succinct. Before you send your e-mail, reread it. Delete unnecessary phrases, words, or sentences.
- Be polite. Think of your e-mail as a short letter, and follow etiquette rules. Use *please* and *thank you*.
- Be suitably formal when writing e-mail. The rule of thumb is to be almost as formal in e-mail as you are in a standard letter.
- Always capitalize the appropriate words, be specific about needs, and use a proper closing.
- Use the subject line that is provided on the e-mail form. This line should be concise but convey the purpose of the message to the reader.
- If you are replying to a message but are changing the subject of conversation, change the subject line also.

- Edit and proofread carefully. Do not send an e-mail that contains inaccuracies or incorrect grammar.
- Use complete sentences and paragraph structure.
- Capitalize and punctuate properly.
- Do not run sentences together; it is difficult to read e-mail constructed in this manner.
- Insert the nature of the message on the subject line.
- Include a salutation.
- Use a colon after the salutation. A comma can be used in a nonbusiness application.
- Check the letter for spelling and grammatical errors.
- Insert a blank line after each paragraph.
- Always include your name and title (if appropriate) when replying to an e-mail.
- Assume that any message you send is permanent. The message can be sitting in someone's private file or in a tape archive.

SELF-REFLECTION

How are my writing skills? What is my experience writing letters? What do I remember from English classes in high school? What was the content that I thought I would never use but now need? How could writing skills have been taught to me when in high school that would have made the information more useful then? Where can I get additional help in writing skills?

E-mail Ethics and Etiquette

There is a growing body of ethical issues in regard to e-mail. Some organizations have developed a code of ethics for using e-mail. This form of communication should follow the same ethical guidelines used for any form of written communication in the massage practice:

- Do not send personal e-mail from your office computer.
- When people send you inappropriate e-mail, let them know politely that you cannot receive it.
- Do not use e-mail to berate or reprimand anyone.
- Do not use e-mail to send information that involves any type of legal action; third parties who should have no knowledge of the action may obtain the information.
- Do not forward junk mail or chain letters.
- Do not forward an e-mail unless you know it is true.
- Do not include credit card numbers or any other information that can contribute to identity theft or that presents a security risk, such as driver's license, social security number, or bank account number.
- Do not forward confidential client information.
- Do not criticize or insult third parties.
- Avoid using different types of fonts, colors, clip art, and other graphics in e-mail. It clutters the message and may be difficult for the reader to view.
- Do not keyboard your message in all uppercase.

- Avoid sending messages when you are angry.
- Observe the Golden Rule in cyberspace; treat others as you would like to be treated.
- Act responsibly when sending e-mail or posting messages to a discussion group.
- Use a style and tone that are appropriate to the intended recipient.
- Before you reply to an e-mail, ask yourself if you really need to reply.
- Answer your e-mail promptly.

The contents of the letter can be retained as a permanent record. Anything you do not want written documentation of should not be entered. Confidentiality must be maintained, and rules of courtesy should be followed. An appropriate closing should be included.

OTHER TYPES OF WRITTEN COMMUNICATION

Other types of written communication routinely used include post cards, interoffice memoranda, and manuscripts. For many of these documents, there are templates available

that aid in formatting and eliminate the steps of setting up the document.

Post Cards

There will be times when it is more practical to send a client a post card than to write a letter. Post cards can be used to announce specials events such as a self-massage class being offered as a promotion for new clients. Figure 9-13 illustrates how a postal card should be addressed and the placement for the message.

Interoffice Memoranda

Although most office correspondence is keyboarded on office letterhead, the *interoffice memorandum* is a time-saving form and is entered on plain paper (Fig. 9-14). This type of communication is often used within a clinic or group practice or within a professional building where several professional offices are located. The form provides space for the name of the department or individual to whom the memorandum is being sent, the date, subject or reference line, and space for the sender's name. The memorandum should be brief, clearly stated, well organized, and

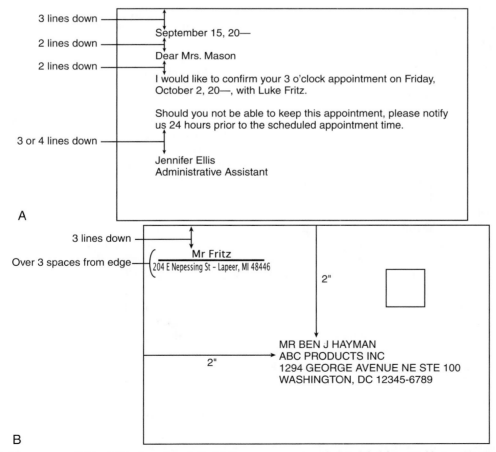

FIGURE 9-13. **A,** Message on a 5.5 by 3.5 inch post card. **B,** Addresses on a post card. (*Modified from Finkbeiner BL, Finkbeiner CA: Practice Management for the Dental Team, ed 6, St. Louis, 2006, Mosby.*)

INTEROFFICE MEMORANDUM

TO: Amy Husted

FROM: Luke Fritz

SUBJECT: Reassignment to business manager position

DATE: October 19, 20--

For some time I have been thinking that we should promote you to the position of office manager. After our discussion last Friday, I would like to confirm this reassignment. Both my father and I feel that you have considerable expertise in client management and have excelled in the recent courses in small business management in which you have been enrolled. Both of us would like to discuss this transition with you.

Let's meet on Friday, October 25, at 2 P.M. to discuss this matter. If this date is inconvenient for you, please let me know.

FIGURE 9-14. Interoffice memorandum.

easy to read. A copy of the memorandum should be made for the office files. If several people are to receive the memorandum, their names are inserted in the space provided, or additional copies are made and the individual names entered on each memorandum.

MANUSCRIPTS

In the first part of this chapter, emphasis was placed on general correspondence. In academic and health environments, you may be asked to write a report or research paper. The massage community is emphasizing the creation of case reports by massage therapists. These reports are being collected and completed to identify trends that indicate the need for further research. The foundation also has an open-access journal in which the case reports may be posted for others to read (Box 9-17). Whether you are writing a business report or an academic report, you should follow standard style when preparing it.

Many styles exist for manuscript preparation, depending on the nature of the report. Each style requires the same basic information. For example, one style may use the term *bibliography*, whereas another uses *references*, and a third prefers *works cited*. Although a publisher may provide the author with a format for a manuscript, a popular documentation style used for research papers is provided by the Modern Language Association (MLA). When preparing a paper, you must adhere to some form of documentation style. Therefore, if none is given, it is wise to select the MLA style, which includes the following:

- Use 8.5 by 11 inch paper.
- Double-space all pages of the paper with 1-inch top, bottom, left, and right margins.
- Indent the first word of each paragraph one-half inch from the left margin.
- At the right margin of each page, place a page number one-half inch from the top margin and 1 inch from the right margin. Double space between the header and the body. Only use Arabic numbers; do not use pp, p, or the # sign.
- On each page, precede the page number with the author's last name.
- When a quotation contains less than six lines, set it off with quotation marks, and keep it within the normal text, followed by the reference. When a quotation contains six or more lines, set it off by indenting it 1 inch from the right and left margins. Check MLA sources for other requirements regarding longer quotes, special circumstances, and quotations within quotations.
- Each figure and table needs to be labeled and numbered. Place the words *figure* or *table* (and the number) a double space before the figure or table. Other materials, such as charts, photographs, and drawings, also need to be labeled and numbered, and they should include a caption.
- No title page is required. Instead, on the first page, place only the author's name on the first line, and double space each successive line, followed by the instructor's name, the course name and number, and the date. This should be in a block at the left margin beginning 1 inch from the top of the page.
- Center the title four line spaces below the date and other related information (e.g., course number). The title's first,

---

BOX 9-17 | The Massage Therapy Foundation

The Massage Therapy Foundation (http://www.massagetherapyfoundation.org/) advances the knowledge and practice of massage therapy by supporting scientific research, education, and community service.

JOURNAL

The Massage Therapy Foundation publishes the electronic journal, *International Journal of Therapeutic Massage & Bodywork: Research, Education, & Practice* (IJTMB). The IJTMB is a peer-reviewed scientific journal for the therapeutic massage and bodywork profession, and it is available free of charge.

The IJTMB takes an open-access approach to scholarly publishing, allowing the reader to access articles online. This approach enables dissemination of scientific findings to a vast number of professionals in the massage and bodywork field.

The IJTMB is published quarterly, and the first edition was launched in the summer of 2008. Three principal sections are planned for the IJTMB:

Research: Quantitative, qualitative, and integrative research papers are published in this section.

Education: This section provides a forum for massage and bodywork educators on topics such as curriculum development, instructional design, and testing.

Clinical Practice: This section represents a venue for practitioners to stay up-to-date on issues such as planning, marketing, managing, and evaluating a successful practice.

MASSAGE THERAPY FOUNDATION PRACTITIONER CASE REPORT CONTEST

The Massage Therapy Foundation is delighted to invite you to participate in our Practitioner Case Report Contest. The Foundation has chosen to encourage the writing of case reports to provide an opportunity for massage therapists and bodyworkers to develop research skills and enhance their ability to provide knowledge-based massage to the public. The Foundation is a philanthropic, nonprofit 501(c)(3) organization that grants money for scientific research and community service projects, and it is a resource for research education to the massage and bodywork professions at large. (See the Foundation's mission and goals in Appendix A.)

Case Report Goals and Guidelines

Case reports play an important role in the professional literature. This contest is intended to enhance professional development skills of the practitioner: writing case reports help develop communication skills, critical thinking skills, and could contribute to future research and clinical practice. Cash and publication recognition will be awarded to practitioners submitting the top reports. (See the awards in Appendix H.)

Continuing Education credit is available through the National Certification Board of Therapeutic Massage and Bodywork (NCBTMB) for submitted reports that follow all guidelines. (See Appendix G for more information.)

Case Report Structure

Practitioners must report on an independent clinical intervention(s) on one client. This includes doing a literature review on the presenting condition; creating and implementing a treatment plan in accordance with the literature, the needs of the client, and the practitioner's expertise; writing up the results; discussing the implications of the outcomes; and offering suggestions for future study.

For complete details, including the referenced appendices, visit the Web site (http://www.massagetherapyfoundation.org/practitionercontest.html).

Modified from http://www.massagetherapyfoundation.org.

---

last, and principal words should be capitalized. Do not underline, italicize, or use all capitals in the title. Do not end with a period. A question or exclamation mark may be used if appropriate.

Place reference citations in the body of the paper in parentheses with the page numbers where the referenced information is located. These parenthetical citations are used instead of footnoting each source at the bottom of the page. Footnotes are used only for explanatory notes. In the body of the paper, use superscripts (raised numbers) to signal that an explanatory note exists. Explanatory notes are optional. If used, the note is placed at the bottom of the page as a footnote or at the end of the paper as an endnote.

MLA style uses the term *works cited* for bibliographic references. These are placed on a separate numbered page. Center the title (Works Cited) 1 inch from the top margin. List references in alphabetical order by each author's last name. Double space all lines. Works cited from books, journals, magazines, newspapers, letters, online sites, and compact disks have their own MLA reference style that should be followed.

MANAGING BUSINESS MAIL

With the increase in written communications, demands for efficient processing and distribution of incoming and outgoing mail need to be addressed.

Processing Outgoing Mail

Outgoing correspondence may be prepared earlier in the day, but it is often organized for mailing at the end of the day as part of the daily routine.

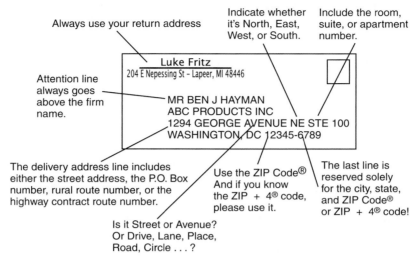

FIGURE 9-15. Guidelines recommended by the U.S. Postal Service for addressing mail correctly. *(Modified from Finkbeiner BL, Finkbeiner CA: Practice Management for the Dental Team, ed 6. St. Louis, 2006, Mosby.)*

CLASSIFICATION OF MAIL

Some of the outgoing mail is sent as first-class mail, some as fourth class, some insured, and some special handling using the address guidelines in Figure 9-15. You need be aware of these classes of mail and be able to select the best classification for the type of item being mailed:

- First-class mail consists of letters, government or private postcards, business reply mail, bills, and statements of accounts.
- Second-class mail includes newspapers and published periodicals.
- Third-class mail includes items such as books, circulars, catalogs, or miscellaneous printed material weighing less than 16 ounces.
- Fourth-class mail, often called parcel post, is used for printed material and packages weighing more than 16 ounces. The rate of postage varies, depending on distance. The United States is divided into zones, and parcel post rates are figured accordingly.

Although mail is classified in one of these four classifications, additional special services may be used. If sent first class, valuable or important items can be registered to provide protection and evidence that the article has been received. A special fee is charged for this service, and a receipt is furnished by the post office. The post office accepts the responsibility if the mail is lost and will pay the sender the insured amount. The fee for registered mail varies according to the declared value.

Special delivery service is available for all classes of mail. The post office delivers special delivery mail as quickly as it reaches the post office of destination. Rates are determined by weight and destination.

Certified mail is available for first-class mail. The sender is provided a receipt, and proof of delivery of the letter is recorded at the post office. No insurance coverage is available on certified mail.

Insured mail service applies to third- and fourth-class mail; articles may be insured up to a value of $200 against damage, theft, or total loss. The fee for insured mail is determined by the amount of the insurance on the package contents.

Special handling service is available only for third- and fourth-class mail. If the mail is marked "special handling," it receives the fastest handling of third- and fourth-class mail, but it is not delivered by special messenger.

Express mail service is provided by the U.S. Postal Service, and delivery occurs within 24 hours. Express mail service is available 7 days per week, 365 days per year (weekend and holiday deliveries are no additional charge) for items that weigh up to 70 pounds and are 108 inches in combined length and girth.

Other questions that arise regarding outgoing mail can be answered by checking with the U.S. Postal Service. Manuals are available from the Superintendent of Documents, Government Printing Office, Washington, DC 20402\MDomestic Mail Manual, 19 and International Mail Manual, 14.

A postage scale is used to determine the weight of outgoing mail and is an asset in the massage business office. Mail sent with insufficient postage may be returned to the sender, causing a delay in service. A postage meter can be a time-saving device. Although various sizes of postage meters are available, a desk model is practical for a private practice. The meters are purchased outright, but the meter mechanism is leased. A meter license is obtained from the U.S. Postal Service. With new electronic models, meter resetting

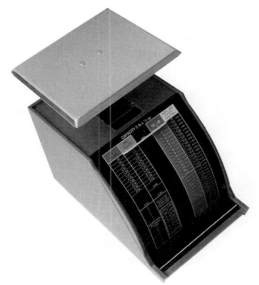

FIGURE 9-16. Postage meter. *(From Finkbeiner BL, Finkbeiner CA: Practice Management for the Dental Team, ed 6, St. Louis, 2006, Mosby.)*

is done by means of a telephone call. An active account with the Postage-By-Phone System and the appropriate meter are needed. No special telephone hookups, computers, or software are required. The customer signs up for the system and then places funds into an account to draw on as postage is ordered. Monthly reports listing the account activities are sent to the customer. In keeping with this new technology, postage scales are available that weigh and automatically determine correct postage rates (Fig. 9-16). The accuracy of electronic scales helps to eliminate overpayment in postage. The meter can also be set for the amount of postage required for packages. The amount is printed on a tape, which is then affixed to the package.

Outgoing mail that is addressed correctly, has the proper amount of postage, and is pre-postmarked goes through the post office faster and will arrive at its destination sooner.

FACSIMILE

Another electronic means of communication is the facsimile (fax) machine. A fax machine is a scanning device that transmits an image of a document over standard telephone lines. It is described in detail in Chapter 10. The massage therapist may find this method of transmitting written communication very effective when it is necessary to have an immediate response. Transmission requires a transmission cover sheet, and transmitted information must be maintained confidentially.

MAILING AND DELIVERY SERVICES

Mailing services are service enterprises that specialize in mail communications. A mailing service is an independent postal service that is a complete business center that processes metered and bulk mail, first-class mail, and air freight.

Shipping providers, such as United Parcel Service (UPS), FedEx, Greyhound Package Express, Purolator Courier, and many others, are gaining popularity with businesses that wish letters or packages delivered the next day. When selecting a provider, it is important to consider the cost, speed of delivery, and convenience. Most shipping providers require the completion of a special form. The following list provides information about delivery services:

- Rates are determined by weight, distance within specified zones, and required time of delivery.
- Maximum weight varies with the carrier.
- Some packages may be insured against loss or damage.
- Packages to be shipped can be picked up at the place of business. Deliveries are made to the exact address indicated on the parcel (Fig. 9-17).
- Deliveries are not made to post office boxes.
- Attempts are made for delivery at no additional charge, except for U.S. Express Freight Services.
- The sender is not charged for return of an undeliverable package.
- Shipping providers are available in most areas.

Processing Incoming Mail

The location of the massage practice may determine whether the mail is delivered to the office by a regular postal mail carrier or a post office box is rented and the mail is picked up at the post office.

When the mail is first sorted, you will need to distinguish between the various types of mail received:

- First-class mail, including priority mail, personal mail, special delivery, registered or certified mail, payments, invoices, and general correspondence
- Printed matter, such as announcements of professional meetings, solicitations for contributions, collegiate newsletters, and other semiprofessional materials
- Magazines and newspapers for the reception room, as well as professional journals and periodicals
- Advertisements
- Samples of massage products
- Supplies ordered from a massage supply company

After the initial sorting, the personal mail receives prompt attention. When payments are received, attach the returned portion of the statement, or note on the envelope the amount of money received. Enclosures should be clipped to the letter, invoice, or statement, and all incoming correspondence should be stamped with the date and time received Fig 9-18.

When discarding the envelopes of incoming mail, be sure the entire contents have been removed and all important

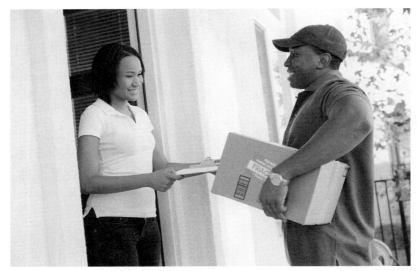

FIGURE 9-17. Package delivery to a place of business. *([2008] © Stephen Coburn. Image from BigStockPhoto.com.)*

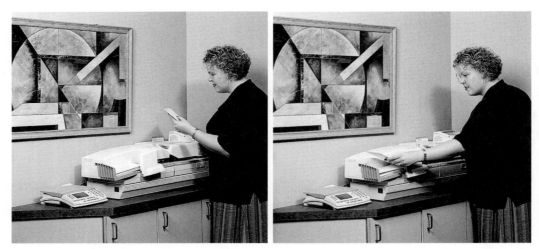

FIGURE 9-18. Automatic time-stamp machine. *(From Young AP:* Kinn's The Administrative Medical Assistant, *ed 5, St. Louis, WB Saunders, 2003.)*

data, such as company name, individual name, postmark date, and time (if significant), have been recorded. You may even need to retain the envelope in some situations. The magazines for the office should be distributed to the reception room and the older issues removed and recycled.

Businesses receive many advertisements, and many of them are regarded as junk mail. If the advertisements are of no value, throw them away.

When massage supplies are received in the office through the mail, they need to be processed as soon as possible. This

Luke Fritz

204 E Nepessing St – Lapeer MI 48446

INTEROFFICE

ROUTING SLIP

Please read the attached _____
and record the date passed on to the persons indicated.

Refer to:	Date Received	Date Passed on
Stephen Austin	_____	_____
Hilda Baker	_____	_____
Blair Downing	_____	_____
Debbie Green	_____	_____
John Mann	_____	_____
Stephanie Powers	_____	_____
Routed by:	_____

FIGURE 9-19. Mail routing slip. ⊜ This letter template is posted on Evolve at http://evolve.elsevier.com/Fritz/business.

Good Stuff from the Government

UNITED STATES POSTAL SERVICE TOOLS
All of the following items can be found at http://www.usps.com.
- Shipping products and services: Send domestic and international packages.
- Print online postage: Print postage and labels online using USPS Click-N-Ship or an authorized provider.
- Supplies: Boxes, scales, labels, and more.
- Mailing products and services: Domestic and international mailing choices.
- Create your own cards: Create unique greeting cards, gift cards, postcards, and more.
- Create direct mail: Learn more about direct mail or create direct mailings online.
- Change of address: Get your mail after you move. Change it online.
- PO box service: Get your mail when and where you want it.
- Hold mail: Have your mail held while you are away.
- Mail service updates: Check updates in your area.
- Missing children: USPS helps find America's missing kids.

procedure is detailed in the inventory chapter (see Chapter 12). Open any samples received in the mail. Most of these samples accompany literature that should remain with the product. If it is not something you intend to use throw it away.

SUMMARY

Different forms of written communication are used within a massage practice. You may have to write a letter to a client regarding payment schedules or to the insurance company. You may use email to confirm client appointments or send a thank you to a client for a referral, and the SOAP notes need to be written correctly and coherently.

For certain types of writing, you will want to use stationary with your name or company name at the top, also be known as letterhead. This paper is usually a heavier quality paper than you would use for everyday copying. Whatever the reason for writing, you need to use correct grammar, punctuation, style, and capitalization. The word processing programs are almost foolproof, so use them.

Be sure to chuck the junk. Your business space needs to be clutter free. Junk mail and old magazines can become clutter and lead to disorganization. Recycle the old magazines, open and discard the junk mail, and take care of the current mail.

Bibliography

Capital Community College Humanities Department: *A guide for writing research papers based on modern language association (MLA) documentation*, Hartford, CT, 2004, Capital Community College, Available at http://www.ccc.commnet.edu/mla/index.shtml (accessed June 2009).

Federal Express Corporation: *FedEx Service Guide*, Memphis, 2004, Federal Express.

Fulton PJ: *General Office Procedures for Colleges*, ed 12, Cincinnati, 2003, South-Western.

Gibaldi J: *MLA Handbook for Writers of Research Papers,* ed 6 (for high school and undergraduate students), New York, 2003, Modern Language Association of America.

Gibaldi J: *MLA Style Manual and Guide to Scholarly Publishing,* ed 2 (for graduate students, scholars, and professional writers), New York, 1998, Modern Language Association of America.

Locker KO: *Business and Administrative Communication,* ed 6, New York, 2003, McGraw-Hill/Irwin.

Modern Language Association: Format, Bibliography, Style Conventions. Available at http://www.mla.org (accessed June 2009).

Netiquette tips: Keying in, *Newslett Natl Business Educ Assoc* 11:2, 2000.

Sabin WA: *The Gregg Reference Manual*, ed 10, New York, 2004, McGraw-Hill/Irwin.

U.S. Postal Service: *The Postal Manual*, Washington, DC, U.S, 2004, Government Printing Office.

Evolve Annotated Web Links

http://evolve.elsevier.com/Fritz/business

Capital Community College, Guide for Writing Research Papers Based on MLA Documentation: http://www.ccc.commnet.edu/mla/index.shtml

Massage Therapy Foundation: www.massagetherapyfoundation.org

Modern Language Association (MLA): www.mla.org, http://www.mla.org/style

U.S. Postal Service: www.usps.com

Workbook

1. List and explain the characteristics of an effective letter.

   _____
   _____
   _____
   _____
   _____

2. Explain the benefits a newsletter may have for a massage practice.

   _____
   _____
   _____
   _____
   _____

3. Outline the acceptable format for addressing envelopes.

   _____
   _____
   _____
   _____
   _____

4. Outline the procedures for sorting incoming mail.

   _____
   _____
   _____
   _____
   _____

5. List and define the four classifications of mail.

_____
_____
_____
_____

6. Discuss the special mail services that can be used by a massage office.

_____
_____
_____
_____

7. Explain the functions of a postage meter.

_____
_____
_____
_____

8. List the advantages of using a commercial delivery service.

_____
_____
_____
_____

9. Explain a situation that can be handled through a fax process.

_____
_____
_____
_____

10. On the computer, create and store in a file a letterhead for Joseph W. Lake, Massage Therapist, and Ashley M. Lake, Massage Therapist. Use the letterhead data found in this chapter for the massage therapists. If desired, add clip art as appropriate.

11. Using the letterhead created in #10 (Font: Times New Roman), keyboard the following letters.

Keyboard the following letter in block style with mixed punctuation. Use the current date, and address a small envelope. Fold the letter to insert into a small envelope. Make a copy for the office files, or store it electronically:

Mrs. Jason Calloway, 2453 Prescott Avenue, Grandville, MI 49302. Dear Mrs. Calloway (P) We have written to Doctor Jack Notman as you requested. He is most interested in your case and will be expecting you to contact his office very soon. (P) When we first corresponded with Doctor Notman, we mailed him a complete set of your client records as requested. We also indicated to him at that time that you are a diabetic. (P) I suggest you contact his office. If we can be of further assistance, do not hesitate to call us. Sincerely Joseph W. Lake, Massage Therapist (reference initials)

Keyboard the following letter in modified block style with open punctuation. Use the current date, and address a large envelope. Fold the letter to insert into a large envelope. Make a copy for the office files, or store it electronically:

Reliance massage tables, 1600 Michigan Avenue, NE, Grand Rapids, MI 49502. Gentlemen (Subject line: massage table defect) (P) I am returning the massage table we ordered for our client, Mr. H. B. Rider. Mr. Rider was impressed with the massage table used in our office and asked if we would be able to order a table for him to have at home. The table arrived at our offices with a crack in the front left table leg. We will be returning the table for replacement and would expect that your company pay for all shipping and handling. We appreciate your cooperation in this matter. Sincerely, Joseph W. Lake, Massage Therapist (reference initials)

Keyboard the following letter in block style with mixed punctuation. Use the current date and an appropriate-size envelope. Make a copy for the office files, or store it electronically:

Mr. Robert Clay, 6690 Jefferson SW, Wyoming, MI 49507. Dear Mr. Clay (P) I know you have been pleased with the work our office has done for you and your wife. We have enjoyed having both of you as clients. (P) We feel sure you have misplaced the last two statements that we have sent to you, but we would appreciate it if you would stop by the office so we can make an arrangement to bring your account up to date. (P) Thank you for your cooperation in this matter. Sincerely, Ashley Lake, Massage therapist.

12. Develop a newsletter to be sent by e-mail to your client list that is announcing new research on the use of massage for pain management. A newsletter can be a valuable marketing tool, but it is not a sales pitch. Instead, it provides information essential to your clients. It educates your clients about your company's position and your commitment to servicing their needs. It is better to have a lean newsletter than one full of fluff that shows you do not value your clients' time.

TELECOMMUNICATIONS

KEY TERMS

Call forwarding
Call holding
Caller ID
Cellular technology

Conference call
Facsimile (fax) machine
Pager
Speed dialing

Telecommunications
Time zones
Voicemail

LEARNING OUTCOMES

Mastery of the content in this chapter will enable the reader to:

- Define key terms
- Define telecommunications
- Explain the application of telecommunications in a massage office
- Describe various types of telecommunication systems commonly used in a massage office
- Practice efficient telephone techniques

- Receive, transmit, and record telephone messages
- Plan and place outgoing telephone calls
- Use the features of special telephone equipment and services
- Describe the best way to manage telephone calls commonly encountered in the massage office

The telephone is the most important piece of equipment in the office. It is the most common and most important communication device in the world because it is the fastest and easiest way to transmit messages.

For 90% of the clients in a massage office, the first contact is made by telephone. Like it or not, first impressions are lasting ones, and telephone management is an area that deserves more attention. Effective communication on the phone requires that you have a broad knowledge of therapeutic massage, possess a high degree of self-confidence, are alert, are able to make decisions, and show good verbal communication skills. Speaking with a smile in the voice, being enthusiastic, and having a cordial manner are essential skills that generate the framework for positive communication. Speaking with hostility or disinterest is sure to influence the client negatively and ensures that future communications, if they still exist, with clients will be more difficult (Fig. 10-1). Always remember that this is a service business.

TELECOMMUNICATIONS IN MASSAGE THERAPY

The term *telecommunications* refers to the science and technology of communication by electronic transmission of impulses, as by telegraphy, cable, telephone, radio, or television. In a practical sense, telecommunications in a massage office refers to the different kinds of telephone systems and communication that result from the use of the telephone lines. In this chapter, you will learn about the various types of telephone systems, such as key systems, cellular phones, hands-free telephones, conference calls, answering machines, and pagers. You will also learn how to manage communication using these systems.

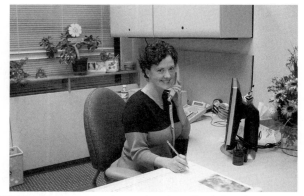

FIGURE 10-1. A voice that makes the caller feel as though a smile is coming through the receiver is a winning voice. *(From Finkbeiner BL, Finkbeiner CA:* Practice Management for the Dental Team, *ed 6, St. Louis, 2006, Mosby.)*

Telephones

With the array of specialized telephone equipment now available, the massage therapist can take advantage of state-of-the-art equipment to become more efficient. For a modest price, massage business owners can buy sophisticated telephone systems that can improve the productivity and profitability of their enterprise. Telephone companies and agencies usually are very accommodating in helping businesses determine their needs for telephone equipment and in making recommendations. Various types of equipment can also be explored at product Web sites using search programs. The equipment and services discussed subsequently can be useful in the massage office.

Integrated business communication systems offer features designed for a small business such as a massage practice. A system such as the one shown in Figure 10-2A automatically redials the last outside number dialed at the touch of a button, easily establishes a three-way conference call with the conference button, and on most system phones, allows you to dial and talk without picking up the handset. It includes basic transfer and hold functions, as well as programming of multiple numbers to allow *speed dialing* of frequently called numbers. Information can be displayed in many languages, which is an important feature in the global community. An expanded version of this system (see Fig. 10-2B) enables you to enlarge the capacity of the model. A massage therapist may feel that only a basic, traditional telephone is required; however, a versatile telephone system with the features described allows more efficient handling of the many telephone calls received daily. This is especially important if you are in a single-person business, which is common for many massage professionals. Communications can be improved from one area of the office or clinic to another through the paging and intercom features. With single-button access, the person to be contacted can be reached quickly. Often, the individual can answer intercom calls without touching the phone or interrupting work.

Plug-in *voicemail* systems are fully integrated messaging systems residing on a plug-in circuit board that is used with the Partner Advanced Communications System. The system provides users in larger massage practices or clinics audio instructions on using personal speed dialing, conferencing, or group paging by dialing into the voicemail. It also offers callers a prompt connection to various departments or areas in a clinic and can record messages in the voicemail. This level of sophistication for telecommunication systems is not typical in the single-person massage practice, but with massage therapists working more often in multidisciplinary heath care systems or large spas, it is important to understand how these systems function. It is common to have to communicate using these complex communication systems.

Personal computer (PC)–linked telecommunications systems let businesses manage incoming and outgoing calls,

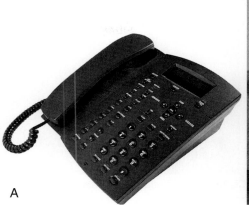
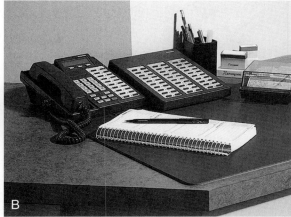

FIGURE 10-2. A, Basic, easy-to-use telephone systems for small businesses include features such as a built-in speakerphone for convenience and the ability to establish three-way conference calls. **B,** A larger model expands the capacity of a phone system. *(From Finkbeiner BL, Finkbeiner CA: Practice Management for the Dental Team, ed 6, St. Louis, 2006, Mosby.)*

organize personal information, and store client information (e.g., telephone numbers) in a database file that can be retrieved for autodialing. It also allows programming of phones from a PC (Fig. 10-3). With this type of computer-telephone integration, incoming calling information can be used to provide an automatic pop-up window on a PC that displays a caller's database file; this allows you to greet the caller by name and have detailed information readily available for answering questions. This system brings the efficiency and productivity of advanced telecommunications technology to small and medium-size businesses.

Cordless telephone systems provide an extended mobility range in the office (Fig. 10-4) and allow you to leave the base station and communicate with other areas without having to use answering machines or voicemail or play telephone tag. Be cautious when using a cordless phone that conversations are not overheard.

A cellular phone, or cell phone, is a portable communication device (Fig. 10-5). When a massage therapist needs to maintain contact with a central location while driving from one place to another, *cellular technology* makes it possible to use a fully functional telephone. This technology breaks down a large service area into smaller areas, called cells. Each cell is served by a low-powered receiver-transmitter. As the mobile caller moves from one cell to another, a switching office automatically moves the call in a corresponding fashion. The mobile telephone switching office communicates with a land-based subscriber to complete mobile calls to fixed locations serviced by telephone lines.

A hands-free telephone allows you to work on the computer, access records, or perform some other task while talking on the telephone. This time-saving device is becoming very popular in clinics and private massage offices. The concept of a hands-free system can be carried into other methods of communication, such as pagers and walkie-talkie types of systems (Fig. 10-6).

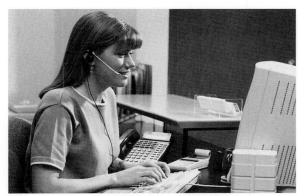

FIGURE 10-3. Telecommunications systems linked to personal computers provide rapid access to client data. *(From Finkbeiner BL, Finkbeiner CA: Practice Management for the Dental Team, ed 6, St. Louis, 2006, Mosby.)*

With these systems, it is never appropriate to take a call while giving a massage. In the rare situation, such as an emergency, when you must take a call, inform the client of the possibility before the massage.

SELECTING A TELEPHONE SYSTEM

Before selecting a system, examine the specifications carefully to determine the cost of the standard features and the cost of each of the optional features. Be sure to consider the cost of operating and maintaining the system.

TELEPHONE FEATURES

Telephones offer a multitude of features, from the very basic to the highly technical. The following paragraphs describe some of the basic features.

The massage therapist may find the hands-free *speakerphone* feature very convenient. With most systems, with a push of a button, the speaker's voice is picked up by a

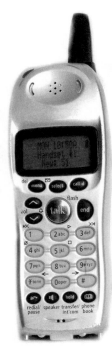

FIGURE 10-4. Cordless phone systems allow extended mobility in the massage office. *(2005 © Cora Purdy. Image from BigStockPhoto.com.)*

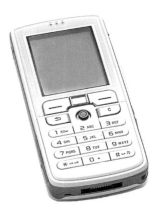

FIGURE 10-5. Cellular phones allow massage therapists and staff members to communicate while outside of the massage office. Some advanced cellular models include additional features such as multimedia access or the ability to capture and send or receive digital images. *(2005 © Cora Purdy. Image from BigStockPhoto.com)*

microphone. Speakerphones are particularly valuable for group meetings.

Voicemail messaging, or phone mail, uses advanced recording and routing functions to combine the features of a telephone, a computer, and a recording device. This feature can be learned quickly and is simple to use. The only equipment needed is a touch-tone telephone.

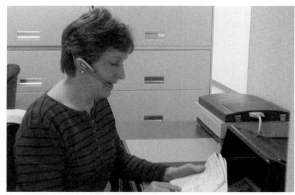

FIGURE 10-6. A hands-free telephone system allows the administrator to perform other tasks while speaking on the telephone. *(From Finkbeiner BL, Finkbeiner CA: Practice Management for the Dental Team, ed 6, St. Louis, 2006, Mosby.)*

Massage office applications include voice-recorded daily updates of appointments available or unavoidable cancelations such as an emergency and directions to the massage office. Alternatives to voicemail include an answering machine or answering service. The stand-alone answering machine differs from voicemail in that it does not have the option of sending messages to various locations. However, callers can leave a message and receive information from the office.

An answering service with operator-answered calls can be used when clients call after office hours, on weekends, or on scheduled days off. The answering service operator informs the caller where the massage therapist can be reached or takes the information from the caller and then notifies the massage therapist. This type of service is seldom used in the massage practice but may be an option if the client base prefers talking to a person rather than electronic equipment. Regardless of whether a voicemail system or a separate automatic answering device is used, some basic courtesies must be observed:

- If an answering machine is used, turn it on before leaving the office.
- In the outgoing message, indicate that the caller has reached an answering system.
- Give clear information about office hours or ways to contact the massage therapist.
- Make sure the caller has adequate time to record a message.
- On returning to the office, check the calls on the voicemail or recorder.
- Take care of any necessary follow-up to the recorded calls. Most systems allow the user to access the answering machine or voice mailbox to receive messages even when off site.
- Update the outgoing messages regularly.
- Avoid nonprofessional messages that are distracting to the caller.

Many features are available on most phone systems:

Text messaging: Text messaging is quickly becoming an important feature for phone applications. It is a quick and efficient way to send and receive information.

Conference calls: If the massage therapist needs to talk to several people in various locations simultaneously, a *conference call* may be placed. The call is arranged through a conference call operator, who is given the names and telephone numbers of the individuals included in the call and the time the call should be made. With special equipment, several people can hear and participate in the call at each location. This feature is becoming invaluable because the ability to schedule face-to-face meetings is costly in terms of time and travel.

Caller ID: The *caller ID* feature can identify a caller before the telephone is answered by displaying the number of the telephone from which the person is calling. You may block your number from appearing by pressing a special key.

Call forwarding: A telephone call can be automatically forwarded to another telephone number with *call forwarding.*

Call holding: The *call holding* feature is frequently used in massage offices, which often receive calls in rapid succession. This feature allows you to answer a second call while the first caller holds on the line. Care should be taken to extend maximum courtesy to the caller asked to hold (Box 10-1).

Music on hold: The music on hold system provides the caller with music or a short narrative about treatment in the massage office while the person is on hold. The system can be personalized to address specific types of treatment in the office and then revert to music periodically. This feature tends to ease the caller's impatience and can offer short educational clips that may market certain aspects of the practice.

Automatic call back: A caller can give instructions to a busy station to call back as soon as the busy station is free.

Automatic call stacking: Calls that arrive at a busy station are automatically answered by a recorded wait message.

Speed dialing: Commonly called numbers can be stored in the telephone's memory, and the call can be made by keying in a one- or two-digit code. Speed dialing cuts down on the time spent dialing frequently called numbers.

Call restriction: Unauthorized long-distance telephone calls can be eliminated with this feature. If an individual is authorized to make a long-distance call, the call is given an authorization code that must be keyed into the telephone before the call can be processed. The telephone may also be programmed not to accept long-distance calls.

Identified ringing: This feature provides distinctive ringing tones for different categories of calls. For example, internal calls may have one long ring, whereas outside calls may have two short rings.

Multiple lines or key telephones: Multiple lines are a standard feature on most telephones in a larger massage business. Special care must be taken when using them to ensure privacy and to avoid interfering with other calls in progress.

If multiple lines are available for receiving or placing calls, one of the lines often is for a number that is not listed in the telephone directory or printed on the business stationery. This line should be used for outgoing calls, leaving the other lines available for incoming calls. A telephone system with multiple lines can be used for inside and outside calls. This can be a very efficient system, but you must remember several key points, which are presented in Box 10-2.

Pagers

A *pager* is a telecommunication device that allows a person to receive accurate messages instantly. The pager can receive numeric messages, including phone numbers and special codes you have devised, or alphanumeric messages. Most pagers, such as the one shown in Figure 10-7, are easy to read, have various alert tones, display the date and time, offer various-size message slots, and retain messages in memory.

Smartphones

A smartphone combines the functions of a cellular phone, a personal digital assistant (PDA), and a handheld computer in a single device (Fig. 10-8). These devises can do so much that they usually are underused because there is so much to learn. They often have a still and video camera, text and e-mail capability, and ability to store documents and music. They are able to enhance the office-on-the-go concept. From the user's point of view, carrying a single device that does everything on the road is much better than having to carry multiple devices and manage their synchronization. The BlackBerry and various smartphone technologies are wireless and allow the user to access mobile communication centers, reply to and forward voicemails, initiate conference calls, and access directories. Users can access e-mail, corporate data, and the Internet. New technology, such as

---

BOX 10-1 | Using Call Holding

■ Excuse yourself from the first caller before answering a second call.
■ Greet the second caller with the standard office greeting.
■ If the second caller requires only a short response, complete the call, and return to the first caller.
■ If the second caller appears to need more extensive assistance, explain that you are on another call, ask the caller if he or she can wait, and place the call on hold. If the caller does not want to wait, ask where the person can be reached and say that you will return the call. Always return the call promptly.
■ In returning to the first caller, always thank the person for waiting before proceeding with the conversation.

BOX 10-2 | Using a Multiple-Line Telephone System

1. Determine which line to answer. It usually is indicated by a ring or buzz, and the button flashes until the line is answered. Depress that line's key before lifting the receiver.

2. If you are placing an outside call, determine which line is available (indicated by an unlighted button). Depress the key for that line, and dial the number. If you accidently select a line that has been placed on hold, depress the hold key again to put the call back on hold.

3. If you place an incoming call on hold, tell the caller that you are doing so. Depress the hold key, which keeps the caller on the line (the hold key then returns to its normal position). The line key remains lighted, which indicates that the line is in use. Other calls then can be placed or received on another line.

4. Before transferring a call, be sure to inform the caller that you are doing so, because the person may not want the call transferred. Give the caller the extension number to which he or she is being transferred in case the call is disconnected. This allows the caller to call the person back directly. To transfer an outside call with the button system, you must first place the call on hold. Then push the button for local, which lights when in use (the local button is for in-office transfers only). Dial or buzz a number in the office telephone system; the telephone is answered on local in another office. Inform the massage therapist of a call on a particular line, and the massage therapist completes the call from that telephone. If you must return to the incoming line, remember which line your caller used. *Hold reminder* is a feature on advanced telephone systems that gives a reminder tone at various intervals to indicate that a caller is still waiting. Depress that button, which opens the line again and allows you to complete the call.

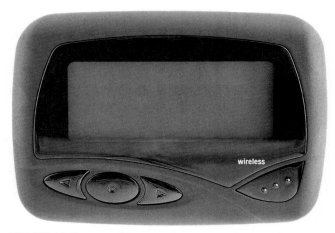

FIGURE 10-7. A portable pager. *(2005 © Carolina Smith. Image from BigStockPhoto.com.)*

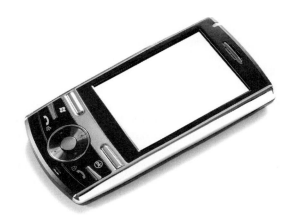

FIGURE 10-8. Smartphone technology is revolutionizing telecommunications. *(2008 © Vitaliy Pakhnyushchyy. Image from BigStockPhoto.com.)*

the smartphone, continues to develop and will revolutionize telecommunications.

Facsimile Communication System

Another electronic means of communication is the *facsimile (fax) machine* (Fig. 10-9). A fax machine is a scanning device that transmits an image of a document over standard telephone lines. The machine operates like a photocopy machine that sends an image by wire. At the receiving end, another fax machine receives the transmitted copy. The message may be a handwritten document (in ballpoint pen), a keyboarded page, or a picture. The cost of transmitting a fax message is the same as a telephone call because the message is transmitted through the telephone lines. Many offices prefer to have a dedicated telephone line for the fax machine rather than using the business telephone number.

A fax machine may be a stand-alone unit or may be incorporated into the office computer. The cost of the fax machine varies greatly, depending on added features.

Calling Card Calls

Many people use calling cards. Calling cards allow calls that the person makes while traveling to be charged to the office. Key 0, the area code, and then the telephone number. When the operator answers and requests your calling card number, key in the number on your card.

Telephone Directories

The telephone directory is a vital tool in the business office. It is important that you look through it and become familiar with the type of information available so that you can use the directory as efficiently as possible. The telephone

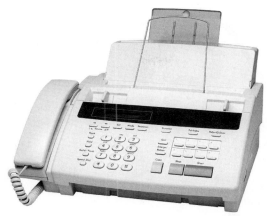

FIGURE 10-9. Facsimile (fax) machine. *(From Finkbeiner BL, Finkbeiner CA:* Practice Management for the Dental Team, *ed 6, St. Louis, 2006, Mosby.)*

directory provides selected area codes for many cities in North America and foreign countries and an illustration of *time zones.* You also may find the following information:

1. A community profile
   Past and present
   Community events
   Things to do and see
   Parks and recreation
   Colleges and universities
   Transportation services
2. Maps
   Overview of the city
   Area maps
   Maps of nearby communities
3. Zip codes
4. Senior citizen information

The front pages of the telephone directory provide important information, such as emergency phone numbers, including the police, fire, ambulance, suicide prevention, and poison control numbers. Page 1 of the front pages has a table of contents. Review this page so that you can quickly find other services listed in the directory.

The white pages of the telephone directory usually are divided into three sections: (1) the residence section, which is an alphabetical listing of the names, addresses, and telephone numbers of individuals; (2) the business white pages, which is an alphabetical listing of the names, addresses, and telephone numbers of businesses; and (3) the blue pages, a section that lists the names, addresses, and telephone numbers of local, state, and federal government offices. An 800 or 888 number allows an individual to call a business toll free. Companies that use this service are listed in the telephone directory with an 800 or 888 number. If you know a company has such a number, but it is not available in the

local directory, the information may be obtained by keying 1-800-555-1212. As with most information services, a fee may be charged for this service.

The yellow pages list the names of particular businesses according to the type of service the business provides. For example, assume you are interested in obtaining laundry service for the office, but you are not familiar with companies in your area that provide this service. The category can be broken down as follows:

Laundries
Laundries—Self-service
Laundry—Equipment—Commercial

The companies specializing in each area are listed alphabetically. Because this section is used as a sales tool, it has additional advertisements and a variety of print styles.

The classic telephone book is giving way to the directory being provided on the Web. In this format, search programs can be used to locate the information.

DEVELOPING EFFECTIVE TELEPHONE ETIQUETTE

Most people take great care to exude a professional business appearance, but few people take as much pride in developing their telephone image. People often forget when using the telephone that the person on the other end of the line is a human being.

You must take time to develop a professional telephone personality. To be effective on the telephone, you must keep a smile in your voice, answer calls promptly, be attentive and discreet, be cordial and responsive, ask questions tactfully, take messages courteously, speak distinctly, place calls properly, avoid sexism, and be considerate to the caller. The techniques for successful telephone contact, which involves a voice-to-voice relationship, are somewhat different from those of successful personal contact, which involves a face-to-face relationship (Fig. 10-10).

Your Speaking Voice

The speaking voice has four separate but interrelated components: loudness, pitch, rate, and quality.

Loudness refers to the volume of your voice. If you speak too loudly, the listener may be uncomfortable. Have you ever talked on the telephone with someone who spoke so loudly you had to hold the receiver away from your ear? If so, you know how unpleasant excessive volume is to the listener. The opposite situation can be equally unpleasant. If you lack confidence, your voice may be so quiet that people will ask you to repeat what you have said. If this happens, you should try to increase your confidence and your volume.

The rate of speaking can determine how well another person understands you. When discussing familiar procedures

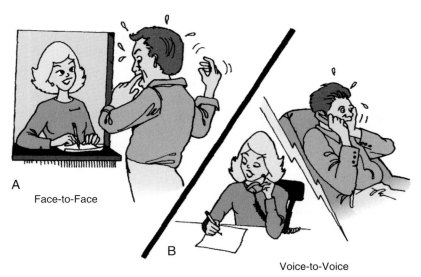

A
Face-to-Face

B
Voice-to-Voice

FIGURE 10-10. A, Face-to-face conversation. Nonverbal cues are apparent; a person smiles or gestures to make a point. Poise, interest, and sincerity provide observable feedback. Facial expressions help to indicate the degree of understanding. Discussion is extemporaneous, and notes typically are not used. **B,** Voice-to-voice conversation. The impression of the person is acquired only through hearing. Interpretation comes only from the tone of voice. The degree of understanding is determined by questioning and by rephrasing statements. Notes are advantageous in this situation. *(Modified from Finkbeiner BL, Finkbeiner CA: Practice Management for the Dental Team, ed 6, St. Louis, 2006, Mosby.)*

with a client, you may tend to speak rapidly, forgetting that this is new material to the client. There is no ideal rate, but a general rule is to speak at a rate that does not detract from the clarity of your message and that is easy and comfortable to listen to for an extended period.

Pitch is the tone of the voice. This is more difficult to change, because after it has been developed, persistent discipline is required to alter it. A low, gravelly voice or a high, squeaky voice may be unpleasant to listen to and is hard on your throat. Many exercises are available from the local telephone company and reference libraries for improving voice pitch.

The quality of your voice is a combination of physical and psychological factors. Changes in each of these alter the effectiveness of your speaking voice. Daily experiences affect this quality, and care should be taken to withhold depression, excitement, and anger from your voice when speaking on the telephone in a business setting.

To achieve a good telephone personality, you should develop the qualities of alertness, expressiveness, interest, naturalness, and distinctness. A client calling the massage office expects to have the call answered promptly. You should answer the phone within the first two rings. This is difficult if you are in a single-person business. This situation can be addressed with effective use of answering systems. Make sure that clients understand that an answering system is used and how often and when you return calls. Schedule enough time between appointments (minimum of 15 minutes) to return calls.

Everyone enjoys being recognized, and you should be attentive to the client's identity and express this in your voice. When a client calling the office identifies himself, you reply, "Yes, Mr. Jones (or first name if appropriate), how may I help you?" Using first names is appropriate for regular clients if a first-name basis has been requested.

When talking on the phone, do not stammer and stutter and say, "Yeah, well, uh, I don't know." Such a response indicates to the client that you are inexperienced. If you do not know the answer to a question or want to investigate more before responding, say, "I will be glad to check" or "Let me gather more information and call you back within the next hour." This type of response indicates you have made a sincere effort to help and lets the client know you are willing to seek an answer if there is a problem. If you promise a client you will call back, do it at the time you promised. Offer to find an answer if you do not know; do not force the client to ask you to seek the information.

Nothing is more boring than listening to a person who speaks in a monotone. Put expression into what you say. Add enthusiasm to your voice by using natural voice inflections. To create a smile in your voice, place a mirror in front of the telephone. This ensures that you put a smile on your face before you answer the telephone. Try it; it works! Act enthusiastically, and you will feel enthusiastic.

Clients calling the massage office have a definite purpose and expect you to be interested in their issues. Give each client your undivided attention. Do not interrupt or become preoccupied with another matter. You can show interest in the client by asking appropriate questions and by not rushing to terminate the conversation.

To be natural, you must be yourself. Do not be a phony. An unnatural voice is easily detected. Keep the breathy "daaarhling," "sweetie," "honey," and "dear" words out of your vocabulary. "Sugar and syrup" have no place in massage business communication, so keep them out of your voice. It is also inappropriate to use slang. Slang is an informal language consisting of words and expressions that are not considered appropriate for formal occasions. Slang is the use of informal words and expressions to describe an object or condition. Slang is vocabulary that is meant to be interpreted quickly but not necessarily literally, because slang words or terms are often a metaphor or an allegory. Slang changes from generation to generation and culture to culture, so it is confusing and often disrespectful.

To speak distinctly, you must pronounce each syllable of the word completely. When using a handheld telephone, speak directly into the transmitter, which should be about 1 inch from your lips. Do not chew gum, bite on a pencil, or cover your mouth with your hand; these actions create mumbled conversation and do not present a good image for the massage office. Some examples of what to say and what not to say include the following:

Avoid	Say
Bye-bye	Good-bye
Huh?	I do not understand.
	Would you please repeat that?
Uh-huh	Yes
	Of course
Yeah	Yes
	Certainly
Okay	I agree
	Yes

SELF-REFLECTION

How do I sound on the phone? When I talk on the phone with someone, what type of voice is most pleasant? What is most irritating? What are my bad phone habits? What are my best phone skills?

Creating a Good Image

In addition to achieving good voice qualities, you must be able to choose the word or phrase that best communicates the message and makes the best impression. In general, to promote better understanding, you should use short, simple, descriptive words that are appropriate to the situation. When using technical massage terms, names, numbers, formulas, or foreign words, the information should be given slowly and distinctly. Suggestions for identifying letters are presented in Box 10-3, and those for identifying numbers are given in Table 10-1.

BOX 10-3 Using Words to Identify Letters

The following words may be used to identify letters for a caller:
A as in Alice
B as in Boy
C as in Charles
D as in Dog
E as in Edward
F as in Frank
G as in George
H as in Hat
I as in Ida
J as in Jack
K as in King
L as in Lion
M as in Mary
N as in Nancy
O as in Old
P as in Peter
Q as in Queen
R as in Robert
S as in Susan
T as in Thomas
U as in Union
V as in Victory
W as in William
X as in X-ray
Y as in Young
Z as in Zero

TABLE 10-1 Pronouncing Numbers Clearly

NUMBER	SOUNDS LIKE	FORMATION OF THE SOUND
0	Zir-o	Well-sounded Z, short I, rolled R, long O
1	Wun	Strong W and N
2	Too	Strong T and OO
3	Th-r-ee	Single roll of the R, long EE
4	Fo-er	Long O, strong R
5	Fi-iv	I changes from long to short; strong V
6	Siks	Strong S and KS
7	Sev-en	Strong S and V, well-sounded EN
8	Ate	Long A, strong T
9	Ni-en	Strong N, well-sounded EN

A variety of words and phrases in the massage office can convey an unfavorable image to the client (Fig. 10-11). These are *red flag phrases*, and replacements are suggested that can create a more positive image (Table 10-2). Each time you speak on the telephone, think about what you are saying. Ask yourself if that is what you intended to say. Put yourself in the client's position to decide whether you are communicating connotations that should be avoided.

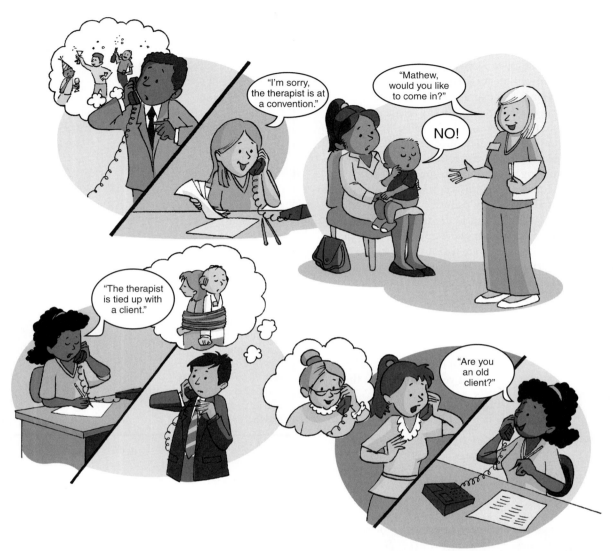

FIGURE 10-11. Red flag words and phrases. *(Modified from Finkbeiner BL, Finkbeiner CA:* Practice Management for the Dental Team, *ed 6, St. Louis, 2006, Mosby.)*

Managing Incoming Calls

Although each call to and from the massage office presents a unique situation, most calls can be placed in specific categories, and certain conditions remain constant in each situation. As a result, you will be able to formulate certain questions and answers for each situation. Care should be exercised not to use these statements in a rote manner, but to incorporate the ideas into your own words and develop a technique that fulfills the philosophy of the massage business.

Examples of typical conversations can illustrate efficient management of the telephone in a massage office. Some suggestions for managing incoming calls are presented in Box 10-4.

Managing Outgoing Calls

As a business professional, you will be placing many outgoing calls. The following tips are helpful for making such calls:

1. Plan ahead. Be sure to have the telephone numbers written correctly. If you are calling a client, list the name with the telephone number; if you are calling another massage therapist's office or business, have that number written or easily accessible. Be sure to consult the telephone directory if you are in doubt about a correct telephone number. Names appear in the telephone directory in alphabetical order; however, some public services or governmental agencies may be listed differently. For

TABLE 10-2 Red Flag Phrases

RED FLAG WORD OR PHRASE	USE INSTEAD
Cancellation	Change in the schedule
Waiting room	Reception room
Thank you for calling (without use of name)	Thank you for calling, Mrs. Main.
Cost	Investment
Remind	Confirm
Hurt, pain	Uncomfortable, discomfort
Old client	Former client
Operatory	Treatment room
Cost, price, charge	Fee
Bill	Account
When would you like to come in?	Do you prefer mornings or afternoons?

BOX 10-4 Telephone Etiquette for Incoming Calls

- Answer promptly.
- Identify yourself and the business.
- Speak distinctly, clearly, and slowly.
- Avoid slang.
- Listen attentively; do not interrupt.
- Do not talk to anyone else while speaking on the phone.
- Speak directly into the transmitter.
- Excuse yourself if you must attend to another call.
- Thank the caller if the person is asked to hold.
- Let the caller hang up first.

---

example, state offices are listed under the state name first and then alphabetically according to office. County and city offices are listed by county or city name first and then alphabetically according to the office. Federal offices are listed under United States Government first and then alphabetically according to the office. Parochial and other private schools are listed alphabetically by the name of the school. Another source for obtaining the correct telephone number for most businesses is the business white pages or yellow pages directory. If you know the name of the business, you can check in the business white pages in alphabetical order. It is becoming common to look up phone numbers using the Internet instead of a paper phone book.

2. If the telephone you are using is a lighted push-button system, make sure the line is free before you place your call (the light signals when the line is in use). As the telephone receiver is lifted, make sure you hear the dial tone before starting to dial (the word *dial* relates to the old rotary phone system).

3. When your call is answered, identify yourself: "Hello, Mr. Jones (or David if appropriate). This is Sandy, your massage therapist."

4. State your reason for calling. If you are changing a client's appointment, have another appointment time available. Indicate why the change is being made, because it may cause a disruption in plans, and the client may also have to adjust another appointment or work schedule. "I am returning your call concerning your request for an earlier appointment."

5. The person who placed the call should also terminate it. It is discourteous to hang up without an indication that the conversation is finished. End the conversation with a courteous "good-bye" and then replace the receiver gently.

6. If you reach a wrong number, apologize for the inconvenience, verify that you dialed the number correctly, and recheck the number before redialing.

Examples of common outgoing calls are given below:

The purpose: Confirmation of a client's appointment for the following day.

The call: When the client answers the telephone, identify yourself, and state the reason for calling: "Hello, Mrs. Thompson, this is Luke, your massage therapist." You may then continue with your message, stating it briefly and completely: "I would like to confirm (not *remind*) your appointment for tomorrow at 1:30 PM." When the client acknowledges it affirmatively, you may say, "We look forward to seeing you tomorrow at 1:30," and then conclude the call by saying, "Good-bye." Wait for the client to hang up.

Sometimes, clients state, "I won't be able to keep the appointment tomorrow, and I'll call you later for another one." Although this may be a legitimate statement and the client does plan to call you at a later date, you should pursue the conversation, because it may be a signal that there has been a lack of communication with the client. Instead of abruptly concluding the conversation, ask the client, "Would it be possible to reschedule your appointment for a week from today?" If the client continues to be noncommittal, say, "I don't understand." Is there a reason for not wanting to make an appointment now?" This usually brings the client to the point of explanation. "My daughter gave me the gift certificate for Mother's Day, and I really do not want a massage." What you do next depends on your policies and procedures, which were described in Chapter 2.

When placing a long-distance call to different time zones, the time difference must be kept in mind. The United States is divided into four time zones: Eastern, Central, Mountain, and Pacific (Fig. 10-12). For example, if it is 2 PM in Grand Rapids, Michigan (Eastern time zone), it is 1 PM in St. Louis, Missouri (Central time zone), 12 PM in Denver (Mountain time zone), and 11 AM in Los Angeles (Pacific time zone). Make sure you know what time it is where you are calling to avoid disturbing someone at an inconvenient time. If you reach an incorrect number when dialing long distance,

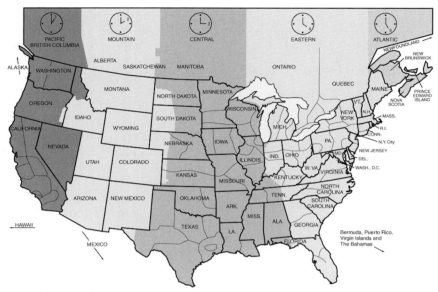

FIGURE 10-12. Time zones in the United States. *(From Young AP:* Kinn's The Administrative Medical You, *ed 5, St. Louis, 2003, WB Saunders.)*

obtain the name of the city, the state, and the number you have reached, and immediately notify the operator of the error so that no charge will be made for the call.

Taking Telephone Messages

Be prepared for incoming calls by keeping a pencil and message pad handy. Obtaining the correct information on messages is of utmost importance. Repeat the message, spelling of names, and the telephone number if a return call is necessary. Take sufficient time to obtain the correct information for the message. Be sure to date the message, indicate the time it was taken. *Do not trust your memory. Write things down.* The message should always be signed by the person taking it in case questions arise later about the information. Forms similar to the one shown in Figure 10-13 may be ordered from most stationery suppliers.

LEARNING ACTIVITY

Pair with someone, and practice taking a message by writing it down. Switch roles. Then place all the messages in a bag, and each person should pull out a message and read it. Discuss how accurate each message is and how it can be improved.

Personal Telephone Calls

The telephone in the massage office is installed as a service to the massage clients and should be maintained as a business telephone. Staff members should refrain from using the telephone for personal calls, and only emergency calls should be made.

Good Stuff from the Government

THE INSTITUTE FOR TELECOMMUNICATION SCIENCES IS THE FUTURE OF TELECOMMUNICATIONS

The telecommunications and information technology planning function represents the highest-level system or network perspective of the Institute for Telecommunication Sciences (ITS) This work includes planning and analyzing existing, new, and proposed telecommunications and information technology systems, especially networks, to improve efficiency and enhance performance and reliability. ITS performs this work for wired and wireless applications. This encompasses work frequently referred to in industry as *systems engineering*. All phases of strategic and tactical planning are conducted in this area, as well as problem solving and implementation engineering. ITS engineers identify users' functional requirements and translate them into technical specifications. Telecommunication system designs, network services, and access technologies are analyzed, as well as information technologies, including Internet and Internet-related schemes.

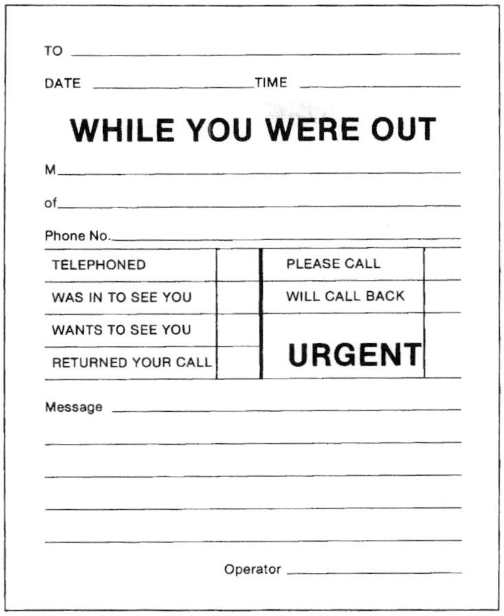
TO
DATE TIME
WHILE YOU WERE OUT
M
of
Phone No.

TELEPHONED		PLEASE CALL	
WAS IN TO SEE YOU		WILL CALL BACK	
WANTS TO SEE YOU		URGENT	
RETURNED YOUR CALL			

Message

Operator

FIGURE 10-13. Message form. *(Courtesy of SYCOM, Madison, WI. In Finkbeiner BL, Finkbeiner CA:* Practice Management for the Dental Team, *ed 6, St. Louis, 2006, Mosby.)*

SUMMARY

Telecommunications include the cell phone, smartphone, Internet, office phone, voicemail, answering system, e-mail, and facsimile. These are important forms of communicating with your new and current clients. You can choose whatever works for your and your clients, including e-mail, telephone systems, and cell phone text messaging. An answering system or voicemail system is an important piece of communication equipment when you are unable to take a call, such as when giving a massage.

Unlike the use of postcards, texting, or the Internet, use of telecommunication methods allows the tone of your voice to project your concern and enthusiastic attitude. Proper etiquette is important when speaking on the phone. You should document your messages or discussions, because this allows for smooth conversation and hinders future frustrations when talking with clients, insurance representatives, or other business personnel.

Bibliography

Fulton PJ: *General Office Procedures for Colleges*, ed 12, Cincinnati, OH, 2003, South-Western.

Rader MH, Kurth LA: *Business Communication*, ed 2, Cincinnati, OH, 1994, South-Western.

Evolve Annotated Web Links

http://evolve.elsevier.com/Fritz/business

Institute for Telecommunication Sciences: Telecommunications and information technology planning (http://www.its.bldrdoc.gov/pub/ntia-rpt/tpr/2007/telecommunications_and_information_technology_planning-07.pdf)

Workbook

1. List and briefly explain five qualities of a good telephone service.

2. Explain the management of the following calls:

   a. Laura Cochran calls the office and tells you she ran a marathon and her muscles are very sore. She needs to see the massage therapist right away.

    b. Mrs. Gross calls the office and states that she is new in town. She wants to make an appointment for her son, Jim, who uses a massage therapist along with a physical therapist.

_____

_____

    c. Mr. Hubbard calls and states that his daughter threw her back out when jumping on the trampoline. He asks, "What do I need to do?"

_____

_____

3. Replace the following statements with statements that would create a better image.

    a. "I'm sorry, the massage therapist is tied up with a client."

_____

_____

    b. "Johnny, would you like to come in now?"

_____

_____

    c. "Laura, this technique won't hurt much."

_____

_____

    d. "I'm sorry, the massage therapist is running late."

_____

_____

4. Complete a message form using the following telephone conversation: Mr. Schultz from Pine Mutual Insurance Company calls the office and wants you to tell the massage therapist he will meet her at the Yacht Club at 4:30 PM today. If this is not agreeable, Mr. Schultz can be reached at 495.8272.

5. List and briefly define four telephone systems or services available for use in a massage office.

_____

_____

_____

6. List and briefly describe various types of information that can be found in a telephone directory.

_____

_____

_____

7. Locate telephone numbers for each of the following. Keyboard the names and telephone numbers in tabular format on a Rolodex-type form provided in the classroom or the office of employment.
    a. Internal Revenue Service
    b. Police Department
    c. U.S. Post Office
    d. State employment commission

8. Using the Yellow Pages, locate one company and telephone number for each of the following. Type the information on a Rolodex form provided in the classroom or the office of employment.
    a. Massage supply company
    b. Cleaning service
    c. Computer repair service

11

APPOINTMENT MANAGEMENT SYSTEMS

KEY TERMS

Appointment book

Appointment book matrix

Appointment call list

Appointment card

Buffer period

Daily appointment schedule

Dovetailing

Prime time

Unit

LEARNING OUTCOMES

Mastery of the content in this chapter will enable the reader to:

- Define glossary terms
- Describe appointment book styles
- Describe appointment software options
- Complete an appointment matrix
- Identify solutions to common appointment scheduling problems
- Make an appointment entry

- Design an appointment schedule list
- Identify common appointment book symbols
- Describe the use of a treatment plan
- Complete an appointment card
- Complete a daily schedule
- Describe a call list
- Explain advanced-function appointment scheduling

Ⓔ Guidelines for the Learning Activities and answers to the Workbook questions are located on Evolve at http://evolve.elsevier.com/Fritz/business.

APPOINTMENT MANAGEMENT SYSTEM

The appointment management system can take the form of a traditional *appointment book* or software installed in the business computer. Some think that electronic appointment scheduling is time consuming and that it makes checking future schedules difficult. This is not true. Box 11-1 lists the advantages of an electronic appointment book. The traditional appointment book is discussed in this text because it is often used by the massage therapist practicing in a small business setting.

You will be able to use an electronic appointment management system once you activate the CD in this text.

The appointment system, which contains lists of all the scheduled clients and events for the massage therapist and staff, is the control center of the business and an important factor in the success or failure of a massage practice. Basic scheduling concepts (Box 11-2) are the same regardless of the type of system used. Only the process of data entry is different.

The massage therapist should analyze his or her business practice and determine an organized system of appointment control that (1) maximizes productivity, (2) reduces staff tension, and (3) maintains concern for the clients' needs.

BOX 11-1	Advantages of an Electronic Appointment System

- Treatment rooms can be color coded.
- Production goals can aid appointment scheduling.
- Production data are visible daily.
- Data entries are easier to read.
- Autoscheduling eliminates paging through the book.
- Various screen-viewing modes are available.
- Cross-referencing saves time and motion.
- Client data are more likely to be accurate.
- Searching for appropriate appointment openings is easier.
- Procedures can be posted to several different records from one entry.
- Client follow-up is easier.
- No manual record filing is necessary.

BOX 11-2	Tips for Efficient Appointment Management

1. Put one person in charge of the appointment system.
2. In a traditional appointment book, make accurate, neat entries.
3. Accommodate the client as much as possible, but maintain control of the appointment schedule.
4. Establish guidelines for problem situations.
5. Make sure the practice is controlled through the appointment system, not by it.

If you practice massage in a large massage clinic, medical facility, chiropractic office, spa, or sport and fitness center, there may be a receptionist who manages the appointment process. If problems with scheduling occur, it may be necessary to review the skills of the receptionist and the type of system used.

Electronic and traditional systems are addressed in this chapter. The concepts presented can be used in an electronic or a manual system because they are the same for both.

Selection of a Traditional Appointment Book

When an appointment book is used, the size and design of the book are determined by the needs of the massage practice. You should review the available styles to determine what is best for the business. Time and motion studies have indicated that the most efficient format for an appointment book is the week-at-a-glance style, in which all days of the week can be seen at one time; this allows you to observe openings in the schedule quickly (Fig. 11-1).

The binding on the appointment book may have three to nine rings or may be spiral. Spiral-bound books appear to withstand a greater amount of use. The books may be printed with or without dates and may have one or more columns (Fig. 11-2).

The individual days are divided into time increments. Some books provide 30-minute increments, others 10- or 15-minute increments. The smallest time increment is referred to as a *unit* (u). Typical massage appointments are 30, 45, 60, and 90 minutes. The 30-minute unit is the most logical for massage scheduling. Fifteen-minute units are also used in the massage practice, especially when the massage therapist works in the health care area and health care insurance is billed for services.

SELF-REFLECTION

What is the best appointment schedule for my style of massage and stamina? How much time do I need between massage sessions to change over the room, take care of restroom needs, and perform other tasks? What if I am working for a business that schedules 60-minute appointments one right after the other? Will that work for me? How will I manage back-to-back 30-minute sessions? What is different about how I would schedule myself from scheduling done by an employer?

Options for the Electronic Appointment Book

With the electronic appointment system, appointments can be entered, canceled, rescheduled, and moved easily with one keystroke. The benefits of the electronic system (see Box 11-1) set it apart from the traditional system. Common electronic software scheduling packages usually have a number of components:

Goal scheduler: This component takes into consideration fixed and variable overhead and the massage therapist's preset goals for the year. In this system, a goal builder window indicates last year's goal and actual production for the same period last year. It then indicates this year's status.

Autoscheduler: This feature allows you to find an opening in a matter of seconds, and information can be viewed in several formats. The daily appointment screen with a find window allows you to find a date and time for a client with minimal keystrokes.

Daily appointment screen: Most systems allow you to color code rooms. The daily appointment screen usually has two viewing modes. The regular view generally shows the treatment rooms in a column format with the client's name. This is helpful when several practitioners are working at the same time in the office. The expanded view on the enclosed CD (Fig. 11-3) shows details for a full week, including the weekend. The find option brings up a calendar and lets you go directly to any specified day or zoom out to the weekly or monthly screen (Fig.11-4).

Client record: The client information screen (Fig. 11-5) in most systems can be divided into different categories, such as demographics, financial data, insurance, recall, and appointments. Client information that can be entered on this record includes the client's complete name, marital status, gender, age, date of birth, work and home phone numbers, current balance, referrals, medical alerts, and appointment time preferences. Other information can be stored in other dialog boxes, such as session, SOAP notes, billing, and insurance billing screen.

Designing the Appointment Book Matrix

An *appointment book matrix,* or outline of the appointment book, functions like the matrix of an amalgam restoration; it provides support. It is the framework around which appointments are made. A matrix should be completed before a new appointment book or electronic system is used. It should include the following elements:

Holidays: In many traditional books, holidays are noted by the manufacturer (Fig. 11-6A). However, you may find it necessary to enter special holidays observed in your locale

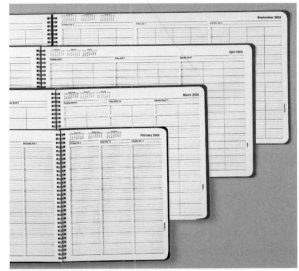

FIGURE 11-1. Week-at-a-glance appointment book in various sizes. *(Courtesy of SYCOM, Madison, WI. In Finkbeiner BL, Finkbeiner CA:* Practice Management for the Dental Team, *ed 6, St. Louis, 2006, Mosby.)*

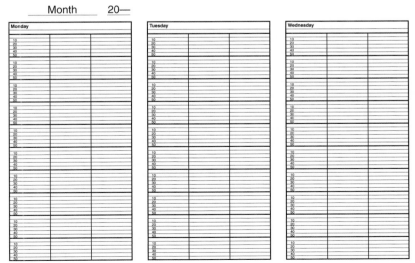

FIGURE 11-2. Undated multiple-column appointment book. *(Courtesy of SYCOM, Madison, WI. In Finkbeiner BL, Finkbeiner CA:* Practice Management for the Dental Team, *ed 6, St. Louis, 2006, Mosby.)*

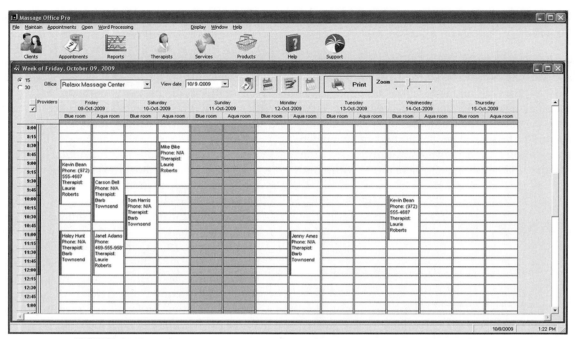

FIGURE 11-3. Daily appointment screen (expanded view). *(Courtesy of Island Software)*

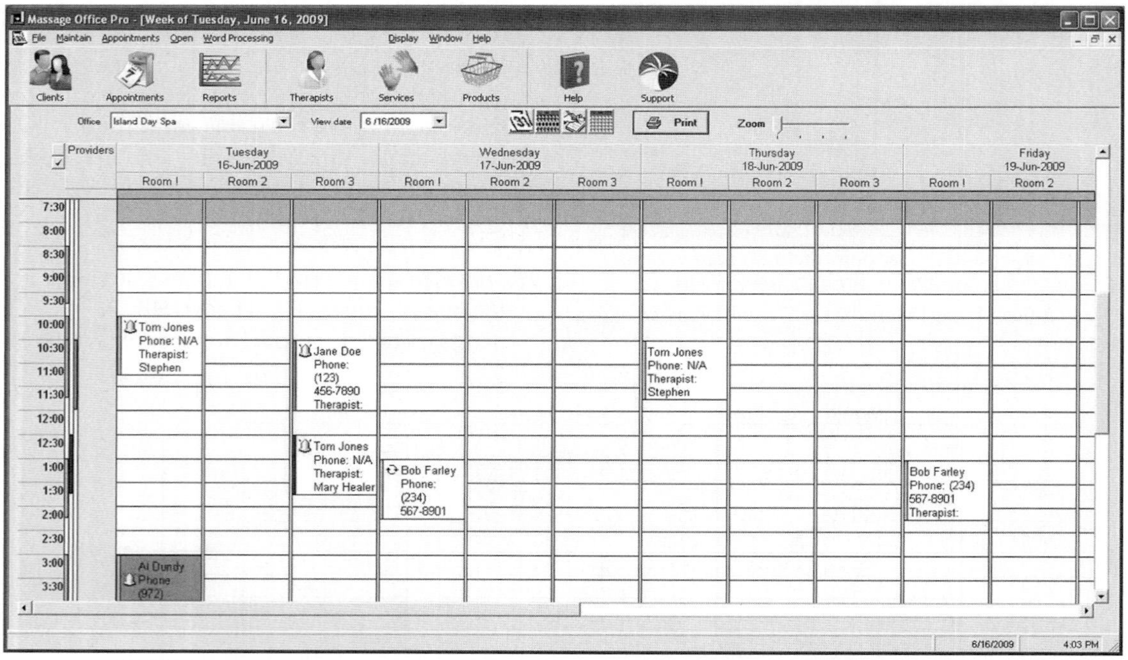

FIGURE 11-4. Quick-glance screen showing a week at a glance. *(Courtesy of Island Software.)*

or business. This can be done by placing an X across the entire day and marking it with the name of the holiday (see Fig. 11-6B).

Lunch hours: Lines may be used to cross out lunch hours. However, a broad, yellow felt-tip marker accomplishes the same task and can be written over legibly (Fig. 11-7). After you become experienced with the appointment book, it will be unnecessary to mark off these hours.

Buffer periods: A *buffer period* is a small amount of time set aside to absorb the hectic workload of the day. Typically, 1-unit increment of time (a 15-minute unit is typical for a massage practice) is set aside in the morning and again in the afternoon. If this space is colored in with a yellow felt-tip pen, an entry can be made without erasing (Fig. 11-8). The buffer period should not be inserted during the busiest periods of the day. If you are a sole

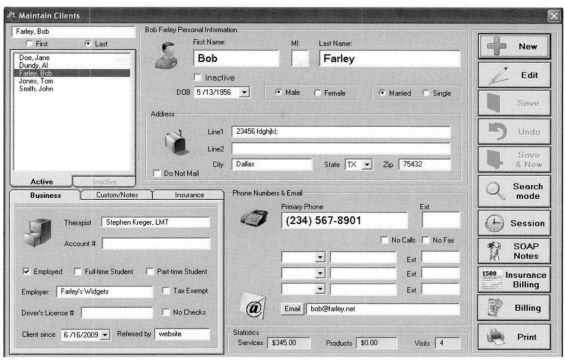

FIGURE 11-5. Client information screen. *(Courtesy of Island Software.)*

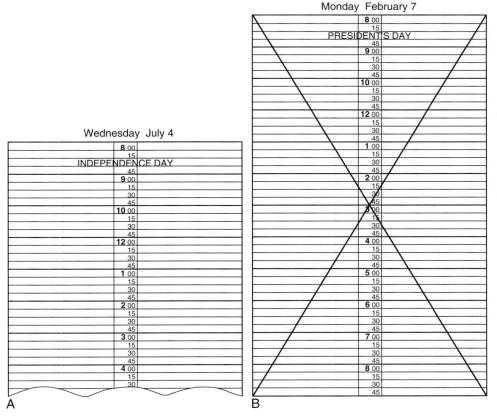

FIGURE 11-6. A, Holiday page from a traditional appointment book. **B,** An X drawn through a page from an appointment book to indicate a holiday or business closure. *(From Finkbeiner BL, Finkbeiner CA:* Practice Management for the Dental Team, *ed 6, St. Louis, 2006, Mosby.)*

		11 00	
		15	
		30	
		45	
LIONS CLUB		12 00	
AT		15	
UNIVERSITY CLUB		30	
Rm. 1005		45	
		1 00	
		15	
		30	
		45	

FIGURE 11-7. Lunch hour highlighted in a traditional appointment book with a felt-tip marker. *(From Finkbeiner BL, Finkbeiner CA: Practice Management for the Dental Team, ed 6, St. Louis, 2006, Mosby.)*

practitioner and managing your own schedule, a buffer system of a 15-minute period twice daily and at least one 30-minute period is recommended. It is also necessary to provide adequate buffer periods between client sessions. Fifteen minutes between appointments is necessary to clean and again set-up the massage area. In addition to providing a massage for the client, you must perform all business responsibilities, cleaning, laundry, and other miscellaneous activities required when operating a successful business practice.

LEARNING ACTIVITY

Create a sample appointment book matrix using the following guidelines.

Professional meetings: A notation about the location and nature of the meeting can be made on the appropriate date, with an X blocking out the specified time (Fig. 11-9).

Staff meetings: Time should be set aside regularly, usually once or twice each month, for all members of the staff to meet and discuss goals for the business. This time should not be scheduled during the lunch period or after business hours; it should be integrated into regular business hours (see Chapter 2 for suggestions on scheduling staff meetings).

Tuesday, April 24

JOHN FLETCHER FR #8

FIGURE 11-8. One-unit buffer highlighted in a traditional appointment book with a felt-tip marker. *(From Finkbeiner BL, Finkbeiner CA: Practice Management for the Dental Team, ed 6, St. Louis, 2006, Mosby.)*

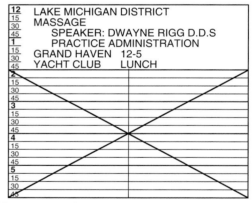

LAKE MICHIGAN DISTRICT
MASSAGE
SPEAKER: DWAYNE RIGG D.D.S
PRACTICE ADMINISTRATION
GRAND HAVEN   12-5
YACHT CLUB   LUNCH

FIGURE 11-9. Time for a meeting is indicated with an X. *(Modified from Finkbeiner BL, Finkbeiner CA: Practice Management for the Dental Team, ed 6, St. Louis, 2006, Mosby.)*

IMPORTANT FACTORS IN SCHEDULING APPOINTMENTS

You will deal with a variety of situations in scheduling appointments. Management of the appointment book requires a well-defined plan, an established appointment sequence, and an ability to maintain strict control over the appointment book while still meeting the needs of clients.

Massage Therapist's Biologic Clock

Some people are early birds, and others are night owls. It is important to understand your body rhythms to best use your time. Not all people are at their best at all times of the

day. Some people do not reach their peak period until 1 or 2 PM, when the early birds who were dynamic at 8 AM have begun to lose energy. Others work best in the evening. This becomes an important factor in determining when to schedule the client. Because massage is a service business, you also need to consider when clients are available for massage sessions. The massage schedule can begin as early as 6 AM and continue well into the evening, depending on when clients are available and how their needs fit with your schedule.

Scheduling for Productivity

Massage therapy is a business, and one of the most effective ways to be profitable is to increase productivity. This is a real concern because massage is very time intensive. Overlapping booking is not possible as it is with spa treatments or medical service; there is a limit on the number of clients one massage therapist can work with in a day. If your body mechanics are effective, you should be able to schedule five massage sessions per day and maintain basic business procedures. A full-time practice for a single massage therapist requires a minimum of 50 scheduled business hours per week, including massage sessions, buffer periods, facility management (e.g., cleaning),

various marketing activities, business activities (e.g., paying bills, billing clients, ordering supplies, returning calls). A typical day begins at 7 AM. Standard massage sessions of 60 minutes are scheduled as shown in the figure below.

An alternative is to begin the business day later and work later into the evening. This type of scheduling works for those practicing massage in an office setting where clients come to them. The buffer time allows for the massage

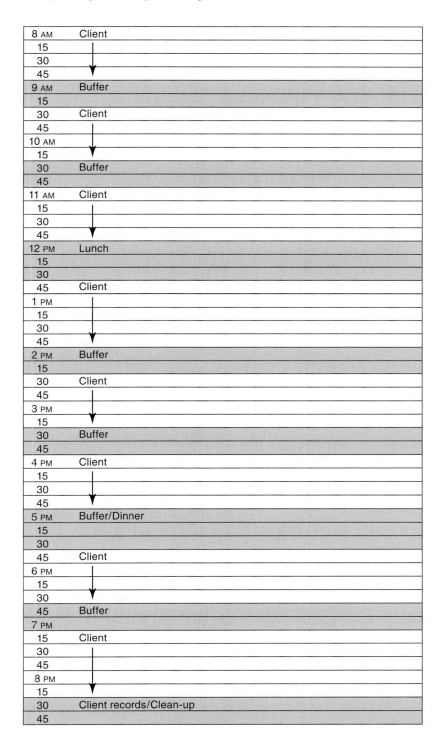

therapist to manage office tasks, clean and setup massage area, collect fees, make the next appointment for the client, and be available to greet the next client. It also allows for a longer appointment for those that may want a 90-minute session and enough time to accommodate the quick turn-over required of the 30-minute sessions.

SELF-REFLECTION

How does my biologic clock influence my workday? What time of day is my down time or up time? How do I set my schedule to best support my inner clock? What happens when I get off my schedule or have to work on a schedule that does not match my biologic clock?

If you are practicing in a setting where you do not have to manage the office (i.e., as an employee in a business with a receptionist), you will need less buffer time. Instead, you will likely be scheduled with two break periods and a lunch or dinner period. You will be expected to stay on schedule so that clients do not have to wait. Sessions are usually scheduled at 30 minutes or 50 minutes, and you must be able to effectively prepare the massage area, wash your hands and arms, and greet the next client.

Business Hours

Most massage businesses develop a schedule that includes extended business hours beyond the traditional workday. They may include early morning, evening time, or week-end days. There is no significant difference in scheduling appointments for this type of practice, but it requires special attention in the selection of an appointment book and in designing the matrix. Care should be taken that the days identified for extended hours include times to cover all the hours the business will be open. This situation may require an unmarked appointment book that allows you to insert the days and times in accordance with the business schedule.

Management of Prime Time

Prime time is the period most often requested by clients; in most businesses, it is the time after 3 PM. Not all who request this time will receive it, and clients must be informed of the need to schedule this time on a rotating basis.

Habitually Late Clients

A small number of clients persist in being late for their appointments. You should stress the importance of being on time for the appointment by explaining, "Mr. Campbell, your massage sessions require all the time allotted, and being on time for your appointment is therefore important to you." Your office policy should address the ramifications of late clients.

Standing Appointments

Because massage is a retention-client business and massage is most beneficial if received regularly, the goal is to have client book standing appointments. This can be on a weekly basis, every other week, or monthly. Occasionally, a client wants two sessions each week. Because massage therapy is paid for by the client (no insurance coverage), the amount of financial resources that can be allocated to massage on a monthly basis must be considered when setting a standing appointment schedule.

Standing appointments should be encouraged and can account for three fourths of the practice. Based on 20 clients each week, this means that 15 sessions would be standing appointments. The most common pattern is an appointment every other week or twice each month. This schedule is most affordable for the most out-of-pocket payers. It is realistic to expect that of the 15 standing appointments, 10 would be of this type. This combination would be 20 different clients: 10 appointments one week and 10 appointments the alternate week. Five weekly standing appointment massage clients is a reasonable business expectation. Some clients will get a massage regularly on a monthly basis. You can expect that five clients per week will be of this type and account for 20 individual sessions. On a weekly basis the standing appointment schedule would look something like this:

Five weekly standing appointments = 5 clients
Ten every-other-week (bimonthly) standing appointments = 20 clients
Five monthly standing appointments = 20 clients
Five appointments open for new clients or special circumstances

If you analyze this, you can see that a full-time massage practice consists of 45 clients who have some sort of standing appointment and another group of 25 to 30 clients who get a massage occasionally. For the sake of profitability and productivity, the massage therapist should foster the standing appointment system.

Clients Who Arrive on the Wrong Day

Clients may arrive on the wrong day or at the wrong time. The error may be the client's, or you might have written the wrong date on the appointment card. You should ask to see the appointment card, and if the client has made the mistake, indicate the actual date and time of the appointment. If you or another staff member made the error, an apology is necessary, and the client should be seen by the massage therapist if at all possible. The built-in buffer system in the daily schedule should make this possible. You may be able to contact the scheduled clients, explain that an "unexpected change has occurred in the schedule," and delay their arrival. Regardless of who is responsible for the error, you should remain tactful and helpful in correcting the mistake.

Drop-Ins

Nothing is more frustrating than to have a client drop by the business and say, "I was just in the area and thought I'd drop in and see I could get a massage." If one of the open (nonstanding) appointments is available, the individual can be seen. Otherwise, tactfully inform the client that you see clients by appointment only, and tell the person when the next appointment is available.

This practice does not apply to the many walk-in (convenience) massage clinics established in the past few years. One of the prime objectives of these clinics is to accommodate clients without appointments.

Broken Appointments

Sometimes, a client absolutely must cancel an appointment or is prevented from keeping the appointment by some unforeseen circumstance. Most clients respect the massage therapist's time, and the massage therapist should be understanding when a cancellation occurs. Other clients, unfortunately, seem always to find an excuse for breaking an appointment. Although most massage therapists' initial reaction is to charge for broken appointments, this becomes difficult to accomplish and results in poor public relations. The client should be informed of the importance of keeping the appointment; for example, "Mrs. Ward (or Shawna), because you have been unable to keep your massage appointment on a regular basis, I can no longer justify keeping you as a standing-appointment client. I do have a few appointments available every week that I reserve for those who cannot commit to a standing appointment schedule. This may be a better option for you."

If the client continues to cancel appointments, she should be told, "I am unable to continue to make appointments for you because of the ongoing cancelations. I have only a few open sessions, and I have people who would like to schedule a massage with me." However, such a policy should be exercised only after all other options have been explored by the massage therapist and client. Therapeutic massage is such a personal business that a disgruntled person can create a lot of negative word of mouth. Just as important, you have to invest your time in clients who are able to meet your business goals, and because there are limits on the number of

clients an individual massage therapist can see, it is important that each client is reliable.

Dovetailing

Dovetailing means working a second client into the schedule during another scheduled client's treatment. Many health care professionals and some service professionals (e.g., cosmetologists) can accomplish this. Massage therapists should not attempt this type of scheduling.

Establishing an Appointment Time

To prevent conflicts with clients over appointment times, do not ask, "What is the most convenient time for you?" or "What is your day off?" or "When does Frank get out of school?" It is wiser to ask, "Is morning or afternoon better for you?" and then present two choices for the client. You will lead the client into making a choice realistically within your schedule, and you will not be forced to say "I'm sorry" to each of the client's suggestions. Encourage clients who understand that massage therapy is the type of health care service that achieves the best benefits with regularly scheduled care. Massage is best at prevention, and prevention is an ongoing process. When clients ask, "How often should I get a massage?" explain the importance of preventative care, and suggest a standing appointment for every week or every other week. Explain that the every-other-week appointments can be effective if clients also do some self-help and that monthly appointments can be supportive if they are willing to do a lot of self-help work on their own. The analogy of housekeeping or car maintenance often helps clients understand the importance of regular massage appointments. After educating the client about the importance of regular massage, explain, "I have a limited number of appointments available each week. It is best if we schedule a standing appointment. I have Tuesdays at 4:30 PM, Saturdays at 11:00 AM available for weekly sessions, and Mondays at 8:00 PM is available for every other week. Will any of these times work for you?

ENTERING APPOINTMENTS

Appointment Book

An entry in the appointment book must be made in pencil. It must be accurate, complete, and legible, and it should include the information shown in Box 11-3.

Because of the limited amount of space available for each entry, symbols must be used to make special notations about a client. Table 11-1 lists several symbols commonly used in the appointment book. Each entry was made in pencil and is accurate, complete, and legible. An appointment sequence is established in coordination with the treatment plan.

SELF-REFLECTION

Do I arrive late for appointments? Have I cancelled an appointment at the last minute or been a no-show? Will I show up on time for client's appointments, or do I have a tendency to be late, cancel, or be a no-show? How would this type of behavior influence client satisfaction and retention?

BOX 11-3	Information to Include in an Appointment Book Entry

- Client's full name, with cross-reference in case of duplication of names
- Home and business phone numbers to confirm the appointment or to reach the client in case of an emergency
- Type of massage, if appropriate
- Length of the appointment, indicated with an arrow
- Special notations (e.g., new client)

TABLE 11-1	Symbols for Traditional Appointment Book Entries

SYMBOL	MEANING
N	New client
*	Client prefers an earlier appointment.
B	Business phone number
H	Home phone number
↓	Length of appointment

Appointment Card

An *appointment card* is a written notification of the client's appointment that the client takes home. After the entry has been made in the appointment book, the information is transferred to the appointment card. It is entered directly from the appointment book in ink and should be easy to read. Recheck the appointment card before giving it to the client to make sure the information in the book and on the card is the same.

A traditional appointment card is made of medium-weight or lightweight stock and measures about 2 by 3.5 inches to fit easily into a wallet. Appointment cards usually are white with black print. However, many businesses are color coding cards, using matching or contrasting ink to carry out a color theme in the business. The information on the card includes the massage therapist's full name, credential initials, address, and phone number, and the business policy on broken appointments. Lines are provided for the client's name and the day, date, and time of the appointment. Figure 11-10 shows a variety of appointment cards that can be used in the massage business. The cards shown in parts A and B of the figure are for only one appointment; the card shown in part C is a series-type appointment card, on which more than one appointment can be listed. The series card saves your time and the cost of additional cards.

In an electronic system, the appointment often is listed on the exit receipt. It also can be listed on a walk-out statement, but many clients seem to like the security of a separate appointment card. The electronic system does eliminate the potential for error in writing on the appointment card.

Clients who schedule standing appointments tend to get in the habit and seldom cancel appointments. There will be times when their schedule may change, such as around the

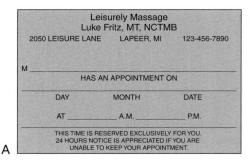

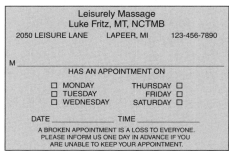

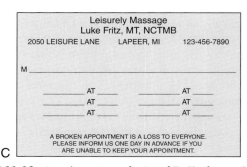

FIGURE 11-10. Appointment cards. **A** and **B,** Single appointment cards. **C,** Series-style appointment card. *(Modified from Finkbeiner BL, Finkbeiner CA:* Practice Management for the Dental Team, *ed 6, St. Louis, 2006, Mosby.)*

holidays or vacation or some sort of unexpected obligation, and the massage therapist should be tolerant of these occasional changes. The benefits of regular standing clients far outweigh some scheduling changes.

DAILY APPOINTMENT SCHEDULE

Each day, you should pull the clinical records for each of the next day's clients and complete a daily schedule. The *daily appointment schedule* is a chronologic listing of the day's activities. If there are openings in the daily schedule, you can attempt to fill the appointment from an appointment call list.

The *appointment call list* is a current list of clients who would like an appointment but do not have a standing appointment or who would like to change appointments on a particular day. The list can include potential new clients that have previously requested an appointment but none was available. The client's name, phone number,

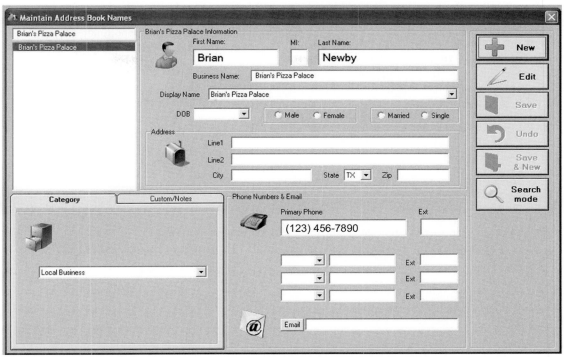

FIGURE 11-11. Electronic address book. *(Courtesy of Island Software.)*

and information are listed in a notebook or at the back of the appointment book, or this data may be entered in the address book of the practice management software (Fig. 11-11). These individuals can be called in an attempt to fill the daily appointment schedule if an opening occurs.

After you have become familiar with the techniques of appointment book management, it can be a very enjoyable part of the business. Using time efficiently can make each day in the business more productive and can reduce tension while still meeting the clients' needs. If the rules in Box 11-2 are followed, the massage business can maintain efficiency.

 Good Stuff from the Government

OFFICE OF SMALL BUSINESS DEVELOPMENT CENTERS: ENTREPRENEURIAL DEVELOPMENT PROGRAM

The Office of Small Business Development Centers (SBDCs) provides management assistance to current and prospective small business owners. SBDCs offer one-stop assistance to individuals and small businesses by providing a wide variety of information and guidance in central and easily accessible branch locations. The program is a cooperative effort of the private sector, the educational community, and federal, state, and local governments. It is an integral component of the Entrepreneurial Development program's network of training and counseling services.

SUMMARY

Scheduling and handling appointment mishaps are important parts of a massage business. Success depends on knowing how to use the appointment book or computer software program. Whether you use two or more buffers throughout the day within your practice, you need to know who is coming in next to know how to prepare. Being prepared helps the flow of the day and keeps appointments on time, which your clients will appreciate. Use the appointment cards to help your clients remember their scheduled times, and use a reminder system for those who need a reminder the day before an appointment.

Your business hours may depend on your biologic clock or the time your clients are available. When are most of your standing appointments, or what is the most popular time for drop-ins? Many service industries, such as cosmetology and medical practices, use dovetailing, which does not work for massage therapy. Our business must dedicate a time slot for just one client. If using a receptionist, a client can come in early to complete paperwork and perform some of the tasks that would require a buffer slot in a single massage practice.

Keep an appointment call list for those waiting for a time slot for massage to help your business to continually grow. Try to be flexible with your open time slots for consistent clients who have unexpected disruptions.

CD Now is the time to watch the tutorial on the enclosed CD at the back of the book on how to use the software. Activate the CD, and begin the tutorial, which is a very detailed step-by-step instruction on how to maximize the use of the practice management software. After the tutorial, use yourself as your first client, set up your first people management page, then set up your first massage appointment. Complete the intake forms. Pretend you had your first massage, fill out the SOAP notes, and then book yourself for a recurring appointment every 2 weeks.

Bibliography

Schumann TC: Top five opportunities to improve your profit, *J Mich Dent Assoc* 87(issue 2):20, February, 2005.

Evolve Annotated Web Links

http://evolve.elsevier.com/Fritz/business

U.S. Small Business Association, Office of Small Business Development Centers: Entrepreneurial Development (http://www.sba.gov/aboutsba/sbaprograms/sbdc/index.html)

Workbook

1. Discuss the types of appointment systems available for use in the massage business.

2. Explain the advantages of an electronic appointment system.

3. Explain the components of an appointment matrix.

4. List the information that should be entered in the appointment book when an appointment is made.

5. What information is included on the following forms?

   a. Appointment card

   b. Appointment daily schedule

   c. Call list

6. List four rules for efficient management of an appointment book.

MARKETING THE MASSAGE THERAPY BUSINESS

KEY TERMS

Advanced appointment
  system
Advertising

Mail recall system
Internet recall system
Marketing

Recall system
Telephone recall system

LEARNING OUTCOMES

Mastery of the content in this chapter will enable the reader to:

- Define key terms
- Explain marketing techniques in massage therapy
- Describe external and internal marketing

- Explain the purpose of a recall system
- Identify different types of recall systems
- Develop a recall system

e Guidelines for the Learning Activities and answers to the Workbook questions are located on Evolve at http://evolve.elsevier.com/Fritz/business.

WHAT IS MARKETING?

One of the greatest needs of any small business is to understand and develop *marketing* programs for their products and services. Because massage is a service business, marketing is an essential concept. Throughout this textbook, the Small Business Association (SBA) has been recommended as a source for success based on the ability to build a growing body of satisfied customers. Modern marketing programs are built around the marketing concept and performance, which focuses on identifying and satisfying the customer's needs. Marketing is about education of potential clients about what you can do for them. Marketing is not about you; it is about how your skills can help clients. Instead of focusing on you (e.g., where you went to school, how many modalities you are trained), market yourself as an innovative problem solver for the client. Emphasize how your massage service helps their nagging issues, pain, or personal dilemmas.

Potential clients are motivated by the following ideas:

Self-interest: People want to know what is in it for them. They are interested what makes something better in their life. Do not talk about you; start talking about them.

Comfort: People do business with people they know and trust. Start a conversation with people by giving them articles, newsletters, or other information that you have created to help them. Especially with massage, you need to appeal to them by offering information through presentations at service groups, health fairs, or other places where they can meet you.

Something unique: Are you effectively communicating the one thing that makes you unique? What can you offer that no other massage business can? In one sentence, describe it. This is your core marketing message. Use it over and over to generate interest and get people talking about you.

Communication: A service business is a relationship. To sustain good relationships (i.e., retention clients), you have to stay in touch with customers. Continue to communicate through phone calls, e-mails, lunch dates, and other opportunities.

Marketing is perceived by lots of business people to mean promotion and *advertising*. However, the term *marketing* covers company culture and positioning, market research, new business or product development, advertising and promotion, and public and press relations.

In a service business, you are marketing yourself—your expertise and capabilities, your reliability, and your commitment to excellent service. Your service technically does not exist until the customer pays for it. Service is not a tangible product, so what you are selling is the promise to deliver what you set out to deliver. Your marketing efforts should focus on communicating that promise to your clientele. All business policies and activities should be aimed at satisfying customers' needs, and to accomplish this, you (or the employer with your help) need to do the following:

- Determine the needs of customers (i.e., market research)
- Analyze competitive advantages (i.e., market strategy)
- Select specific markets to serve (i.e., target marketing)
- Determine how to satisfy those needs (i.e., market mix)

Marketing research is an organized way of finding objective answers to questions every business must answer to succeed. Every small business owner-manager must ask the following questions:

- Who are my customers and potential customers?
- What kind of people are they?
- Where do they live?
- Can and will they buy?
- Am I offering the kinds of goods or services they want and doing so at the best place, at the best time, and in the right amounts?
- Are my prices consistent with what buyers view as the value of the products or services?
- Are my promotional programs working?
- What do customers think of my business?
- How does my business compare with my competitors?

Marketing should be a natural habit that is practiced at all times. It is important to educate clients about the massage practice and procedures; provide quality treatment in a comfortable, safe environment; offer outstanding customer service; and make clients want to tell their family and friends about their great massage therapist and staff. To market a massage practice effectively, the massage therapist needs a specific set of skills that can aid him or her in promoting the practice. The next section will help you refine these questions and provide direction in how to uniquely answer them for yourself.

THE MARKETING PLAN

An effective marketing plan is key to the success of your massage business. If you are an employee, you need to be assured that the business owner will market you in an effective way. The marketing plan should include market research, location, the customer group targeted, competition, positioning of the service, pricing, advertising, and promotion.

Massage is effectively promoted for a niche market. A niche market is a small, focused target population interested in your services. The idea of appealing to a niche market revolves around being unique and in demand. With this in mind, it makes sense that the first step in mastering the identified niche market is determining what makes you uniquely qualified to serve the client. What makes you different from other massage therapists? You must be able to provide clients with a great massage that meets their needs, and you have to do it in a way that allows them to justify the investment of time and money. To find your niche target market, you need to understand potential clients' interests. There are three main reasons why people are attracted to therapeutic massage services:

- Massage satisfies a basic need for touch and connection.
- Massage solves a problem for the client, such as reducing stress, improving sleep, or increasing productivity.
- Massage feels good, and it makes the client feel good.

SELF-REFLECTION

This is a very important question to ask yourself: What makes me unique?

UNDERSTANDING MARKETING

Mass marketing strategies do not work well for service businesses. You are constrained by the amount of clients you can service well. To please your clients, you can focus only on a certain number of accounts or customers to sustain your business. If you decide to get as many clients as possible, there is the risk that you will spread yourself too thin and that the quality of your work will suffer.

There are several effective ways to attract clients:

Referrals: The recommendation of satisfied clients or professional colleagues is often the most effective way of bringing in new clients. You may give them promotional materials, such as business cards or brochures, that they may share with others.

Client relations: Clients will patronize your service repeatedly if they are satisfied. It is therefore important to cultivate your existing client base and bond with them. Because massage therapy is more than a product-based business, you need to practice excellent customer service every second that you deal with a client. Your business depends on it.

Participation in organizations: Networking is the key promotional technique in marketing a service business, and participating actively in organizations is the best way to network. There are many different service and community organizations, such as Lions Clubs International, Kiwanis International, Optimist International, Rotary International, and Zonta International.

You must stay current with the trends in massage, massage research, and business. To stay current in massage skills, you need to invest in continuing education and to read massage therapy research. To remain current in business, you need to read business articles (Box 12-1).

BOX 12-1 | Staying Informed

The Massage Therapy Foundation (http://www.massagether apyfoundation.org/) advances the knowledge and practice of massage therapy by supporting scientific research, education, and community service.

AllBusiness (AllBusiness.com) is an online media and e-commerce company that operates one of the premier business sites on the Web. The site has received critical acclaim and attention from *The Wall Street Journal, Forbes, Business 2.0, Fortune, The New York Times, US News & World Report, USA Today,* and other publications. AllBusiness helps business professionals save time and money by addressing real-world business questions and presenting practical solutions. The site offers resources, including how-to articles, business forms, contracts and agreements, expert advice, blogs, business news, business directory listings, product comparisons, business guides, and a business association.

Business professionals can access the AllBusiness group's content and services through a number of channels, including the AllBusiness.com Web site, RSS feeds, e-mail, newsletters, and through its partnerships with leading Web properties. AllBusiness is a wholly owned subsidiary of Dun & Bradstreet and is based in San Francisco, CA.

ArticlePlanet provides marketing articles available on its Web site (http://www.articleplanet.net/).

COMMON METHODS OF MARKETING

Certain approaches to marketing have proved successful. The sign in front of your office remains one of the most effective marketing strategies. It is common to have a Web site. Networking with others and word of mouth information are the best ways to market your business.

Business Signage

Signs are one of the most efficient and effective means of communication. Signs help people find you, they reach people who are passing by, and they present an image of your business. In short, signs tell people who you are and what you are selling.

A sign is the most direct form of visual communication available. So many people use signs without a second thought that it is easy to overlook their importance. Signs perform three major communication functions for your business: They give information and direction, provide a format for street advertising, and build your image.

On-premises signs are your most effective and efficient means of commercial communication because they are inexpensive, available, practical, easy to use, always on the job, and directly oriented to the trade area of your business. Your sign is an integral part of your advertising program.

Signs are inexpensive. When compared with the cost of advertising in some other media, the on-premises sign is very inexpensive. Unless your trade area encompasses an entire city or region, in which case you must rely on broad-based media coverage, there is no better advertising dollar value than your on-premises sign.

Signs are available to every shop owner. There is no need to schedule the use of your sign. Your sign is available to you whenever you need it, and it can be used however you please.

Signs are easy to use. No special skills or resources are needed to operate a sign after it has been installed. If it is an illuminated sign, all you need to do is flip the switch, and that may not be necessary with the use of timing equipment. After the initial expenditures are made, no special resources or professional services are needed. You need only to operate and maintain your sign.

A sign must be noticeable. After a while, a sign becomes part of the landscape. It loses some of its ability to attract attention. If you periodically change some small design element or use changeable copy, your sign can continue to attract interest. A sign needs to be large enough to read. You need to know how far a person is from your store when he first sees your sign and the speed of traffic on your street. With this information, a competent sign company can use a formula to calculate the necessary size for your design and build you an effective sign.

Decide on a message that is clear and simple. Focus on key words. Choose one or two words that describe your business. Clever or strange names may attract only certain customers. Be brief. The cleaner and clearer the message, the more impact it has. Lists or unclear names or symbols confuse rather than communicate. The design of your sign is very important. Your sign tells people a lot about your business. Stark, simple design and materials may suggest discount prices and no frills. Elegant and expensive sign materials may suggest luxury goods and services.

You should consider several factors when deciding on the cost of your on-premises sign. A sign is an investment because it is one of the most permanent parts of your business. It is exposed to weather and constant use. The average life of signs is 5 to 11 years, depending on type of materials used, construction, and other factors. Find out how many years of service to expect from your sign. It pays to purchase good materials if you intend to use the sign over a period of years. No business can afford to have a sign that is falling apart. A dilapidated sign tells the public that you do not care about your business image or their visual environment.*

Web Site

Another important tool in marketing your service business is a Web site. For the price of an advertisement in the yellow pages, you can have a Web site that can serve as a brochure,

direct mail piece, and newsletter rolled into one. The Web is an avenue that should never be ignored. Many different Web sites on the Internet offer you a Web site for a fee, and some Internet service providers (ISPs) even provide a small Web site free of charge if you use their Internet service (Box 12-2). The American Massage Therapy Association (AMTA) and Associated Bodywork and Massage Professionals (ABMP) offer options to members for building their own Web sites. The specifics of choosing a Web site provider can be found by searching on the Web or contacting the organizations directly. Chapter 5 provides detailed information regarding the Internet.

Business Trademark

The massage therapist needs to create an identity. What makes the practice different? Large corporations such as 3M, Sony, Starbucks, Microsoft, and Amazon.com all have an identity. For instance, a massage therapist may sum up the practice's identity by using words such as *thorough*, *caring*, or *leading edge*. The word *thorough* denotes that each client will be given quality time. *Caring* suggests old-fashioned commitment to the client, regardless of business pressure. The phrase *leading edge* indicates that the massage therapist is progressive and keeps abreast of new materials and techniques.

Enthusiastic Attitude

The single most important characteristic for business success is an enthusiastic attitude. The individual with an enthusiastic attitude shows up for work every day on time, is willing to help others, maintains a cheery disposition all day, and ensures that clients come first. This enthusiastic attitude means the "no whining rule" is always in place, because whining is contagious. The enthusiastic attitude means the client's problems come first and personal problems are kept to yourself or shared with a friend in private.

Seizing Opportunities

There are many ways to get the word out about a massage practice. For instance, when a new client makes an appointment, you could say, "Mrs. Timmons, we are looking forward

---

BOX 12-2	Web Site–Hosting Web Sites

www.abmp.com
www.amtamassage.org
www.smallbusiness.yahoo.com
www.googlewebhosting.net
www.bluehost.com
www.inmotionhosting.com
www.ncbtmb.org

---

*Source: U.S. Small Business Administration.

to seeing you at 3 PM on Wednesday. By the way, would you like to make an appointment for any other members of the family at this time?"

Practice Ambassadors

Each member of the massage practice or larger organization such as a spa is expected to be an ambassador for the practice. Each staff member should be provided with his or her own business cards and should promote the practice to family and friends. It may be possible to suggest that the office be used after hours for community group meetings or self-help classes if office space is adequate.

MARKETING FORMS

Marketing can be divided into two forms: internal and external.

Internal Marketing

Internal marketing is what the massage professional does within the business to retain clients. Internal marketing is the first impression. Internal marketing is how you retain clients after you have attracted them to the practice.

Successful internal marketing meets the needs of the client. After the client is on the massage table (or mat or chair), you will have only this chance to prove your professional skills. This is a critical time in practice development. In the massage practice, the goal is to develop a retention-client base in which people receive massage on some sort of regular schedule (e.g., weekly, monthly). Whereas external marketing gets people in the door, satisfaction and client return is your sole responsibility. If clients do not rebook appointments, it is necessary to take an objective inventory of what occurred from the moment the client walked in the door until the follow-up call a couple of days after the first massage. Determine what went right and what went wrong. Although the occasional client may be visiting from out of town or received a gift certificate and just did not like massage, most of the time, the responsibility for retention or lack of it depends on the interaction between the massage therapist and the client.

After an objective and honest evaluation of yourself, consider any other staff or coworkers who interacted with the client, and evaluate the environment. Was the restroom clean? Was the massage area warm enough? Was the office really noisy? Something or someone made the massage session uncomfortable and unsatisfactory for the client. It may be helpful to do a follow-up call and ask sincerely for feedback. People often avoid situations of potential conflict, or they do not want to hurt your feelings, but you may be fortunate enough to find someone who will risk telling you the truth. When this occurs, be genuinely thankful.

In Figure 12-1, notice that most of the ideas for internal marketing for client retention are staff-oriented. Clients who

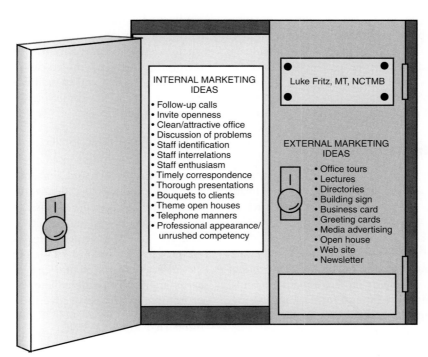

FIGURE 12-1. Internal and external marketing ideas. *(Modified from Finkbeiner BL, Finkbeiner CA:* Practice Management for the Dental Team, *ed 6, St. Louis, 2006, Mosby.)*

know that the massage therapist cares about them and does not consider them case numbers or blank checks will return to the practice and, more importantly, will refer friends and colleagues.

External Marketing

External marketing focuses on getting people in for the first massage; after they are in the door, internal marketing takes over. The key to successful external marketing is to determine who your prospective clients are and the best method to attract them. The massage therapist must identify his or her objectives, define the strengths of the practice, determine the budget, and review all the sources for external advertising. Some forms of marketing can be as simple as offering lectures to local organizations or as complex as media advertising. Figure 12-1 illustrates other potential sources of external marketing.

ADVERTISING

The process of advertising is often thought to be the same as marketing, but advertising is only one aspect of a marketing plan. Advertising is an activity used to attract public attention to a service, product, or business. Most often advertising is in the form of paid announcements in the print, broadcast, or electronic media.

Methods of advertising include banners at sporting events, billboards, Internet Web sites, logos on clothing, magazines, newspapers, radio spots, and television commercials. Although advertising may seem like the perfect way to get a message out about your massage business, it does have several limitations. Marketing focuses on individuals, and general forms of advertising are unable to focus on an individual's specific needs. Most forms of advertising cannot provide in-depth information about a service or product without being cost prohibitive. Advertising is expensive.

Forms of Advertising for the Massage Business

Advertising can take a number of forms. Some forms of advertising are effective for a service business such as massage.

COMPARATIVE ADVERTISING

Comparative advertising compares one brand of a product directly or indirectly with one or more competing brands. In the spa industry, this is a common form of advertising. One drawback of comparative advertising is that customers have become skeptical about claims made by a company about its competitors, because accurate information has not always been provided. If you engage in comparative advertising, be careful not to misinform the public about a

competitor. It will ultimately hurt your business, and it does not serve the profession as a whole to suggest that competitors have poor products. Incorrect or misleading information may trigger a lawsuit by the competitor or regulatory action by a governmental agency such as the Federal Trade Commission (FTC).

COOPERATIVE ADVERTISING

Cooperative advertising is a system that allows two parties to share advertising costs. This form of advertising is recommended for the massage business because of shared interest in the education of the public and increased awareness about massage. Cooperative advertising is especially appealing to small business owners who could not afford to advertise adequately on their own.

DIRECT-MAIL ADVERTISING

Direct-mail advertising uses catalogs, flyers, letters, and postcards mailed to potential clients. There are a few advantages to this form of advertising because it can be included in a specific area for distribution or can be targeted to a demographic, such as those retired. Direct mail is not recommended for advertising massage services. It is expensive, considered junk mail, and paper mail is rapidly being replaced by electronic media.

OUTDOOR ADVERTISING

Billboards and messages painted on the side of buildings are common forms of outdoor advertising, which are often used when quick, simple ideas are being promoted. Signage (discussed earlier) can be considered a form of outdoor advertising. Because repetition is the key to successful promotion, outdoor advertising is most effective when located along heavily traveled city streets and when the product being promoted can be purchased locally. It is recommended that you spend time developing and placing your sign because it can be your single most effective form of advertising.

PERSUASIVE ADVERTISING

Persuasive advertising is used after a product is known and to build selective demand. For example, your massage business can produce special advertisements promoting the stress-reduction benefits of massage in a stressful world, and your business design and facilities can enhance this effect. This type of advertisement allows you to charge more for massage services because of the perceived higher quality of the massage environment. Persuasive advertising is likely a better approach to differentiate your business from a competitor than comparative advertising.

PRODUCT ADVERTISING

Product advertising pertains to nonpersonal selling of a specific service or product. An example is a television commercial promoting a specific soft drink rather than all types of sodas. The primary purpose of the advertisement is to promote a specific type of massage, such as sports massage or reflexology. Although massage as a product can be advertised in this way, it should be accompanied with information that indicates the individualized attention to the client's needs that only you can provide.

REMINDER ADVERTISING

Reminder advertising is used for products or services that have become common in the minds of the public. The advertisements are designed to remind clients to receive a massage and to maintain awareness about the business. For example, a text, e-mail, or newsletter can be sent to remind clients that massage provides the most effective benefits if received on a regular basis.

POINT-OF-PURCHASE ADVERTISING

Point-of-purchase advertising uses displays, demonstrations, or other promotional items near the product or service that is being sold. The primary motivation is to attract clients to the display so that they will purchase the product. For example, a display about the addition of essential oils or an ongoing DVD playing in the reception room about a form of hydrotherapy that is offered in conjunction with the massage can be used to encourage the client to add the additional product or service (for an additional fee) to the basic massage. This form of advertising is effective if the products or services offered are quality and add to the benefits of massage.

SPECIALTY ADVERTISING

Specialty advertising is a form of sales promotion designed to increase public recognition of a business by putting the business name on a variety of items, such as caps, gym bags, jackets, key chains, and pens. The value of specialty advertising depends on how practical and visible the item is. This form of advertising can successfully increase public recognition, especially when large groups are targets, such as at a health fair or a city summer festival.

For advertising to be effective, it must encourage customers to make an initial purchase of a massage and keep current clients returning for massage on a regular basis. This usually is done by providing new and different information about massage that is designed to build client loyalty.

Advertising Expense

Advertising is expensive. A larger advertising budget is required to achieve high advertising frequency. It is estimated that a consumer needs to come in contact with an advertising message nine times before it will be remembered. Without aggressive advertising, potential clients will not become aware of your massage business and how it is different from other massage businesses in the area.

Determining Advertising Strategy

A new business requires considerably more advertising to make customers aware of its existence. As your business becomes recognized, fewer advertising resources are needed.

You should decide on the best method to maximize consumer interest in and awareness of the massage business. Massage is a best advertised on a local basis to a target market. People typically travel only 30 minutes to get a massage. If you are providing massage services at the client's location, it is common to limit the travel time to no more than 60 minutes. You therefore know the target location by identifying the perimeter limited by these travel distances.

After your target area is determined, you must determine what type of individual you want to reach. Do you want to target a population such as local business owners or a senior citizen exercise groups, or do you want a very mixed demographic? The answer determines whether you will advertize by direct mail, a newspaper insert, or a phone book. If you are targeting a population, it may be better to go to a location such as the local sports center or a support group meeting, do a demonstration, and hand out a flyer. Phone book advertising is now provided electronically, and it can be used to target specific populations and areas in ways that paper phone books cannot. Radio and television also target local areas or populations and can be more affordable by using special offers by the station. This often occurs in conjunction with some sort of community event, such as a charity run or parade.

One advertising strategy is to run ads during the holidays to promote season-specific offers, such as a discount on a gift certificate for Mother's Day. You may be able to take advantage of group advertising rates in a special advertising blitz offered by the local newspaper to promote local businesses during a special event or holiday. Figure 12-2 shows a press release that was put out with the hope that a local paper would pick up the story. If a newspaper decides to run your story, a representative likely will call you to obtain more information regarding your business, and in the process, you will receive free advertising. A press release must be written in an inviting and enticing manner. There are many examples found on the Internet, and templates may be found within your personal computer software. After you complete your press release, you want to get it out to as many newspapers, radio stations, or television stations as possible. This can be done by e-mail, fax, or hand delivery.

The best form of advertising for a service business such as massage is to meet potential clients in their environment. Offer to speak at community events, clubs, and support group meetings. Be visible and involved in your community. Do demonstrations. Provide massage at an introductory fee for the police department, fire department, and other government bodies. Network with other health professionals

---

RELAXATION BEGINNINGS

Contact: Luke Fritz

204 W Nepessing St
Phone (123) 456-7890
Email hec@sbcglobal.net

PRESS RELEASE

Relaxation Beginnings is providing a 15-minute chair massage
for each Mother's Day gift certificate purchase

Relaxation Beginnings recognizes their current
clients and future clients with 15-minute chair massages

Lapeer, MI, May 1, 2009: Owner Luke Fritz wants to send out a BIG thanks to all his clients and all his future clients by offering them a free 15-minute chair massage for every 1-hour Mother's Day gift certificate purchase. He wants the public to know how beneficial massage can be and to show his gratitude to all the moms out there who work so hard and need relief from stress. One lucky visitor will win a Spa package worth $150.00
Relaxation Beginnings Open House is May 10, 2009, from 10 AM to 5 PM. Refreshments and hors d'oeuvres will be provided. Come check out the serenity and peacefulness of Relaxation Beginnings. Friends, family, and children welcome.

FIGURE 12-2. Press release.

---

who may refer their clients to you. These forms of advertising within the full marketing plan are effective, cost efficient, and easy to implement, regardless of whether you are opening your own business or supporting your employer in an advertising campaign.

Marketing is a client-centered process. You are telling potential clients that you have a service that will benefit them. If people do not perceive a need for the service or receive benefit from a service, they will not become sustaining clients for you. Remember—it is all about the client.

When using any source of advertising, the massage therapist must realize that the results will not be immediate and that a consistent and repetitive message must be directed to prospective clients to obtain results. You must be able to produce what you claim. No matter where or how much the massage therapist advertises, if quality care is not delivered in a caring, sensitive manner, the client will not return. A good motto to remember is this: you may attract them, but you won't keep them. Chapter 18 helps to target this general marketing information to you specifically.

LEARNING ACTIVITY

Develop an internal and external marketing plan, and list the highlights in the space provided.

_____
_____
_____
_____
_____
_____

KEEPING CLIENTS INFORMED

A *recall system* notifies clients of the timing of routine therapeutic massage care. A recall system helps to support a retention-client base. It helps to achieve one of the primary objectives of massage therapist—helping clients maintain health for a lifetime.

The success of a recall system depends on three factors: client educated about massage benefits, motivation, and consistent follow-up. When you help clients develop a sense of responsibility for their own health and inform them about how regular massage is part of a total health program, everyone benefits. Because recall systems are common in many health care professions such as dentistry and chiropractic, clients often are familiar with how a recall system works. Motivation of clients, which is critical to the effectiveness of the recall system, is the responsibility of the massage therapist and her or his support staff.

After a client has been educated and motivated to accept a recall system, you are responsible for maintaining the system efficiently. The importance of this step cannot be overemphasized. If you ignore the recall system even for 1 month, the effect on the client flow becomes noticeable, and clients begin to feel ignored.

SELF-REFLECTION

How do I feel when I receive reminder calls for appointments? When do reminders become annoying? How can reminders be done so they do not bug someone? How can a reminder call expand into a client motivation and support call?

BOX 12-3	Advanced Appointment System

Advantages
■ No cost involved
■ No time required
■ Simple to use
Disadvantage
■ Clients do not know what their future commitments may be.

BOX 12-4	Suggestions for Using the Telephone Recall System

1. Do not call too early in the morning.
2. Make sure your voice conveys a positive attitude; do not make calls if you are tired or grumpy.
3. Make the calls in private, out of hearing by other clients.
4. Do not pester clients. If they say they will call back, record it on the recall file cards, and wait 2 to 3 weeks before contacting them again. If they do not respond after three calls, ask them if they wish to remain on your active recall program.
5. Have the client's recall record in front of you so that you will be well informed.
6. Try calling on inclement days; clients are likely to be indoors on such days.
7. If you reach an answering machine, speak clearly, and leave a complete message, including the reason for the call, the times the office is open, the telephone number, and a cordial "thank you."

Types of Recall Systems

Several types of recall systems can be used. Most massage therapists find that no one system is perfect; therefore, you will likely use more than one. The three most common recall systems are the advanced appointment system, the telephone recall system, and the mail recall system.

Advanced Appointment System

With the *advanced appointment system*, recall appointments are scheduled before the client leaves the office. A variation is the standing appointment system (discussed previously). Because massage provides the most benefits when received on a regular basis, it is easy to schedule clients to standing appointments. The most common schedule is every other week (e.g., second and fourth Tuesdays at 5:00 PM). The next most common pattern is the weekly standing appointment (e.g., every Saturday at 10:00 AM). The monthly massage appointment is also common (Box 12-3).

Telephone Recall System

The *telephone recall system* allows the most immediate response, because you contact each client by telephone to schedule a recall appointment. This can be a good practice builder for a new practitioner, but it can be an exhausting and time-consuming task in a large, well-established practice and is not needed for clients with standing appointments after they become acclimated to the schedule. In the beginning, reminder calls are important. If a client misses a scheduled appointment without notifying you, it is important to call and confirm whether they wish to continue with the standing appointment schedule.

Because many people have answering machines or voicemail, which allows you to leave messages, the telephone system can be an effective technique that provides personal contact with the client. Text messaging and e-mail can be used as well. Box 12-4 lists a few suggestions for successfully using the telephone in a recall system. The advantages and disadvantages of the telephone system are listed in Box 12-5.

BOX 12-5	Telephone Recall System

Advantages
■ Immediate response from the client
■ Practice builder
Disadvantages
■ May get no answer
■ May be unable to reach the client
■ May disturb the person called
■ Time consuming in a large practice

Mail Recall System

With the *mail recall system*, the client is responsible for making the appointment, and it sometimes is considered a reminder system. Clients receive a card that asks them to contact the office to schedule a massage appointment or that gives them an appointment time and asks them to confirm it (Fig. 12-3). The card should emphasize the importance of regular massage to maximize benefit. The massage therapist or receptionist can address the card, or the client addresses the card, and it will be sent before the next visit. The latter arrangement can be especially effective, because clients recognize their own handwriting when they receive the card, and this may confirm their interest in the recall system. Despite some drawbacks (Box 12-6), the mail recall system can be advantageous when contacting clients who schedule only occasionally for massage and are unwilling to commit to standing appointments.

Internet Recall System

The client may be an avid user of the Internet and may use an e-mail system. An *Internet recall system* can be useful for notifying a client regarding open appointments and can

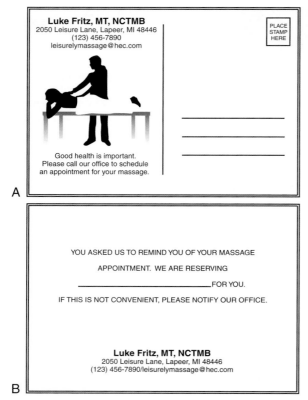

A

B

YOU ASKED US TO REMIND YOU OF YOUR MASSAGE

APPOINTMENT. WE ARE RESERVING

_____ FOR YOU.

IF THIS IS NOT CONVENIENT, PLEASE NOTIFY OUR OFFICE.

Luke Fritz, MT, NCTMB
2050 Leisure Lane, Lapeer, MI 48446
(123) 456-7890/leisurelymassage@hec.com

FIGURE 12-3. A, Recall notice to inform a client of the need to schedule an appointment. **B,** Recall card sent to client for confirmation. *(Modified from Colwell, Division of Patterson Companies, Champaign, IL.)*

BOX 12-6	Mail Recall System

Advantages
- Places responsibility on the client
- Provides a visible reminder

Disadvantages
- Possible to ignore notice
- Cost of postage
- Lack of immediate response

provide a means of confirming an upcoming appointment. If using this system, you need to give the client a date and time that you will hold this appointment open until. If not notified by the specified date and time, the open appointment time will be given to someone else.

There are many types of recall systems, and you need to find what works for certain clients and use that system with that client. Figure 12-4 shows one style of recall card that you can put your message on regarding an upcoming appointment or "haven't seen you in a while" message, which can be generated from the practice management software at the back of this book.

LEARNING ACTIVITY

Compare and contrast the pros and cons of the various types of recall systems. Which ones would be best for a small business, large business, spa business, or on-site business?

_____

_____

_____

ESTABLISHING A RECALL SYSTEM

After the recall system has been determined, you should set up a recall file that is simple, efficient, and accurate. The most efficient recall system is managed electronically.

Electronic Recall Files

The computer is a valuable component of recall management. The practice management software generates a list of clients who need to be contacted (Fig. 12-5). The computer also can produce the letter or card or create mailing labels for pre-prepared cards. If the office uses a telephone recall system, you can generate a master list of clients and their telephone numbers.

Follow-Up

Clients must be recalled routinely. Clients need to be informed about how the recall system works and how they will be notified before they leave the office. The administrative personnel or massage practitioner must maintain flawless records and manage the system to ensure that the client returns to the office in a timely manner.

Purging the System

Periodically, as with any records management system, the recall records should be purged. To avoid the possibility of litigation for negligence, the therapeutic massage office should inform the client that the record is being removed from the system. A letter should be sent to the client (and included in the client's record) informing the person that you are removing him or her from the recall system; this protects the practice and reminds the client one last time of the importance of a maintaining regular massage appointments.

The main focus of a recall system is to support clients in receiving regular massage care. It is more than a reminder call for a scheduled appointment. It is an educational system that helps clients remain motivated in their self-care. Using a recall system is beginning to become popular in the massage business setting. A recall system is a method of informing, educating, supporting, and encouraging clients to maintain a regular pattern of massage care. Recall systems have been

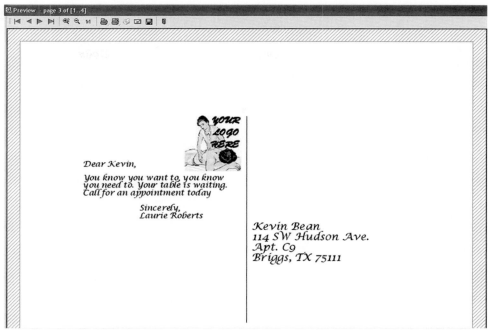

FIGURE 12-4. Recall card example. *(Courtesy of Island Software.)*

Process	ID	Name	Recall Date	NPA	NRA
☑	19	Madison G. Abbott	1/30/2008		
☑	20	Mark Abbott	12/18/2007		
☑	25	Bryan Abernathy	12/18/2007		
☑	72	Bryan A. Abernathy	2/23/2008		
☑	43	Jeremy Adam	12/19/2007		
☑	42	Jedidah Adam	1/30/2008		
☑	45	Jesse Adam	1/30/2008		
☑	6	Scott Alexander	12/1/2007		
☑	32	Richard Ballard	12/18/2007		
☑	33	Megan Ballard	1/30/2008		
☑	68	Jim Carson	12/18/2007		
☑	61	Kelly Davies	12/1/2007		
☑	57	Matthew Dickson	1/30/2008		
☑	12	Jody Farkas	1/30/2008		
☑	23	Carl Malone	1/30/2008		
☑	50	Eugene Partridge	2/20/2008		
☑	67	Cole Walden	2/20/2008		

Recalls to Process — OK — Cancel — Mark All — Clear All

Patients to be processed: 17   E-mails to be processed: 0   Total Pages: 1

FIGURE 12-5. An electronic file generates a list of all clients due for recall in a specific month. *(Courtesy of Island Software.)*

Assessment	Value (1 = worst; 10 = best)/date
Gait	7 / 8-7-09, 9 / 8-26-09
Sleep habits	5 / 8-7-09, 6 / 8-26-09
Increased ROM	8 / 8-7-09, 9 / 8-26-09
Anxiety	9 / 8-7-09, 9 / 8-26-09

FIGURE 12-6. Improved Health Assessment Card is used for a recall system.

used in many health service professions, such as chiropractic, dentistry, physical therapy, and mental health. They are also used in other service professions, such as cosmetology and health and fitness centers. The increasing focus on the total spa experience and massage franchise clinic will increase the use of recall systems to maintain full appointment schedules. Recall systems keep you in touch with clients and support the professional relationship. Figure 12-6 shows data that can be printed on the back of one of your recall cards to remind the client of the progress he or she has been making.

Good Stuff from the Government

U.S. SMALL BUSINESS ADMINISTRATION PUBLICATIONS

Marketing Series

1. Creative Selling: The Competitive Edge, MT-1: Explains how to use creative selling techniques to increase profits.
2. Marketing for Small Business: An Overview, MT-2: Provides an overview of marketing concepts and contains an extensive bibliography of sources covering the subject of marketing.
3. Researching Your Market, MT-8: Learn inexpensive techniques that you can apply to gather facts about your customer base and how to expand it.
4. Selling by Mail Order, MT-9: Provides basic information on how to run a successful mail order business, and includes information on product selection, pricing testing, and writing effective advertisements.
5. Advertising, MT-11: Advertising is critical to the success of any small business. Learn how you can effectively advertise your products and services.
6. Signs: Showcasing Your Business on the Street, MT-12: For most businesses, good signage is the most economical and efficient form of attracting customers.

Marketing and Outreach

The Office of Marketing and Customer Service (OMCS) in the Office of Communications and Public Liaison creates, implements, and evaluates the overall marketing and outreach program to meet the broad needs of the U.S. Small Business Administration (SBA) and its network of field offices serving small business interests across the country. The OMCS ensures the proper branding of SBA as "Your Small Business Resource." SBA's marketing efforts include development of a wide variety of print and audio-visual materials and fostering alliances with associations, corporations, and government agencies.

Energy Star (http://www.sba.gov/energy/index.html)

The Federal Government helps small businesses increase their energy efficiency through the ENERGY STAR for Small Business Program, an effort tailored to meet the special needs of small business owners. ENERGY STAR, a joint program of the Environmental Protection Agency and the Department of Energy, is completely voluntary and provides free technical support and expertise.

Delivering Success Video Series

The U.S. Small Business Administration and the U.S. Postal Service bring you Delivering Success—video interviews with successful entrepreneurs who share the lessons they have learned about owning a small business (http://www.sba.gov/tools/audiovideo/deliveringsuccess/index.html). Pick the topic that interests you, or sit back and spend less than an hour viewing the entire series. Discover how these successful entrepreneurs met the challenges of small business ownership.

- Entrepreneurial Spirit: Learn what it takes to turn a passion into a business.
- Getting Started: How to overcome obstacles when starting a business.
- Financing: Discover how SBA-backed financing helped these entrepreneurs start their businesses.
- Planning & Research: Critical components of success explained by owners who know how.
- Marketing 101: Explore a variety of marketing techniques to build your customer base.
- Hiring & Developing Employees: These owners let you in on what worked for them.
- Promoting & Growing Your Business: Learn innovative techniques to increase your business.
- Business Reality Check: Be prepared to change course from small business owners who had to do just that.

From http://www.sba.gov.

SUMMARY

There can be confusion about marketing. Marketing is not advertising unless the advertising has an educational and informational quality. Marketing is about the clients and the information they need to determine whether the massage services are of enough benefit to them to justify the cost and time they will invest. Marketing never ends in a retention business. Massage professionals need to constantly attend to the clients' education and understanding of the value of massage therapy and products being sold.

The recall system has many benefits. It can be thought of as an automatic message system that provides a means of promoting health by maintaining ongoing massage appointments. For this system to work, the client needs to be aware of the effectiveness of ongoing massage appointments. Clients are the most important persons in the massage business operation, and when they are satisfied, they are your best form of marketing.

Different types of recall systems can work for the massage business. The most common are advanced appointment systems, telephone recall systems, postal mail, and Internet recall systems.

You should perform a routine inventory check of the recall records, and clients should be notified when they will be purged from your recall system. This keeps the records current and may indicate how well you are enforcing the importance of regular massage therapy.

Bibliography

Fritz S: *Mosby's Fundamentals of Therapeutic Massage*, ed 4, St. Louis, 2008, Mosby.

Salvo S: *Massage Therapy Principles and Practice*, ed 3, St. Louis, 2007, Saunders.

Schwab D: What your staff needs to know about marketing your practice, *Dent Econ* 89:51–53, 1999.

Evolve Annotated Web Links

http://evolve.elsevier.com/Fritz/business

AllBusiness (www.AllBusiness.com)

American Massage Therapy Association (www.amtamassage.org)

ArticlePlanet: Marketing information (http://www.articleplanet.net/marketing)

Associated Bodywork & Massage Professionals (www.abmp.com)

AT&T Yahoo: Small business Web hosting (http://www.att.net/s/s.dll?ep=16504&only=y&ch=wh&_lid=677&_lnm=yahoo+small biz+webhosting&site=attportal)

BlueHost: Web hosting solutions (www.bluehost.com)

Google Web Hosting (www.googlewebhosting.net)

InMotion Hosting (www.inmotionhosting.com)

Massage Therapy Foundation (http://www.massagetherapyfoundation.org/)

National Certification Board for Therapeutic Massage & Bodywork (www.ncbtmb.org)

U.S. Small Business Association & U.S. Postal Service: Delivering Success video series (http://www.sba.gov/tools/audiovideo/deliveringsuccess/index.html)

U.S. Small Business Association: Marketing and outreach (http://www.sba.gov/marketingoutreach/index.html)

U.S. Small Business Association: Marketing series (http://www.sba.gov/tools/resourcelibrary/publications)

Workbook

1. Explain two basic types of marketing procedures that could be used in a massage practice.

2. What is marketing?

3. What ideas can be implemented in a practice to increase marketing for existing clients? What can be done to attract new clients?

4. Explain the value of a recall system to a client and to the massage therapist.

5. What determines the success of a recall system?

6. Explain the functions of the three basic recall systems.

_____

_____

_____

_____

_____

7. Explain the advantages and disadvantages of each of the three basic recall systems.

_____

_____

_____

_____

_____

8. What effect would a computer have on a recall system in a therapeutic massage office?

_____

_____

_____

13

INVENTORY SYSTEMS AND SUPPLY ORDERING

KEY TERMS

Back-order memo

Capital supplies

Credit memo

Expendable supplies

Inventory system

Invoice

Nonexpendable supplies

Packing slip

Purchase order

Retail stock

Statement

LEARNING OUTCOMES

Mastery of the content in this chapter will enable the reader to:

- Define key terms
- Identify three types of massage supplies
- Explain various types of inventory systems
- Establish an inventory system
- Explain factors determining supply quantity

- Describe a technique for receiving supplies
- Describe a computerized ordering system
- Identify common supply forms
- Explain the storage of hazardous materials

e Guidelines for the Learning Activities and answers to the Workbook questions are located on Evolve at http://evolve.elsevier.com/Fritz/business.

You may not think of maintaining an inventory of supplies as an important aspect of a massage business, but after you run out of clean linens or disinfecting solution, you will change your mind. You are responsible for maintaining the inventory system in the massage office. Because the massage practice has a business side and a clinical side, you need to maintain an adequate inventory in both areas. It is necessary to have a system that notifies you if supplies are low. For example, in the business office, you can place a card that says *order now* on top of the last ream of copy paper. For clinical supplies, you can keep two containers of lubricant on the shelf, and every time you remove a bottle or tube, you know you need to order another.

It is important to establish a simple inventory system that can be easily maintained. This system may be manual or computerized.

TYPES OF SUPPLIES AND RETAIL PRODUCTS

Supplies

Supplies can be divided into three categories: expendable supplies, nonexpendable supplies, and capital supplies. *Expendable supplies* are single-use items such as paper towels, stationery, massage lotions, and cleaning supplies. *Nonexpendable supplies* are reusable items that do not constitute a major expense; this category includes linens, pillows, blankets, uniforms, and magazines. *Capital supplies* are large, costly items that are seldom replaced, such as a computer, massage table, and office furniture.

Retail Products

The massage therapist may have an inventory of retail products that clients may purchase. Most common are self-massage tools, massage lubricate, essential oils, music, health-related books and magazines, and other products that clients may be interested in.

Not all materials can be purchased from one supplier, and buying from several suppliers may be more economical. Shopping locally promotes good relations and stimulates the local economy, but for economic reasons, a massage therapist may order supplies or products from a larger catalog or discount house. Purchasing office supplies from the dealers in your area is convenient, but many large wholesale supply houses provide quick service and special rates. Cleaning supplies and paper products, such as paper cups, tissues, and paper towels, can be purchased locally from a discount warehouse store and ordered in bulk. Another option for ordering is the Internet, and supply companies are increasingly merchandising online.

LEARNING ACTIVITY

Make an inventory list for a wellness massage business structure with three massage therapists working 30 hours each and completing between 10 and 20 massage sessions per week. Include expendable supplies, nonexpendable supplies, and capital supplies.
Expendable supplies

_____

_____

Nonexpendable supplies

_____

_____

Capital supplies

_____

_____

DESIGNING AN INVENTORY SYSTEM

An *inventory system* is a list of the stock and assets in the massage office. This list is divided into two or three parts: capital equipment and expendable and nonexpendable supplies. If the massage therapist plans to retail products to clients, the inventory system also needs to track stock.

Capital Equipment Inventory Control

A spreadsheet or card file can be used to maintain an inventory of capital equipment. For a spreadsheet, a form such as Excel or Access can be used, and all the major categories of supplies can be listed as headings. The card shown in Figure 13-1 is filled out for each capital item with important information about the item, including maintenance data. The card and spreadsheet systems can save much time and guesswork about servicing equipment and can be helpful to the accountant in determining depreciation for tax purposes. This information should be reviewed frequently for necessary preventive maintenance service, such as for a copy machine.

Expendable and Nonexpendable Supplies Inventory Control

Massage offices usually do not keep a large stock of nonexpendable supplies on hand; however, a list may be included in an inventory system if the massage therapist wishes. Because the expendable supplies require more attention, an inventory of these items is important. The inventory can be automated on a computer or maintained manually.

PRODUCT: Facial Massage Table		
MANUFACTURER: Paragon		MODEL: FIM10
SERIAL NUMBER: 00967-87534	PURCHASE DATE: 4/17/—	
SUPPLIER: Spa Equipment	COST: $700.	
COLOR: Taupe	WARRANTY EXPIRATION: 1/15/10	
DATE OF SERVICE	SERVICED BY	NATURE OF PROBLEM

FIGURE 13-1. Capital equipment inventory card. *(Modified from Finkbeiner BL, Finkbeiner CA:* Practice Management for the Dental Team, *ed 6, St. Louis, 2006, Mosby.)*

Retail Stock

The amount of *retail stock* that is maintained for various products in inventory varies. Items that have expiration dates need to be managed more tightly that items that do not. For example, a foot massage roller can last on the retail shelf indefinitely, whereas essential oil products do not. Items that have a short shelf life (i.e., are dated with an expiration time) need to be ordered in smaller quantities and more often so that the product is fresh and of high quality. The inventory can be automated on a computer or maintained manually.

Computerized Inventory Systems

A computerized inventory system can be created through a special software package or a database you create. The system can be simple or complex. A simple system is adequate for a small massage practice but may not be for a large, multidisciplinary business, such as a medical spa.

ⓔ See the Evolve site for screen shots of the computerized inventory system on your practice CD.

Manual Inventory Systems

For a small massage practice, a manual system is sufficient. A card system or an alphabetical list may suffice for an inventory system in many offices.

CARD SYSTEM

The card system requires a separate card for each product (Fig. 13-2). The cards list complete information about each product and its supplier, and they are placed in alphabetical order according to the product name. They are kept in a file drawer or notebook. As it becomes necessary to order an item, the card is placed in a section of the file marked *To be ordered*. After the item has been ordered, the card is moved to the *On order* section of the file. When the item arrives from the supplier, the card is replaced in its original alphabetical position in the file. If the item is out of stock and has been placed on back-order by the supplier, the card is placed in the *On back-order* section of the file.

A modification of this system leaves all the cards in the alphabetical section at all times, and the status of the item is indicated with a colored tag (Fig. 13-3). A red label may indicate *To be ordered*; blue, *On order*; and yellow, *On back-order*. This system eliminates moving the cards and the chance of misfiling, and it indicates at a glance the status of the items.

ALPHABETICAL LIST

Box 13-1 shows an example of an alphabetical list of materials for inventory. This master list includes a code number for each supplier, the name of each product, and columns for the maximum on-hand level and the minimum reorder point. This list is kept in a protective celluloid cover, and when the reorder point is reached, you place a red check mark in the appropriate space with a waxed pencil. When the items are ordered, the red check marks are erased with a tissue.

MAINTAINING THE INVENTORY SYSTEM

Identifying Reorder Points

Several techniques can be used for reordering supplies. Colored tape may be used to indicate the reorder point on small items (Fig. 13-4), or a tag can be placed on the item (Fig. 13-5). For stationery supplies, a paper tab can be inserted into the stack of materials to indicate the reorder point (Fig. 13-6).

PRODUCT: BIOTONE Lotion

Brand: Advanced Therapy Massage Crème

Supplier: BannerTherapy.com   Phone: 123.456.7890

Minimum	Maximum	Amount Ordered	Date Ordered	Unit Price

FIGURE 13-2. Inventory card. (*Modified from Finkbeiner BL, Finkbeiner CA:* Practice Management for the Dental Team, *ed 6, St. Louis, 2006, Mosby.*)

PRODUCT: BIOTONE Lotion

Brand: Advanced Therapy Massage Crème

Supplier: BannerTherapy.com   Phone: 123.456.7890

Minimum	Maximum	Amount Ordered	Date Ordered	Unit Price

FIGURE 13-3. Colored tag *(arrow)* on an inventory card. (*Modified from Finkbeiner BL, Finkbeiner CA:* Practice Management for the Dental Team, *ed 6, St. Louis, 2006, Mosby.*)

Determining Supply Quantity

In deciding how to maintain an inventory system, you must decide the minimum and maximum amounts of each item you wish to keep in stock. Certain factors can help determine these amounts:

Rate of use: Buying large quantities of infrequently used items is not cost efficient. However, buying bulk quantities of supplies used frequently is economical. For example, buying paper products in large quantities is a good idea if storage space is available.

Shelf life: Some supplies or retail product begin to deteriorate after a certain period. Manufacturers indicate an expiration date on the box. Do not purchase a large quantity of items that cannot be used before their expiration date.

Amount of capital outlay: In addition to prices, the amount of cash available often determines whether an item is purchased in bulk amounts.

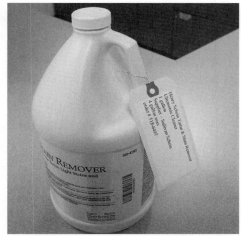

FIGURE 13-5. Tag on a bottle. *(From Finkbeiner BL, Finkbeiner CA:* Practice Management for the Dental Team, *ed 6, St. Louis, 2006, Mosby.)*

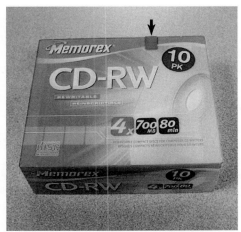

FIGURE 13-4. Colored tape *(arrow)* on small items. *(From Finkbeiner BL, Finkbeiner CA:* Practice Management for the Dental Team, *ed 6, St. Louis, 2006, Mosby.)*

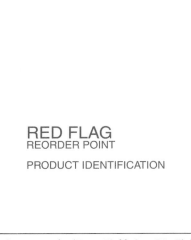

RED FLAG
REORDER POINT

PRODUCT IDENTIFICATION

FIGURE 13-6. Paper tab. *(From Finkbeiner BL, Finkbeiner CA:* Practice Management for the Dental Team, *ed 6, St. Louis, 2006, Mosby.)*

Length of delivery time: Delivery time affects the minimum quantity you wish to have in stock. With the Web-based suppliers and increasing use of delivery services, it is likely that most items ordered will arrive in 2 to 3 days. For additional charges, orders can be processed, shipped, and received in 24 hours. The phrase used to describe this is *just in time inventory.* Using these types of system is efficient for items that expire or are rarely used and when maintaining an inventory on hand is not cost efficient. If several days are required to receive an order for a frequently used item, you may wish to increase the minimum amount on hand.

Amount of storage space: In some offices, storage space is a crucial factor, and lack of it prohibits the purchase of large supplies. Consequently, a large storage space is a benefit economically and increases your efficiency. Keep this in mind when deciding on the facilities and design of the massage business.

Manufacturer's special offers: Manufacturers routinely offer special rates on various materials. However, a special price is not cost efficient if the item stays on the shelf and collects dust.

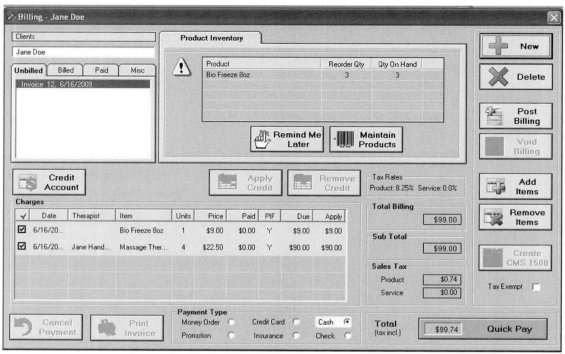

FIGURE 13-7. Record of invoice. *(Courtesy of Island Software.)*

Receiving Supplies

All incoming materials should be handled and stored safely. Every order that arrives in the office should have an invoice, a packing slip, or both. A *packing slip* is an enumeration of the enclosed items. An *invoice* is a list of the contents of the package, the price of each item enclosed, and the total charge. Some companies use the invoice as a *statement* and indicate on the form that it is the statement from which you are to pay the account. Make sure that each item listed coincides with the original order, that each item on the invoice is in the package, and that the total amount listed on the invoice is accurate. Then put the invoice in the *To be paid* file. Record all invoices in the practice management software (Fig. 13-7).

At the end of the month, you will receive a statement, or a request for payment, from the supplier. Each invoice should be checked against the entries on the statement to ensure accuracy before payment is sent. Ensure all changes to the inventory are recorded in the practice management software (Fig. 13-8).

The check is made payable to the supplier (see Chapter 16). The check number is indicated on the retained portion of the statement, the invoices are attached, and these documents are filed in the appropriate subject file.

The paper check is fast becoming a thing of the past as more businesses pay their bills electronically. Various systems are available, but the most common one used by a massage therapist is an automatic transfer of funds from the massage business's account to the supplier's account. This automatic pay and deposit system is convenient, but make sure there

are sufficient funds to cover the transfer. Double check that the invoice was paid, that the amount was correct, and that there was not a "double payment" of the same invoice.

Receiving Credit

Sometimes supplies must be returned for credit. In such cases, the massage supplier sends a *credit memo*, which indicates that the massage therapist's account has been credited for the cost of the returned item. This amount appears as a credit on the statement at the end of the month and should be recorded in the practice management software (Fig. 13-9).

Back-Ordered Supplies

Sometimes an item ordered is not in stock at the supply house, and you will receive a *back-order memo*. The supplier notifies you that the article is back-ordered, or this fact may be noted directly on the invoice. If you need the product immediately, you should attempt to obtain it from another supplier or make an alternative selection.

Purchase Orders

In large institutions, supplies are ordered through a purchasing agent. All items are listed on a requisition, and the order is keyed into a *purchase order*, a standardized order form for supplies. Each purchase order is given a number and sent to the appropriate supplier, who enters this number on all invoices when shipping the supplies.

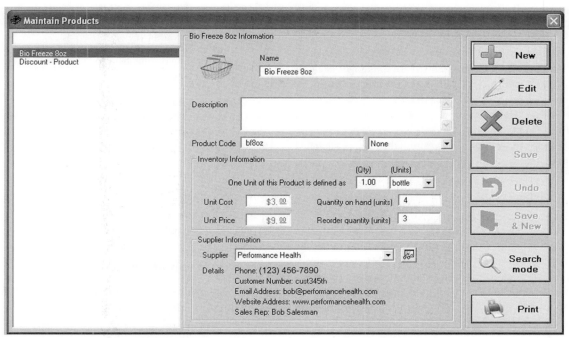

FIGURE 13-8. Inventory record. *(Courtesy of Island Software.)*

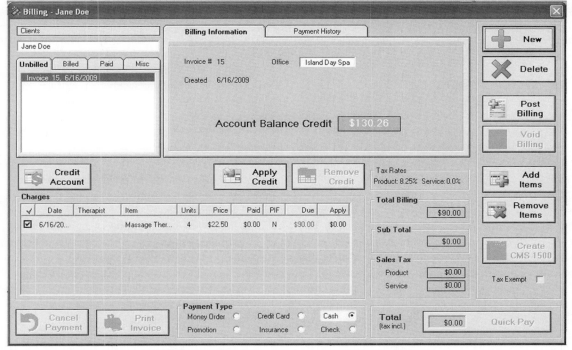

FIGURE 13-9. Credit memo. *(Courtesy of Island Software.)*

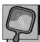

SELF-REFLECTION

How does the system of inventory management fit with my basic personality strengths? Where are challenges likely to occur? Do I tend to wait until I am completely out of something before I purchase, or am I the type of person who wants to have at least one of everything on the shelf at all times? Do I prefer to buy in bulk and overstock, or do I tend to understock? What are my strengths for this aspect of business management?

BOX 13-2	Questions to Consider in Inventory Evaluation

1. Does the system distinguish expendable, nonexpendable, and capital items?
2. Is it simple to use?
3. Does everyone understand the system?
4. Can you identify supply sources for various materials?
5. Can you determine when an item has been ordered, back-ordered, and received?
6. Is stock always current?
7. Are supplies stored safely?

Storage of Supplies

All supplies should be stored in an organized manner that allows quick and easy retrieval. Certain materials require a cool, dry, or dark location. When new materials are received, they should be stocked behind older supplies so that the older supplies are used first. When stationery supplies or large boxes are stored, a label describing the contents should be placed on the outside of each box.

Inventory Evaluation

Box 13-2 provides seven useful questions to aid the evaluation of an inventory system in a massage office.

Good Stuff from the Government

In many businesses, the cost of purchasing merchandise for resale (i.e., retailing) or the costs of purchasing and converting materials into finished products (i.e., manufacturing) represent the business's most significant expenditures. Keeping track of merchandise and materials, known as *inventory*, is important because of the considerable costs involved. This can be accomplished through a good inventory record keeping system.

INVENTORY RECORD KEEPING

Inventory record keeping establishes and maintains information on current inventory, the additions and withdrawals to inventory, and inventory balances at the end of specified periods (e.g., week, month). These records identify the products or materials, the quantities, and the value (i.e., cost) of these products or materials.

PERPETUAL INVENTORY

The perpetual inventory method starts with a physical inventory (i.e., actual count) and then adjusts this inventory for additions and withdrawals. The inventory at the end of the period is calculated by subtracting the number of units sold from the total of the beginning inventory and by adding the additional units produced, as shown in this example (activity value in units):

Beginning inventory	100
Sales	−75
Production	+95
Ending inventory (calculated)	120

The perpetual inventory method is used when reliable sales and production information is readily available and the frequent taking of physical inventories would be burdensome. However, physical inventories must be periodically taken (e.g., quarterly, annually) to check the calculated inventories. The inventory records are then adjusted to agree with the physical inventories. The financial effect of these adjustments is reflected in the balance sheet and the profit and loss statement of the business.

PERIODIC INVENTORY

The periodic inventory starts with the physical inventory taken at the end of each period. Sales or production amounts are then calculated based on the beginning and ending physical inventories. This method is used when reliable sales or production data are not readily available.

INVENTORY CONTROL

Inventory control is the management of inventory, and it relies heavily on information provided by the inventory record keeping system. Inventory is required to support the operations of the business, whether it is a retailing or manufacturing business. The proper management of inventory helps the business achieve its objectives in sales, costs, and profits. The business plan must recognize and define the role inventories will play in achieving the business objectives.

- Setting objectives for inventory: the type, quantity, cost, and order or production point (i.e., what quantity will initiate action for resupply) of products or materials
- Recording and reporting actual results (i.e., done by the inventory keeping system)
- Comparing actual results with objectives and analyzing the differences

Good Stuff from the Government—cont'd

■ Taking action to correct problems or improve business performance

Inventory supports the sales activity. This means having what the customer is willing to buy, when he or she needs it, at a price that provides an acceptable profit to the business. Inventory control is integrated with systems that track sales, production, and purchasing activities.

Inventory Strategies

Every business competes within an industry and each industry has a life cycle. The strategies employed by the business depend on where in the life cycle the industry is. The management of inventories is influenced by this life cycle. There are four stages in the life cycle of an industry:

Development: Uniquely new products are being developed and market tested. Products must be available for market testing. There is little concern about inventory investment, other than to be sure products are available for market testing and development.

Growth: The product has been demonstrated to have significant market potential, and the business strives to gain a major market share. Investment in inventory is heavy to ensure product availability to gain a significant market share.

Maturity: Growth has leveled off. Inventories are very closely controlled to keep investment in them just sufficient to maintain the market share.

Aging: A period of retrenchment occurs as competitive industries take away or eliminate markets. Inventories decline as unprofitable and marginally profitable segments of the business are weeded out.

The proper control of inventories is essential to the success of any business in which investment in inventories is significant. Awareness of the competition and the state of new product development is just as important as a finely honed record-keeping system. Although the record-keeping system is important, how it is applied will determine the success of the business.

Modified from Anderson DW, editor: Handbook for Small Business, ed 6, Hyannis, MA, SCORE Chapter 225, 1989. Available at http://www.sba.gov/idc/groups/public/documents/sba_homepage/pub_mp31.pdf (accessed June 2009).

CD Review the part of the tutorial on the CD about maintaining inventory. Then make up an inventory management file for three products or supplies (e.g., massage lotion, paper towels, disinfectant). Pretend that you have used one of the items in your practice, and then readjust your inventory.

Continue to explore all of the features of the software program.

SUMMARY

Maintaining inventory is important for your massage business. For example, if you run out of massage lotion before a client's appointment, the shortage is not a good representation of your business skills. Choose an inventory system that will work for you. Whether it is a computer software program, index card method, or a list of where you keep supplies, keep the system current. The amount of any supplies you keep on hand is determined by volume of use and expiration dates of massage lotions or oils. As your massage business changes, so may your usual ordering process. You may need to order more or less often or perhaps change quantities of order. You must determine payment procedures, a filing system for supply receipts, and a system of purchase orders. The storage area may determine the quantity of supplies that are kept on hand and may determine your inventory system. A label on the outside of boxes is mandatory to ensure efficient ordering. An inventory system is an important aspect of a smoothly running massage therapy business.

Bibliography

Tomey AM: *Guide to Nursing Management and Leadership*, ed 8, St. Louis, 2009, Mosby.

⊜ Evolve Annotated Web Links

http://evolve.elsevier.com/Fritz/business

U.S. Small Business Administration, Handbook for Small Business (http://www.sba.gov/idc/groups/public/documents/sba_home page/pub_mp31.pdf)

1. Explain the following terms: expendable, nonexpendable, capital items, invoice, statement, credit slip, and back-order inventory.

_____
_____
_____
_____
_____
_____
_____
_____
_____
_____
_____
_____

2. Explain the processing of an item from the time it is ordered until it is received in the office and the statement is paid.

_____
_____
_____
_____
_____
_____
_____
_____
_____
_____
_____
_____
_____
_____

4. Make a master supply list of 10 common expendable massage supplies, and indicate the maximum and minimum levels, based on the factors that determine supply amounts discussed in this chapter. Identify the manufacturer and, if possible, the most cost-effective supplier of these products in your area.

_____
_____
_____
_____
_____
_____
_____
_____
_____
_____
_____
_____

5. The item was purchased as capital equipment. Make out a card or enter into a database the following information: A massage table was purchased on October 17, 2009, from Apex Massage Supply for $375. It has a 12-month warranty from the date of purchase.

INSURANCE REIMBURSEMENT FOR MASSAGE THERAPY SERVICES

KEY TERMS

Administrator
Alternative benefit plan
Cafeteria plan
Capitation
Claim form
Closed panel system
Copayment
Covered services
Customary fee

Deductible
Direct reimbursement
Fee schedule
Health Insurance Portability and
   Accountability Act of 1996
   (HIPAA)
Health maintenance organization
   (HMO)
Insurer

Limitations
Medicaid
Preferred provider organization (PPO)
   plan
Premium
Reasonable and customary (R&C)
   plan
Reimbursement
Usual fee

LEARNING OUTCOMES

Mastery of the content in this chapter will enable the reader to:

- Define key terms
- Describe massage as a reimbursable treatment for complementary and alternative medicine (CAM)

- Explain health insurance benefits programs and how claims are made

Ⓔ Guidelines for the Learning Activities and answers to the Workbook questions are located on Evolve at http://evolve.elsevier.com/Fritz/business.

The eligibility of therapeutic massage for health insurance benefits continues to be a controversial issue. This textbook does not attempt to take a position on the benefits or difficulties of various forms of insurance *reimbursement*. Instead, circumstances such as state regulations, type of massage business (e.g., spa services, hospital), and the nature of the client's goals will determine whether the massage application qualifies for insurance compensation. There is a trend toward increasing access for coverage for complementary and alterative health care services, but the process remains confusing, and continuity among providers does not exist. The Internet allows access to health information on general and alternative therapies, empowering consumers to seek a variety of approaches to healing and wellness.

As massage therapy becomes more common in health care settings that typically used health insurance for service compensation, it is important to understand how the health insurance system functions. It is not necessary for massage therapists to accept health care insurance reimbursement for the massage services they offer. The client cash-pay system has many advantages. Many health care practitioners that used to take insurance payments are now or considering opting out and returning to a cash-for-services-rendered system. You may choose a career path that requires you to bill insurance directly or maintain necessary documentation so that the insurance biller can adequately request payment for service, and clients will ask questions about the availability of health care insurance reimbursement for massage.

COMPLEMENTARY AND ALTERNATIVE MEDICINE

The globalization of society and the interweaving of cultural diversity have influenced the demand for a variety of healing practices. Escalating costs and decreasing patient satisfaction have encouraged many to explore multidisciplinary health care services.

When surveys conducted in the 1990s discovered how many Americans were using complementary and alternative medicine (CAM) and how many were willing to pay out-of-pocket expenses for these additional products and services, *insurers* felt some pressure to include at least some of these treatments in their plans. This occurred despite the fact that scientific evidence did not uniformly support their effectiveness (and still does not).

Millions of Americans use complementary and alternative health care approaches every year, often in conjunction with conventional medical care. However, because qualified integrated care is not covered by Medicare or Medicaid and other insurers, it is not equally available to all Americans. The Integrated Healthcare Policy Consortium (IHPC) is a broad coalition of health care professionals and organizations driving public policy to ensure all Americans access to a safe, high-quality, health care system that includes conventional, complementary, and alternative approaches, practiced by qualified providers working in respectful collaboration to offer effective patient-centered care.

The Academic Consortium for Complementary and Alternative Health Care (ACCAHC) was formed in 2004 under the auspices of IHPC's Education Task Force. Because ACCAHC has a strong commitment to public safety and accountability, it works only with health care professions that have established clear regulatory mechanisms in the United States or are in the process of doing so. The fully regulated CAM professions in the United States include the following:

- Acupuncture and Oriental medicine
- Chiropractic medicine
- Direct-entry midwifery
- Massage therapy
- Naturopathic medicine

IHPC has documented notable events in the development of integrative health care in the United States (http://ihpc. info/resources/timeline.shtml). The following reports from 2001 through 2006 reflect of progress of integrative health care development. The links and brief description of each report are provided on the Evolve Web site. It would be prudent in your professional development to review these documents:

National Policy Dialogue Final Report, 2001 (http://ihpc. info/resources/NPDFR.pdf)

White House Commission on Complementary and Alternative Medicine Policy Final Report, 2002 (http://ihpc.info/ resources/WHCCAM.pdf)

Institute of Medicine Report on Complementary and Alternative Medicine in the United States, 2002 (http://ihpc. info/resources/IMRCAM.pdf)

Mapping the Emergence of Integrative Medicine, 2003 (http://ihpc.info/resources/Clohesy2003.pdf)

National Education Dialogue Progress Report, 2005 (http:// ihpc.info/resources/NEDPR.pdf)

Coalition for Patients' Rights Statement, 2006 (http://ihpc. info/resources/statement.shtml)

These initiatives and developments have and will continue to have implications for massage therapy practice as part of an integrated health care system. You need to

SELF-REFLECTION

What type of CAM health care services do I use? How do I pay for it? How much do I pay? Am I willing to pay additional premiums for health insurance to have benefits that cover CAM health care? How much am I willing to pay? What types of coverage do I want? What does integrated health care mean? Is health care the same or different from medical care?

be able to function as a massage professional within these environments, especially when considering health insurance coverage for massage services.

The increasing research on the benefits of therapeutic massage and the establishment of the underlying physiologic mechanisms related to these benefits are beginning to influence the insurance providers. Coverage of CAM is largely determined on a state-by-state basis, but certain plans are more flexible than others. Clients need to inquire regarding their insurance reimbursement options. Some CAM-friendly states, such as Connecticut or Washington, where "naturopathic doctors" are state-licensed are setting the example. One example of a CAM-friendly managed care company is Oxford Health Insurance, based in Connecticut.

Most health care plans cover chiropractic and osteopathic manipulation. Acupuncture has gained licensure in many states and is becoming more routinely covered. Some plans also cover treatments such as massage. One popular area of CAM that is almost never covered by insurance is the use of dietary and herbal supplements.

Some insurers include CAM providers in their networks, offering discounted fees. Other insurers may pay part of the cost of CAM treatments if they are ordered by a medical doctor. For the most part, insurance plans that cover CAM treatments have high deductibles, and people must pay a higher amount out of pocket before the insurance steps in to help cover costs. Most insurers pay only for a limited number of visits, which is usually far fewer than the number recommended for complete treatment. Some insurance carriers offer a policy rider, which is extra insurance (for an extra fee) that covers CAM treatments. These are available from a number of reputable insurance companies.

Health spending accounts, also known as health savings accounts (HSAs), are savings accounts specifically set aside to pay for health care services that are often offered outside traditional health insurance plans. Individuals are able to pay for most CAM treatments with HSA funds. The money put in these accounts is tax deductible, which can mean great savings.

MASSAGE AS A REIMBURSABLE TREATMENT

A common question is whether massage therapy should be covered by health insurance as a medical treatment. There is agreement that massage is a valuable heath service. The question is whether it is a medical treatment. Massage application that is result oriented and treatment that is specifically directed to resolve conditions that have been diagnosed and supervised by a physician are most likely to be eligible for insurance coverage. The focus of the massage treatment is on the areas of the body related to the medical diagnosis and prescription, and massage usually is billed in

15-minute segments using current procedural terminology and adhering to the usual and customary reimbursement *fee schedule*.

For massage therapists to state that they are treating someone, they must first be able to legally determine what it is that they are treating. Because it is beyond massage therapists' scope of practice to diagnose and prescribe, they must work from a doctor's prescription if they are claiming to treat a specific condition. The massage therapist must also follow the prescribing physician's treatment orders. The only requirement for being eligible to provide massage that qualifies for insurance payment is that massage therapists are practicing legally in their jurisdictions. There is no specific certification for so-called medical massage that increases the chances that massage will be covered.

Four states mandate that massage be included in health insurance coverage. According to the Council for Affordable Health Care (see Evolve Annotated Web Links at the end of this chapter), they are Washington, New Hampshire, Utah, and Maryland. Other states such as Florida and New York have regulations providing for reimbursement of services for therapeutic massage. The therapists must be licensed in that particular state, and to be licensed, they must have met the state's required educational standards. Because these regulations change, check with the regulatory agencies and individual insurance companies to confirm ability to receive coverage (Box 14-1). Figure 14-1 shows the sources of U.S. health care financing.

Many states allow licensed therapists to bill for personal injuries (e.g., car accidents) if there is a referring physician involved in the case. Some of these states also allow for workers' compensation reimbursement. In some unlicensed states, a person who practices massage therapy without a license may be able to bill insurance for personal injury to a client, such as a car accident, but these are determined on an individual basis. The health insurance world is very complex, and most providers rely on specially trained insurance billers to handle these matters.

HEALTH INSURANCE BENEFITS PROGRAMS

The insurance carrier's method of reimbursement depends on the plan design. The two basic models of benefits programs are indemnity and capitation, although many variations of each model exist (Fig. 14-2).

Indemnity

Indemnity programs are most often referred to as fee-for-service programs. This type of program provides payment on a service-by-service basis, and reimbursement may be made to the enrollee or, by assignment, to the service provider. The following list describes types of fee-for-service programs:

EXPERT Outlook

The owner and director of the College of Integrative Healthcare in Oceanside, California, Dr. Randy Snyder, gives his perspective on the role of massage in health care.

There is currently an increased trend in health care to move more services into the purview of vocationally trained individuals. Some of the reasons include greater cost effectiveness and greater access to larger pools of trained individuals. This will help the massage profession in many ways, as massage therapists are one of the few vocationally trained professionals in the complementary and alternative health care arena. Your services will continue to grow in demand, and your skills will continually need to be updated and enhanced to accommodate this growth. Health care will become a team approach, requiring you to work and communicate more effectively in a variety of environments and under the supervision of other healthcare professionals. You will have opportunities you never expected if you expand your knowledge and thinking and become a lifelong learner!

I work as a utilization manager for an insurance company and have reviewed many treatment plans submitted by massage therapists. Although managed care is new to most massage therapists, it is not new to most health care providers. There are several things you must know about insurance reimbursement. First, realize that most insurance companies have resources that allow you to access information about clinical reasoning and treatment planning. These resources are generally provided through an operations manual or by electronic access via a CD or the Internet. Often we tend to overlook this because we want to speed through the process as easily as possible. This often hinders our ability to work adequately within the system and can cause frustration. Think of it this way: if you're going to play the game, you need to learn the rules.

It is important to have certain information presented through medical records or insurance forms (now mostly electronic) that give the patient's complaints and medical history. The frequency and duration of complaints, as well as the mechanism of injury, if available, should be described. This is usually recorded on a patient intake form by the patient and includes biographical information such as name, address, date of birth, and so forth. In addition, you will need to provide assessment information in the form of postural evaluation, gait, and/or palpation. These findings can be further clarified using graded information (mild, moderate, severe) with regard to range of motion, tenderness, muscle tone, and trigger points. Although it is not necessary to have all this information recorded for every complaint, you should provide enough findings to adequately evaluate all complaints. If you intend to treat something, you need assessment findings that justify the treatment plan, and are reasonable based on the magnitude of the complaints. Once you have assessed the patient, your treatment frequency and duration should be based on the particular needs of the patient, taking all historical and assessment information into consideration. This information should include any historical information about comorbidities (e.g., diabetes, fibromyalgia) that might influence how the patient responds to care. It is not necessary to have a physician's referral with all insurance companies, but referral and comanagement to or from another health care professional must be recorded when indicated. All these things have to do with the accountability factors in health care that other health care professionals must adhere to. The documentation should support and justify your treatment request in a rational manner based on the available evidence-based literature and/or consensus of the profession. Outcomes measurements and tools should be used to gauge client progress.

If someone else is going to pay the bill, they have the right and obligation to review this information. In fact, it goes farther than that. It is also based on health and safety concerns for which the insurance company is held accountable by regulators and accreditation agencies. As our government wrestles with a health care reform bill, there is much talk of comparative effectiveness research where treatments will be compared to one another. This is to help determine which treatments (including massage therapy) are safest as well as most therapeutic and cost effective.

Think, learn, and grow. Don't just graduate and remain stagnant. In this day and age, you will never succeed in any profession unless you stay actively involved in professional development.

BOX 14-1	Regulation of Insurance Billing for Therapeutic Massage

The information covers who may treat and the procedures and the authorization requirements for outpatient therapy services.

Who may perform physical, occupational, or massage therapy?

QUALIFICATIONS	Physical Therapist (PT)	Occupational Therapy (OT)	Massage Therapy (MT)
Must be	Licensed physical therapist	Licensed occupational therapist	Licensed massage practitioner (LMP)
May be	PT assistant under the direction of a licensed PT	OT assistant under the direction of a licensed OT	Not applicable

BOX 14-1	Regulation of Insurance Billing for Therapeutic Massage—cont'd

Who else may perform these services?

■ Medical or osteopathic physicians who are board qualified or board certified in medicine and rehabilitation

■ Attending physicians who are not board qualified or board certified in physical medicine and rehabilitation. Special payment policies apply. See the Physical Medicine chapter in the Payment Policies book (http://www.lni.wa.gov/ClaimsIns/Files/ProviderPay/FeeSchedules/2008FS/Marfsall.pdf).

Can I get paid for services performed by other personnel?

No. The department of labor and industries (L&I) does not pay for services provided by

■ Exercise physiologists

■ Kinesiologists

■ Athletic trainers

■ Students

■ Aides

■ Other unlicensed personnel

Do I need to obtain authorization for the first 12 (PT/OT) or 6 (MT) visits?

No, but the services need to be ordered by the injured worker's attending doctor, physician assistant, or nurse practitioner.

What needs to be done to treat beyond the first 12 (PT/OT) or 6 (MT) visits?

You must do the following:

■ Document improvement in the worker's condition

■ Document continued referral from the attending physician

■ Obtain authorization

Further treatment may be denied by the claim manager if documentation is not available or authorization is not obtained.

How do I obtain authorization for additional (outpatient) visits?

For state fund claims, effective July 1, 2007, the following rules apply:

Standard outpatient and work conditioning services: action required

No. of Visits	PT Only or OT Only	PT/OT Combined
Visits 1-12	No authorization is needed.	If fewer than 12 visits for both disciplines, no authorization is needed.
Visits 13-24	Fax OT/PT Treatment Authorization Fax Request (F248-055-000) form for authorization. (http://www.lni.wa.gov/FormPub/Detail.asp?DocID=1657)	If visits are between 13 and 24 for either discipline, fax OT/PT Treatment Authorization Fax Request (F248-055-000) form for authorization. (http://www.lni.wa.gov/FormPub/Detail.asp?DocID=1657)
Visits beyond 24	Request Utilization Review from Qualis directly. Claim manager will authorize or deny. (http://www.lni.wa.gov/ClaimsIns/Providers/Treatment/UtilReview/Therapy/requestUR.asp)	If more than 24 visits for either discipline, request Utilization Review from Qualis directly. Claim manager will authorize or deny. (http://www.lni.wa.gov/ClaimsIns/Providers/Treatment/UtilReview/Therapy/requestUR.asp)

Visit counts are the total number of visits per claim. New referrals, restart of therapy after surgery, or treatment of new conditions on the same claim do not start again at visit 1. Physical and occupational therapy visits accumulate separately. If work conditioning is provided by PT and OT and more than 24 visits have previously occurred for either therapy discipline, utilization review is required. If work conditioning is denied, L&I will allow up to 12 visits for the discipline that has not reached 12 visits.

Work Hardening	Action Required
All services	Request authorization from claim manager. Claim manager will authorize or deny.

Massage (MT)	Action Required
Visits beyond first 6	Use the Massage Practitioner Treatment Authorization Fax Request (F248-357-000) form (http://www.lni.wa.gov/FormPub/Detail.asp?DocID=2229), or make a referral to the claim manager using the Provider Hotline 1-800-848-0811.

For Self-Insured claims, contact the self-insured employer's claim manager.

From Washington State Department of Labor and Industries.

Usual, customary, and reasonable (UCR) plan: Payment for covered benefits is based on a combination of usual, customary, and reasonable fee criteria.

Reasonable and customary (R&C) plan: Payment for covered benefits is based on *reasonable and customary fee* criteria.

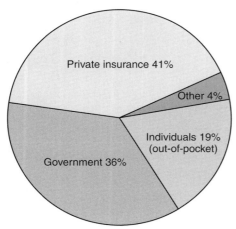

FIGURE 14-1. Sources of financing for health care. *(From Yoder-Wise PS:* Leading and Managing in Nursing, *ed 4, St. Louis, 2007, Mosby.)*

Preferred provider organization (PPO) plan: A participating massage therapist agrees to accept discounted fees for *covered services* rendered to plan enrollees.

Exclusive provider organization (EPO) plan: Benefits are provided only if care is rendered by institutional and professional providers with whom the plan contracts. Some exceptions may be allowed for emergency and out-of-area services.

Point of service plan: Benefit carrier reimbursement levels are determined by the participation status of the massage therapist rendering treatment.

Table of allowances plan: Covered services have an assigned dollar amount that represents the total dollar amount payable for each service.

Open panel system: Any service provider may participate, enrollees may receive massage treatment from any licensed massage therapist, benefits may be payable to the enrollee or the massage therapist, and the massage therapist may accept or refuse any enrollee.

Closed panel system: Enrollees can receive benefits only when services are provided by massage therapists who have signed an agreement with the benefit plan to provide treatment to eligible clients.

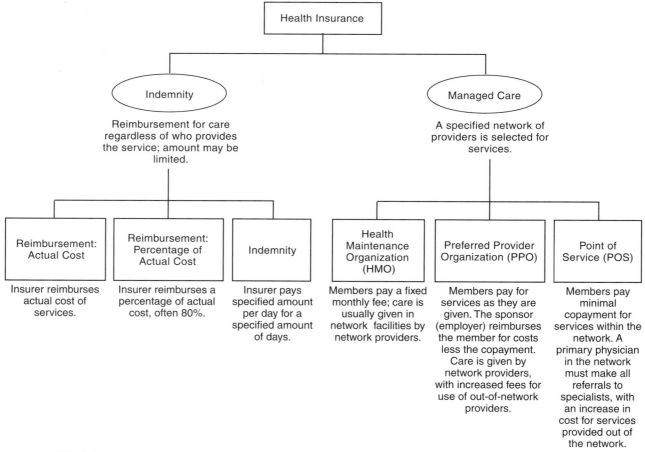

FIGURE 14-2. Forms of health insurance. *(From Gerdin J:* Health Careers Today, *ed. 4, St. Louis, Mosby, 2007.)*

Capitation

Capitation is a benefits delivery system in which a health care professional contracts with the program's sponsor or *administrator* to provide all or most of the health services covered under the program in return for a fixed monthly payment per covered person (per capita). Such a program is also called a *health maintenance organization* (HMO), and it typically is a closed panel system; that is, enrollees select a primary care physician from a list of participating providers, and they go to that office for all their health care unless the primary care physician provides a written referral to a specialist. Some exceptions are made for emergency and out-of-area services. Enrollees usually have no out-of-pocket costs for routine services.

Alternative Benefit Plans

Employers or associations may elect to offer an *alternative benefit plan* for supplemental massage coverage. In most cases, the enrollee pays the massage therapist directly. Examples of this type of plan include discount cards, HSAs, and direct reimbursement.

Large employers or associations may contract with massage clinics to deliver massage services to their enrollees for a discounted rate (i.e., use of a discount card). Many massage benefit carriers recruit massage therapist to participate in their programs. Although the massage therapist may be required to discount fees to enrollees, participation is a proven method for obtaining clients contributing to practice building. When massage therapists sign a participation contract with a benefits carrier, they agree to certain terms and conditions of payment for services rendered to enrollees. Each carrier has a unique set of terms of participation.

HSAs allow individuals to create a tax-free savings account that can be used to pay for deductibles or medical expenses not covered by a health insurance plan. The federal government allows eligible employers to offer their employees a pre-tax salary savings account for payment assistance with health care–related expenses. The maximum amount employees can contribute is $4000 per year for eligible medical, dental, vision, and prescription expenses. Massage may be covered. Contributions to the account are made by payroll deduction, and employees save money because no federal or state taxes or Federal Insurance Contributions Act (FICA) withdrawals are taken out of their earnings. As of January 1, 2004, millions of Americans younger than 65 years old had access to HSAs, which promise to revolutionize health care in America. An HSA is a tax-free savings account that works like an Individual Retirement Account (IRA), except that the money is intended to be used for qualified health care costs. Most rules and procedures that apply to IRAs also apply to HSAs. Massage may be a qualified expense if a physician or chiropractor recommends it, but not if clients decide to seek it on their own. More information is provided in IRS Publication 502 (Box 14-2)

Direct reimbursement plans offer another alternative. An employer or organization can set up a self-funded program for reimbursing covered individuals based on a percentage of the amount spent for massage care (Box 14-3).

BOX 14-2   The Basics of Health Savings Accounts

What is a health savings account?

A health savings account (HSA) is an alternative to traditional health insurance. It is a savings product that offers a different way for consumers to pay for their health care. HSAs enable you to pay for current health expenses and save for future qualified medical and retiree health expenses on a tax-free basis.

You must be covered by a high-deductible health plan (HDHP) to take advantage of HSAs. An HDHP usually costs less than traditional health care coverage, and the money that you save on insurance can be put into the HSA.

You own and you control the money in your HSA. Decisions on how to spend or invest the money are made by you without relying on a third party or a health insurer. You decide what types of investments to make with the money in the account to make it grow.

What is a high-deductible health plan?

You must have an HDHP if you want to open an HSA. Sometimes referred to as a "catastrophic" health insurance plan, an HDHP is an inexpensive health insurance plan that usually does not pay for the first several thousand dollars of health care expenses (i.e., your deductible) but does cover your medical expenses after that. The savings part of your policy is available to help you pay for the expenses your plan does not cover.

To qualify to open an HSA in 2008, your HDHP minimum deductible had to be at least $1100 (self-only coverage) or $2,200 (family coverage). The annual out-of-pocket (including deductibles and copays) for 2008 cannot exceed $5500 (self-only coverage) or $11,200 (family coverage). HDHPs can have first-dollar coverage (no deductible) for preventive care and apply higher out-of-pocket limits (plus copays and coinsurance) for non-network services.

How can I get a health savings account?

Consumers can sign up for HSAs with banks, credit unions, insurance companies, and other approved companies. Your employer may also set up a plan for employees.

How much does an HSA cost?

An HSA is a savings account into which you can deposit money on a tax-preferred basis. You purchase an HDHP, an inexpensive plan that will cover you if your medical expenses exceed the funds you have in your HSA.

From United States Department of the Treasury, http://www.ustreas.gov/offices/public-affairs/hsa/faq-basics.shtml

BOX 14-3   Employment-Based Health Insurance Surveys

DEFINITIONS OF HEALTH INSURANCE TERMS

In February 2002, the federal government's Interdepartmental Committee on Employment-Based Health Insurance Surveys approved the following set of definitions for use in federal surveys collecting employer-based health insurance data. The U.S. Bureau of Labor Statistics (BLS) National Compensation Survey uses these definitions in its data collection procedures and publications. The definitions are periodically reviewed and updated by the Committee.

Administrative Services Only (ASO): An arrangement in which an employer hires a third party to deliver to the employer administrative services, such as claims processing and billing; the employer bears the risk for claims. This is common in self-insured health care plans.

Coinsurance: A form of medical cost sharing in a health insurance plan that requires an insured person to pay a stated percentage of medical expenses after the deductible amount, if any, was paid. After any deductible amount and coinsurance are paid, the insurer is responsible for the rest of the reimbursement for covered benefits up to allowed charges; the individual also may be responsible for any charges in excess of what the insurer determines to be "usual, customary, and reasonable." Coinsurance rates may differ if services are received from an approved provider (i.e., a provider with whom the insurer has a contract or an agreement specifying payment levels and other contract requirements) or if received by providers not on the approved list. In addition to overall coinsurance rates, rates may also be different for different types of services.

Copayment: A form of medical cost sharing in a health insurance plan that requires an insured person to pay a fixed dollar amount when a medical service is received. The insurer is responsible for the rest of the reimbursement. There may be separate copayments for different services. Some plans require that a deductible first be met for some specific services before a copayment applies.

Deductible: A fixed dollar amount during the benefit period, usually a year, that an insured person pays before the insurer starts to make payments for covered medical services. Plans may have per-individual and family deductibles. Some plans may have separate deductibles for specific services. For example, a plan may have a hospitalization deductible per admission. Deductibles may be different if services are received from an approved provider or received from providers not on the approved list.

Flexible spending accounts or arrangements (FSA): Accounts offered and administered by employers that provide a way for employees to set aside, out of their paycheck, pretax dollars to pay for the employee's share of insurance *premiums* or medical expenses not covered by the employer's health plan. The employer may also make contributions to an FSA. Typically, benefits or cash must be used within the given benefit year, or the employee loses the money. Flexible spending accounts can also be provided to cover childcare expenses, but those accounts must be established separately from medical FSAs.

Flexible benefits plan (cafeteria plan or IRS 125 Plan): A benefit program under Section 125 of the Internal Revenue Code that offers employees a choice between permissible taxable benefits, including cash, and nontaxable benefits such as life and health insurance, vacations, retirement plans, and child care. Although a common core of benefits may be required, the employee can determine how his or her remaining benefit dollars are to be allocated for each type of benefit from the total amount promised by the employer. Sometimes, employee contributions may be made for additional coverage.

Fully insured plan: A plan in which the employer contracts with another organization to assume financial responsibility for the enrollees' medical claims and for all incurred administrative costs.

Gatekeeper: Under some health insurance arrangements, a gatekeeper is responsible for the administration of the patient's treatment; the gatekeeper coordinates and authorizes all medical services, laboratory studies, specialty referrals, and hospitalizations.

Group purchasing arrangement: Any of a wide array of arrangements in which two or more small employers purchase health insurance collectively, often through a common intermediary who acts on their collective behalf. Such arrangements may be called cooperatives, alliances, or business groups on health. They are different from one another along a number of dimensions, including governance, functions, and status under federal and state laws. Some are set up or chartered by states, whereas others are entirely private enterprises. Some centralize more of the purchasing functions than others, including functions such as risk pooling, price negotiation, choice of health plans offered to employees, and various administrative tasks. Depending on their functions, they may be subject to different state and federal rules. For example, they may be regulated as Multiple Employer Welfare Arrangements (MEWAs).

Association health plans: This term is sometimes used loosely to refer to any health plan sponsored by an association. It also has a precise definition under the Health Insurance Portability and Accountability Act of 1996 that exempts from certain requirements insurers that sell insurance to small employers only through association health plans that meet the definition.

HEALTH CARE PLANS AND SYSTEMS

Indemnity plan: A type of medical plan that reimburses the patient or provider as expenses are incurred.

Conventional indemnity plan: An indemnity that allows the participant the choice of any provider without effect on reimbursement. These plans reimburse the patient or provider as expenses are incurred.

Preferred provider organization (PPO) plan: An indemnity plan by which coverage is provided to participants through a network of selected health care providers (e.g., hospitals, physicians). The enrollees may go outside the network but would then incur larger costs in the form of higher deductibles, higher coinsurance rates, or nondiscounted charges from the providers.

Exclusive provider organization (EPO) plan: A more restrictive type of preferred provider organization plan under which employees must use providers from the specified network of physicians and hospitals to receive coverage; there is no coverage for care received from a non-network provider, except in an emergency situation.

BOX 14-3	Employment-Based Health Insurance Surveys—cont'd

Health maintenance organization (HMO): A health care system that assumes the financial risks associated with providing comprehensive medical services (i.e., insurance and service risk) and the responsibility for health care delivery in a particular geographic area to HMO members, usually in return for a fixed, prepaid fee. Financial risk may be shared with the providers participating in the HMO.

Group Model HMO: An HMO that contracts with a single multispecialty medical group to provide care to the HMO's membership. The group practice may work exclusively with the HMO, or it also may provide services to non-HMO patients. The HMO pays the medical group a negotiated, per capita rate, which the group distributes among its physicians, usually on a salaried basis.

Staff Model HMO: A type of closed-panel HMO (in which patients can receive services only through a limited number of providers) in which physicians are employees of the HMO. The physicians see patients in the HMO's own facilities.

Network Model HMO: An HMO model that contracts with multiple physician groups to provide services to HMO members; it may involve large single and multispecialty groups. The physician groups may provide services to both HMO and non-HMO plan participants.

Individual Practice Association (IPA) HMO: A type of health care provider organization composed of a group of independent practicing physicians who maintain their own offices and band together for the purpose of contracting their services to HMOs. An IPA may contract with and provide services to both HMO and non-HMO plan participants.

Point-of-service (POS) plan: A POS plan is an HMO/PPO hybrid, sometimes referred to as an open-ended HMO when offered by an HMO. POS plans resemble HMOs for in-network services. Services received outside of the network are usually reimbursed in a manner similar to conventional indemnity plans (i.e., provider reimbursement based on a fee schedule or usual, customary, and reasonable charges).

Physician-hospital organization (PHO): Alliances between physicians and hospitals to help providers attain market share, improve bargaining power, and reduce administrative costs. These entities sell their services to managed care organizations or directly to employers.

Managed care plans: Managed care plans usually provide comprehensive health services to their members and offer financial incentives for patients to use the providers who belong to the plan. Examples of managed care plans include HMOs, PPOs, EPOs, and POSs.

Managed care provisions: Features within health plans that provide insurers with a way to manage the cost, use, and quality of health care services received by group members.

Examples of managed care provisions include:

  Preadmission certification: An authorization for hospital admission given by a health care provider to a group member before their hospitalization. Failure to obtain a preadmission certification in non-emergency situations reduces or eliminates the health care provider's obligation to pay for services rendered.

  Utilization review: The process of reviewing the appropriateness and quality of care provided to patients. Utilization review may take place before, during, or after the services are rendered.

  Preadmission testing: A requirement designed to encourage patients to obtain necessary diagnostic services on an outpatient basis before non-emergency hospital admission. The testing is designed to reduce the length of a hospital stay.

  Non-emergency weekend admission restriction: A requirement that imposes limits on reimbursement to patients for non-emergency weekend hospital admissions.

  Second surgical opinion: A cost-management strategy that encourages or requires patients to obtain the opinion of another doctor after a physician has recommended that a non-emergency or elective surgery be performed. Programs may be voluntary or mandatory in that reimbursement is reduced or denied if the participant does not obtain the second opinion. Plans usually require that such opinions be obtained from board-certified specialists with no personal or financial interest in the outcome.

  Maximum plan dollar limit: The maximum amount payable by the insurer for covered expenses for the insured and each covered dependent while covered under the health plan. Plans can have a yearly or a lifetime maximum dollar limit. The most typical maximum is a lifetime amount of $1 million per individual.

  Maximum out-of-pocket expense: The maximum dollar amount a group member is required to pay out of pocket during a year. Until this maximum is met, the plan and group member shares in the cost of covered expenses. After the maximum is reached, the insurance carrier pays all covered expenses, often up to a lifetime maximum (see previous definition).

Medical savings accounts (MSAs): Savings accounts designated for out-of-pocket medical expenses. In an MSA, employers and individuals are allowed to contribute to a savings account on a pretax basis and carry over the unused funds at the end of the year.

Minimum premium plan (MPP): A plan in which the employer and the insurer agree that the employer will be responsible for paying all claims up to an agreed-on aggregate level, with the insurer responsible for the excess. The insurer usually is also responsible for processing claims and administrative services.

Multiple Employer Welfare Arrangement (MEWA): MEWA is a technical term under federal law that encompasses any arrangement not maintained pursuant to a collective bargaining agreement (other than a state-licensed insurance company or an HMO) that provides health insurance benefits to the employees of two or more private employers. Some MEWAs are sponsored by associations that are local, specific to a trade or industry, and exist for business purposes other than providing health insurance. Such MEWAs most often are regulated as employee health benefit plans under the Employee Retirement Income Security Act of 1974 (ERISA),

(Continued)

BOX 14-3	Employment-Based Health Insurance Surveys—cont'd

although states generally retain the right to regulate them, much the way states regulate insurance companies. They can be funded through tax-exempt trusts known as Voluntary Employees Beneficiary Associations (VEBAs), and they can and often do use these trusts to self-insure rather than to purchase insurance policies. Other MEWAs are sponsored by Chambers of Commerce or similar organizations of relatively unrelated employers. MEWAs are not considered to be health plans under ERISA. Instead, each participating employer's plan is regulated separately under ERISA. States are free to regulate the MEWAs themselves. These MEWAs tend to serve as vehicles for participating employers to buy insurance policies from state-licensed insurance companies or HMOs. They do not tend to self-insure.

Multi-employer health plan: An employee health benefit plan maintained pursuant to a collective bargaining agreement that includes employees of two or more employers. These plans are also known as Taft-Hartley plans or jointly administered plans. They are subject to federal but not state law (although states may regulate any insurance policies that they buy). They often self-insure.

Premium: Agreed on fees paid for coverage of medical benefits for a defined benefit period. Premiums can be paid by employers, unions, employees, or shared by the insured individual and the plan sponsor.

Premium equivalent: For self-insured plans, the cost per covered employee or the amount the firm would expect to reflect the cost of claims paid, administrative costs, and stop-loss premiums.

Primary care physician (PCP): A physician who serves as a group member's primary contact within the health plan. In a managed care plan, the primary care physician provides basic medical services, coordinates, and if required by the plan, authorizes referrals to specialists and hospitals.

Reinsurance: The acceptance by one or more insurers, called reinsurers or assuming companies, of a portion of the risk underwritten by another insurer that has contracted with an employer for the entire coverage.

Self-insured plan: A plan offered by employers who directly assume the major cost of health insurance for their employees. Some self-insured plans bear the entire risk. Other self-insured employers insure against large claims by purchasing stop-loss coverage. Some self-insured employers contract with insurance carriers or third-party administrators for claims processing and other administrative services; other self-insured plans are self-administered. Minimum Premium Plans (MPPs) are included in the self-insured health plan category. All types of plans (i.e., conventional indemnity, PPO, EPO, HMO, POS, and PHOs) can be financed on a self-insured basis. Employers may offer self-insured and fully insured plans to their employees.

Stop-loss coverage: A form of reinsurance for self-insured employers that limits the amount the employers have to pay for each person's health care (individual limit) or for the total expenses of the employer (group limit).

Third-party administrator (TPA): An individual or firm hired by an employer to handle claims processing, pay providers, and manage other functions related to the operation of health insurance. The TPA is not the policyholder or the insurer.

TYPES OF HEALTH CARE PROVIDER ARRANGEMENTS

Exclusive providers: Enrollees must go to providers associated with the plan for all non-emergency care for the costs to be covered.

Any providers: Enrollees may go to providers of their choice with no cost incentives to use a particular subset of providers.

Mixture of providers: Enrollees may go to any provider, but there is a cost incentive to use a particular subset of providers.

Usual, customary, and reasonable (UCR) charges: Conventional indemnity plans operate based on UCR charges. The UCR charge is the provider's *usual fee* for a service that does not exceed the customary fee in that geographic area and that is reasonable based on the circumstances. Instead of UCR charges, PPO plans often operate based on a negotiated (fixed) schedule of fees that recognize charges for covered services up to a negotiated fixed dollar amount.

SOURCES

Survey definitions are available from the National Compensation Survey (BLS), the Medical Expenditure Panel Survey (AHRQ), and the National Employer Health Insurance Survey (NCHS). Definitions also are available from other federal agencies and surveys, such as the Current Population Survey (BLS/Census) and the Employee Retirement Income Security Act of 1974 (ERISA) (from U.S. Department of Labor—Pension and Welfare Benefits Administration).

Glossaries and informational papers from the Web sites of OPM's Federal Employees Health (http://www.dol.gov/ebsa/), Benefit Plans (glossary and specific plan booklets) (http://www.opm.gov/INSURE/HEALTH/), Blue Cross/Blue Shield (http://www.individual-health-plans.com/bluecrossblueshield.htm?source=google), the National Center for Policy Analysis (http://www.ncpa.org/), and the Health Insurance Association of America (http://www.ahip.org/).

Several publications are available.

From Lafferty WE et al: Insurance coverage and subsequent utilization of complementary and alternative medicine providers. *Am J Manag Care* 12:397-404, 2006.

PREPARING MASSAGE CLAIM FORMS

A *claim form* is used to apply for benefits and can be submitted on paper or electronically. With both formats, the same information is required on all claim forms. The trend for paperless business transactions supports the electronic claim process.

Paper Claim Form

There are no standardized forms for massage therapy insurance claims (Fig. 14-3).

Electronic Claim Form

In computerized offices with access to the Internet, claim forms can be filed electronically. Under a provision of the *Health Insurance Portability and Accountability Act of 1996* (HIPAA), effective October 2002, all health care providers, health plans, and health care clearinghouses that transmit data electronically must use a universal language and a standard format. Claims can be filed electronically through a clearinghouse or directly with the carrier.

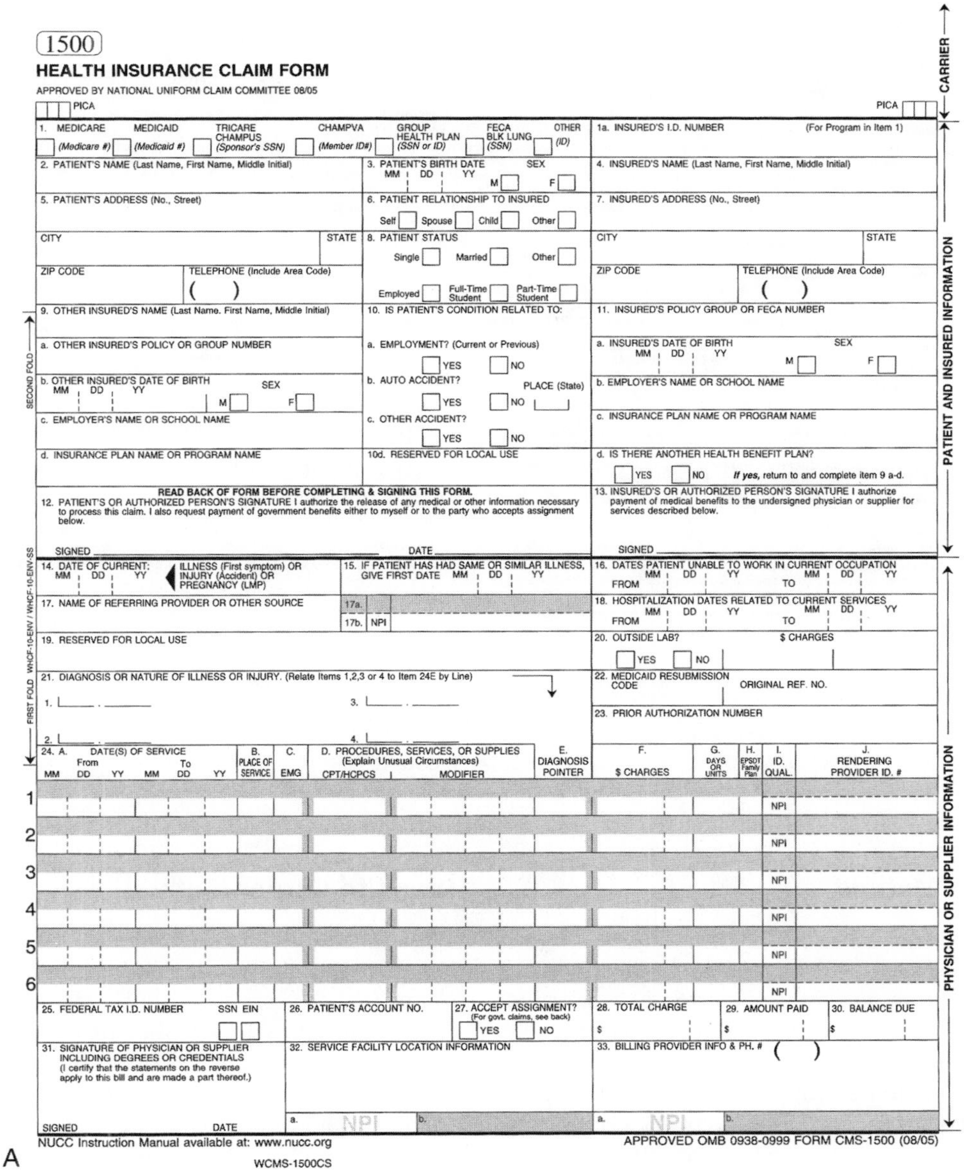
1500
HEALTH INSURANCE CLAIM FORM
APPROVED BY NATIONAL UNIFORM CLAIM COMMITTEE 08/05
PICA PICA
CARRIER

1. MEDICARE (Medicare #) MEDICAID (Medicaid #) TRICARE CHAMPUS (Sponsor's SSN) CHAMPVA (Member ID#) GROUP HEALTH PLAN (SSN or ID) FECA BLK LUNG (SSN) OTHER (ID)
1a. INSURED'S I.D. NUMBER (For Program in Item 1)
2. PATIENT'S NAME (Last Name, First Name, Middle Initial)
3. PATIENT'S BIRTH DATE MM DD YY SEX M F
4. INSURED'S NAME (Last Name, First Name, Middle Initial)
5. PATIENT'S ADDRESS (No., Street)
6. PATIENT RELATIONSHIP TO INSURED Self Spouse Child Other
7. INSURED'S ADDRESS (No., Street)
CITY STATE
8. PATIENT STATUS Single Married Other
CITY STATE
ZIP CODE TELEPHONE (Include Area Code) ( )
Employed Full-Time Student Part-Time Student
ZIP CODE TELEPHONE (Include Area Code) ( )
9. OTHER INSURED'S NAME (Last Name, First Name, Middle Initial)
10. IS PATIENT'S CONDITION RELATED TO:
11. INSURED'S POLICY GROUP OR FECA NUMBER
a. OTHER INSURED'S POLICY OR GROUP NUMBER
a. EMPLOYMENT? (Current or Previous) YES NO
a. INSURED'S DATE OF BIRTH MM DD YY SEX M F
b. OTHER INSURED'S DATE OF BIRTH MM DD YY SEX M F
b. AUTO ACCIDENT? PLACE (State) YES NO
b. EMPLOYER'S NAME OR SCHOOL NAME
c. EMPLOYER'S NAME OR SCHOOL NAME
c. OTHER ACCIDENT? YES NO
c. INSURANCE PLAN NAME OR PROGRAM NAME
d. INSURANCE PLAN NAME OR PROGRAM NAME
10d. RESERVED FOR LOCAL USE
d. IS THERE ANOTHER HEALTH BENEFIT PLAN? YES NO *If yes,* return to and complete item 9 a-d.
READ BACK OF FORM BEFORE COMPLETING & SIGNING THIS FORM.
12. PATIENT'S OR AUTHORIZED PERSON'S SIGNATURE I authorize the release of any medical or other information necessary to process this claim. I also request payment of government benefits either to myself or to the party who accepts assignment below.
SIGNED DATE
13. INSURED'S OR AUTHORIZED PERSON'S SIGNATURE I authorize payment of medical benefits to the undersigned physician or supplier for services described below.
SIGNED
PATIENT AND INSURED INFORMATION
SECOND FOLD
14. DATE OF CURRENT: MM DD YY ILLNESS (First symptom) OR INJURY (Accident) OR PREGNANCY (LMP)
15. IF PATIENT HAS HAD SAME OR SIMILAR ILLNESS, GIVE FIRST DATE MM DD YY
16. DATES PATIENT UNABLE TO WORK IN CURRENT OCCUPATION MM DD YY FROM TO
17. NAME OF REFERRING PROVIDER OR OTHER SOURCE 17a. 17b. NPI
18. HOSPITALIZATION DATES RELATED TO CURRENT SERVICES MM DD YY FROM TO
19. RESERVED FOR LOCAL USE
20. OUTSIDE LAB? YES NO $ CHARGES
21. DIAGNOSIS OR NATURE OF ILLNESS OR INJURY. (Relate Items 1,2,3 or 4 to Item 24E by Line)
1. 2. 3. 4.
22. MEDICAID RESUBMISSION CODE ORIGINAL REF. NO.
23. PRIOR AUTHORIZATION NUMBER
24. A. DATE(S) OF SERVICE From To MM DD YY MM DD YY | B. PLACE OF SERVICE | C. EMG | D. PROCEDURES, SERVICES, OR SUPPLIES (Explain Unusual Circumstances) CPT/HCPCS MODIFIER | E. DIAGNOSIS POINTER | F. $ CHARGES | G. DAYS OR UNITS | H. EPSDT Family Plan | I. ID. QUAL. | J. RENDERING PROVIDER ID. #
1 NPI
2 NPI
3 NPI
4 NPI
5 NPI
6 NPI
25. FEDERAL TAX I.D. NUMBER SSN EIN
26. PATIENT'S ACCOUNT NO.
27. ACCEPT ASSIGNMENT? (For govt. claims, see back) YES NO
28. TOTAL CHARGE $
29. AMOUNT PAID $
30. BALANCE DUE $
31. SIGNATURE OF PHYSICIAN OR SUPPLIER INCLUDING DEGREES OR CREDENTIALS (I certify that the statements on the reverse apply to this bill and are made a part thereof.)
SIGNED DATE
32. SERVICE FACILITY LOCATION INFORMATION a. NPI b.
33. BILLING PROVIDER INFO & PH. # ( ) a. NPI b.
PHYSICIAN OR SUPPLIER INFORMATION
FIRST FOLD WHCF-10-ENV / WHCF-10-ENV-SS
NUCC Instruction Manual available at: www.nucc.org
APPROVED OMB 0938-0999 FORM CMS-1500 (08/05)
WCMS-1500CS

A

FIGURE 14-3. Front (A) and back (B) of an insurance claim form.

(Continued)

BECAUSE THIS FORM IS USED BY VARIOUS GOVERNMENT AND PRIVATE HEALTH PROGRAMS, SEE SEPARATE INSTRUCTIONS ISSUED BY APPLICABLE PROGRAMS.

NOTICE: Any person who knowingly files a statement of claim containing any misrepresentation or any false, incomplete or misleading information may be guilty of a criminal act punishable under law and may be subject to civil penalties.

REFERS TO GOVERNMENT PROGRAMS ONLY

MEDICARE AND CHAMPUS PAYMENTS: A patient's signature requests that payment be made and authorizes release of any information necessary to process the claim and certifies that the information provided in Blocks 1 through 12 is true, accurate and complete. In the case of a Medicare claim, the patient's signature authorizes any entity to release to Medicare medical and nonmedical information, including employment status, and whether the person has employer group health insurance, liability, no-fault, worker's compensation or other insurance which is responsible to pay for the services for which the Medicare claim is made. See 42 CFR 411.24(a). If item 9 is completed, the patient's signature authorizes release of the information to the health plan or agency shown. In Medicare assigned or CHAMPUS participation cases, the physician agrees to accept the charge determination of the Medicare carrier or CHAMPUS fiscal intermediary as the full charge, and the patient is responsible only for the deductible, coinsurance and noncovered services. Coinsurance and the deductible are based upon the charge determination of the Medicare carrier or CHAMPUS fiscal intermediary if this is less than the charge submitted. CHAMPUS is not a health insurance program but makes payment for health benefits provided through certain affiliations with the Uniformed Services. Information on the patient's sponsor should be provided in those items captioned in "Insured"; i.e., items 1a, 4, 6, 7, 9, and 11.

BLACK LUNG AND FECA CLAIMS

The provider agrees to accept the amount paid by the Government as payment in full. See Black Lung and FECA instructions regarding required procedure and diagnosis coding systems.

SIGNATURE OF PHYSICIAN OR SUPPLIER (MEDICARE, CHAMPUS, FECA AND BLACK LUNG)

I certify that the services shown on this form were medically indicated and necessary for the health of the patient and were personally furnished by me or were furnished incident to my professional service by my employee under my immediate personal supervision, except as otherwise expressly permitted by Medicare or CHAMPUS regulations.

For services to be considered as "incident" to a physician's professional service, 1) they must be rendered under the physician's immediate personal supervision by his/her employee, 2) they must be an integral, although incidental part of a covered physician's service, 3) they must be of kinds commonly furnished in physician's offices, and 4) the services of nonphysicians must be included on the physician's bills.

For CHAMPUS claims, I further certify that I (or any employee) who rendered services am not an active duty member of the Uniformed Services or a civilian employee of the United States Government or a contract employee of the United States Government, either civilian or military (refer to 5 USC 5536). For Black-Lung claims, I further certify that the services performed were for a Black Lung-related disorder.

No Part B Medicare benefits may be paid unless this form is received as required by existing law and regulations (42 CFR 424.32).

NOTICE: Any one who misrepresents or falsifies essential information to receive payment from Federal funds requested by this form may upon conviction be subject to fine and imprisonment under applicable Federal laws.

NOTICE TO PATIENT ABOUT THE COLLECTION AND USE OF MEDICARE, CHAMPUS, FECA, AND BLACK LUNG INFORMATION
(PRIVACY ACT STATEMENT)

We are authorized by CMS, CHAMPUS and OWCP to ask you for information needed in the administration of the Medicare, CHAMPUS, FECA, and Black Lung programs. Authority to collect information is in section 205(a), 1862, 1872 and 1874 of the Social Security Act as amended, 42 CFR 411.24(a) and 424.5(a) (6), and 44 USC 3101;41 CFR 101 et seq and 10 USC 1079 and 1086; 5 USC 8101 et seq; and 30 USC 901 et seq; 38 USC 613; E.O. 9397.

The information we obtain to complete claims under these programs is used to identify you and to determine your eligibility. It is also used to decide if the services and supplies you received are covered by these programs and to insure that proper payment is made.

The information may also be given to other providers of services, carriers, intermediaries, medical review boards, health plans, and other organizations or Federal agencies, for the effective administration of Federal provisions that require other third parties payers to pay primary to Federal program, and as otherwise necessary to administer these programs. For example, it may be necessary to disclose information about the benefits you have used to a hospital or doctor. Additional disclosures are made through routine uses for information contained in systems of records.

FOR MEDICARE CLAIMS: See the notice modifying system No. 09-70-0501, titled, 'Carrier Medicare Claims Record,' published in the Federal Register, Vol. 55 No. 177, page 37549, Wed. Sept. 12, 1990, or as updated and republished.

FOR OWCP CLAIMS: Department of Labor, Privacy Act of 1974, "Republication of Notice of Systems of Records," Federal Register Vol. 55 No. 40, Wed Feb. 28, 1990, See ESA-5, ESA-6, ESA-12, ESA-13, ESA-30, or as updated and republished.

FOR CHAMPUS CLAIMS: PRINCIPLE PURPOSE(S): To evaluate eligibility for medical care provided by civilian sources and to issue payment upon establishment of eligibility and determination that the services/supplies received are authorized by law.

ROUTINE USE(S): Information from claims and related documents may be given to the Dept. of Veterans Affairs, the Dept. of Health and Human Services and/or the Dept. of Transportation consistent with their statutory administrative responsibilities under CHAMPUS/CHAMPVA; to the Dept. of Justice for representation of the Secretary of Defense in civil actions; to the Internal Revenue Service, private collection agencies, and consumer reporting agencies in connection with recoupment claims; and to Congressional Offices in response to inquiries made at the request of the person to whom a record pertains. Appropriate disclosures may be made to other federal, state, local, foreign government agencies, private business entities, and individual providers of care, on matters relating to entitlement, claims adjudication, fraud, program abuse, utilization review, quality assurance, peer review, program integrity, third-party liability, coordination of benefits, and civil and criminal litigation related to the operation of CHAMPUS.

DISCLOSURES: Voluntary; however, failure to provide information will result in delay in payment or may result in denial of claim. With the one exception discussed below, there are no penalties under these programs for refusing to supply information. However, failure to furnish information regarding the medical services rendered or the amount charged would prevent payment of claims under these programs. Failure to furnish any other information, such as name or claim number, would delay payment of the claim. Failure to provide medical information under FECA could be deemed an obstruction.

It is mandatory that you tell us if you know that another party is responsible for paying for your treatment. Section 1128B of the Social Security Act and 31 USC 3801-3812 provide penalties for withholding this information.

You should be aware that P.L. 100-503, the "Computer Matching and Privacy Protection Act of 1988", permits the government to verify information by way of computer matches.

MEDICAID PAYMENTS (PROVIDER CERTIFICATION)

I hereby agree to keep such records as are necessary to disclose fully the extent of services provided to individuals under the State's Title XIX plan and to furnish information regarding any payments claimed for providing such services as the State Agency or Dept. of Health and Human Services may request.

I further agree to accept, as payment in full, the amount paid by the Medicaid program for those claims submitted for payment under that program, with the exception of authorized deductible, coinsurance, co-payment or similar cost-sharing charge.

SIGNATURE OF PHYSICIAN (OR SUPPLIER): I certify that the services listed above were medically indicated and necessary to the health of this patient and were personally furnished by me or my employee under my personal direction.

NOTICE: This is to certify that the foregoing information is true, accurate and complete. I understand that payment and satisfaction of this claim will be from Federal and State funds, and that any false claims, statements, or documents, or concealment of a material fact, may be prosecuted under applicable Federal or State laws.

According to the Paperwork Reduction Act of 1995, no persons are required to respond to a collection of information unless it displays a valid OMB control number. The valid OMB control number for this information collection is 0938-0999. The time required to complete this information collection is estimated to average 10 minutes per response, including the time to review instructions, search existing data resources, gather the data needed, and complete and review the information collection. If you have any comments concerning the accuracy of the time estimate(s) or suggestions for improving this form, please write to: CMS, Attn: PRA Reports Clearance Officer, 7500 Security Boulevard, Baltimore, Maryland 21244-1850. This address is for comments and/or suggestions only. DO NOT MAIL COMPLETED CLAIM FORMS TO THIS ADDRESS.

B

FIGURE 14-3, cont'd

Clearinghouse Method

With the clearinghouse method, batches of claims are transmitted to a clearinghouse, which scans the forms for errors or missing information and transmits error-free claims to the appropriate carrier. Claims with errors are electronically returned to the massage office for correction and resubmission. The clearinghouse prints and mails a paper claim for the few carriers unable to accept electronic claims. The advantages of using a clearinghouse are verification of claims and distribution of batches to multiple carriers. The disadvantage is the per-claim charge.

Direct to Carrier Method

With the direct to carrier method, the massage office staff members sort claims according to carrier and transmit the claims for each carrier separately. The carrier receives electronic claims the same day they are transmitted, and because the claims enter the carrier's processing system directly, turnaround time is reduced by an average of 2 to 4 days. Claim payment statements usually are available from the carrier's Web site, which can be accessed only by submitting a password. Many carriers also offer electronic funds transfer (i.e., direct deposit) of claim payments to the massage office's bank account. If both of these electronic systems are used, the benefit payment can reach the massage office's bank account within 24 to 48 hours of transmission of the claim.

Procedural Codes

The American Medical Association (AMA) produces a manual containing thousands of codes for known medical procedures. Because of the ever-changing field of medicine, this manual is revised yearly. Combined with the World Health Association's International Classification of Disease (ICD) codes, the Current Procedural Terminology (CPT) codes offer a concise and accurate description of the medical professional's actions. CPT codes are developed, maintained, and copyrighted by the AMA. As the practice of health care changes, new codes are developed for new services, current codes may be revised, and old, unused codes are discarded. There are thousands of codes in use, and they are updated annually. Development and maintenance of these codes is overseen by AMA editorial boards, and the publication of all the software, books, and manuals needed by those who use them brings an estimated $70 million to the AMA each year.

Healthcare Common Procedure Coding System Codes

These Healthcare Common Procedure Coding System (HCPCS) numbers are the codes used by Medicare (Centers for Medicare and Medicaid Services [CMS]). There are two sets of codes. The first set, HCPCS level I, is based on and identical to the CPT codes described previously. Level II HCPCS codes are used by medical suppliers other than physicians, such as ambulance services or durable medical equipment suppliers. They are typically not costs that get passed through a physician's office, so they must be dealt with by Medicare or Medicaid differently from the way a health insurance company would deal with them (Box 14-4). The insurance biller is the expert on how to code for insurance reimbursement.

Massage therapists may be able to use a few codes from the Physical Medicine and Rehabilitation section of the CPT manual. It is questionable whether this is an appropriate use of the codes because they typically apply to physical therapists; ****97140 Manual Therapy Techniques is the code used.

In chiropractic practice, CPT code 97124 is used for Massage. Chiropractic Manipulative Treatment (CMT) codes are 98940 through 98943. CPT code 97124 describes work including effleurage, pétrissage, or tapotement (e.g., stroking, compression, percussion), each for 15 minutes. Massage (CPT code 97124) describes a service that is separate and distinct from those described by Chiropractic Manipulative Treatment, Osteopathic Manipulative Treatment, and Manual Therapy Techniques. Massage, unlike those techniques, is often considered totally passive in nature. The patient did not participate in the procedure, and the various massage techniques are applied to the patient.

Massage is applied to a large area, often crossing over several types of soft tissue and several areas of soft tissue, and it is used primarily for its restorative effects. In some cases, massage may be used for stimulating soft tissue (i.e., tapotement). The expected outcomes of massage are more general in nature and may be what the patient can tolerate at the more acute stage of their treatment plans. This includes goals such as increasing circulation, decreasing muscle soreness, and decreasing muscle spasm. The research available on massage techniques and their impact on the recovery of muscle function after exercise and on any one of the physiologic factors related to the recovery process shows that these techniques have very little impact. Its greatest influence is on the broad factors of pain modulation, muscle tightness, and blood flow to the related tissues.

The goal of therapeutic massage is to increase circulation and promote tissue relaxation to the muscles. It is of particular value when used in conjunction with other therapeutic procedures on the same day; the treatment plan is designed to restore muscle function, reduce edema, improve joint motion, and provide relief of muscle spasm. Therapeutic procedures can include superficial, effleurage,

---

BOX 14-4	Learn more about CPT and HCPCS Codes

Each year in the United States, health care insurers process more than 5 billion claims for payment. For Medicare and other health insurance programs to ensure that these claims are processed in an orderly and consistent manner, standardized coding systems are essential. The HCPCS level II code set is one of the standard sets of codes used for this purpose.

The HCPCS is divided into two principal subsystems: level I and level II. Level I of the HCPCS is composed of Current Procedural Terminology (CPT), a numeric coding system maintained by the American Medical Association (AMA). The CPT is a uniform coding system consisting of descriptive terms and identifying codes that are used primarily to identify medical services and procedures furnished by physicians and other health care professionals. These health care professionals use the CPT to identify services and procedures for which they bill public or private health insurance programs. Decisions regarding the addition, deletion, or revision of CPT codes are made by the AMA. The CPT codes are updated annually by the AMA. Level I of the HCPCS, the CPT codes, does not include codes needed to separately report medical items or services that are regularly billed by suppliers other than physicians.

Links to more information about CPT and HCPCS codes are available on the Evolve Web site (http://evolve.elsevier.com/Fritz/business).

From http://www.cms.hhs.gov/MedHCPCSGeninfo/.

pétrissage, percussion, pressure-point work (i.e., acupressure and shiatsu), trigger-point work, and deep-tissue techniques. Also included in the CPT code 97124 is the use of a Genie Rub, Thumper, G5, or other device, so long as it is manually applied. Use of handheld tools or probes includes the application of manual pressure, which would likely fall under the massage description. Massage usually is applied to a large area, often crossing over several types of soft tissue and several regions. The code requires that the doctor or therapist be hands-on and constantly attending to the patient, and massage beds, tables, or chairs do not qualify for this code description; for those units, the unlisted modality code would be more appropriate.

Manual Therapy (CPT 97140) describes multiple manually applied services, including manual traction, myofascial release, joint mobilization, manual lymphatic drainage, and manipulation (nonchiropractic). For myofascial release work, the targeted region is a specific muscle or other soft tissue. Findings usually involve an adhesion or area of fibrosis exhibited by a painful band or "knot" within the muscle and subsequent limited range of motion. This code describes manually applied techniques that increase active pain-free range of motion and increase extensibility of myofascial tissue, with the goal of restoring function of the muscle or soft tissue. A variety of active manual techniques that achieve these goals can reasonably be coded with 97140. The specific technique usually is described as active or passive, or both. *Active* or *passive* indicates the method of stretching or elongation of the soft tissue. This procedure is typically considered painful and may need some analgesia before and after service. When documenting the service, the interaction between the patient and therapist should be reported. The chart notes should clearly indicate what style or procedure was performed, with the appropriate reporting of the targeted soft tissue, the technique used, time spent, goals, and the response to the treatment.

Neuromuscular Re-education (CPT 97112) is intended to identify therapeutic exercise designed to retrain a body part (i.e., re-educate the muscle) to perform some task that the body part was previously able to do. This usually is in the form of some commonly performed task for that body part. It is most commonly used for patients after a stroke or surgery. Specific goals typically include work to improve balance, coordination, kinesthetic sense, posture, and proprioception. The idea is that the motor system needs to be "repatterned" for normal activities. Also included are services to retrain poor static or dynamic sitting or standing balance and loss of gross or fine motor coordination. Neuromuscular re-education techniques are usually applied progressively by using active movements under a variety of mechanical conditions. Examples include proprioceptive neuromuscular facilitation, Janda, Feldenkrais, Bobath, Alexander, and cross-crawl techniques. Balance boards and similar equipment also can be documented under this code.

SELF-REFLECTION

How do I feel as I read all of this information? Excited? Interested? Overwhelmed? Frustrated? Nothing? Do I want to be accountable for the record keeping necessary to receive health insurance reimbursement for massage services? If I work for a business that has a biller who does the paperwork, what are my responsibilities? Would that make a difference in my opinion of insurance billing for massage services?

Because massage therapists do not diagnose conditions, the ICD code must be acquired from a prescribing medical specialist. The easiest and most reliable way to obtain the correct codes for massage is to check directly with the insurance company to be billed. Codes can change yearly; do not assume that codes will remain the same.

INSURANCE PAY SYSTEM

Organization

The insurance pay system has four parts:

1. Client
2. Group or program sponsor (e.g., employer, union, business association)
3. Insurance benefits carrier, which may be an insurer, a third-party administrator (TPA), or insurance service corporation
4. Prescribing physician and massage therapist

For the process to succeed, a system of communication and information sharing must connect all four parties. The massage therapist communicates regarding services, coding, and fees for treatment with the client to verify carrier information, benefits, and payment acceptance and with the carrier for billing, payment, and benefit information. This job requires organization, perseverance, and strict attention to detail. The following points can assist in organizing the process. Document each subscriber's scope of coverage (excluding maximums, *limitations*, and deductibles), and obtain the complete mailing address and telephone number for claims and inquiries. Note any special information the carrier requires.

- Keep these materials organized in a notebook or file.
- Inform each client about his or her benefits and the amount for which the client is responsible.
- Set aside a specific time to complete the claim forms or prepare each claim form at the completion of treatment.
- Keep a current file or computer record of outstanding claims, and review it regularly.

- When required, request preauthorization for treatment.
- Regularly verify and update clients' general information.
- Maintain an adequate supply of claim forms.
- Be accurate, and answer all questions on the claim form completely, providing details as required. If a question does not apply, leave it blank.
- Whenever possible, attend seminars presented by benefits carriers to keep current on billing practices.

Insurance Fraud

It is illegal to misrepresent treatment or to inaccurately report fees and dates of service to benefits carriers. The following actions, whether deliberate or unintentional, constitute fraud:

- Billing the benefits carrier for higher fees than the client is charged
- Billing before completion of service
- Predating or postdating services on claim forms
- Improperly reporting treatment (e.g., physical therapy instead of massage therapy)
- Billing for services not rendered

Accuracy and honesty are crucial. Those defrauding benefits carriers may be liable for legal prosecution (Box 14-5).

LEARNING ACTIVITY

Review this chapter, and make a list of the activities involved in billing insurance companies for massage services. Using your practice management software, add a new client into the system. You can base the "client" on someone you know or make up a client. This client will receive insurance coverage for massage. Fill out the proper documents for insurance reimbursement. Continue to update the scheduling and history information and SOAP documentation for a total of 6 sessions for this client, then run a summary report of progress as an update on the progress of the client to be transmitted to the insurance company.

SUMMARY

All parties involved with insurance—the client, massage therapist, the group or program sponsor of the insurance, and the insurance benefits carrier—must communicate effectively to have a successful insurance relationship. The success comes from correctly coding the insurance claims and getting to the appropriate party. Whether the plan is an

BOX 14-5 | **Abstract: Insurance Coverage and Subsequent Utilization of Complementary and Alternative Medicine Providers**

Background: Since 1996, Washington State law has required that private health insurance cover licensed complementary and alternative medicine (CAM) providers.

Objective: To evaluate how insured people used CAM providers and what role this played in health care utilization and expenditures.

Study Design: Cross-sectional analysis of insurance enrollees from western Washington in 2002.

Methods: Analysis of insurance demographic data, claims files, benefit information, diagnoses, CAM and conventional provider utilization, and health care expenditures for 3 large health insurance companies.

Results: Among more than 600,000 enrollees, 13.7% made CAM claims. This included 1.3% of enrollees with claims for acupuncture, 1.6% for naturopathy, 2.4% for massage, and 10.9% for chiropractic. Patients enrolled in preferred provider organizations and point-of-service products were notably more likely to use CAM than those with health maintenance organization coverage. The use of CAM was greater among women and among persons 31 to 50 years of age. The use of chiropractic was more frequent in less populous counties. The CAM provider visits usually focused on musculoskeletal complaints except for naturopathic physicians, who treated a broader array of problems. The median per-visit expenditures were $39.00 for CAM care and $74.40 for conventional outpatient care. The total expenditures per enrollee were $2589, of which $75 (2.9%) was spent on CAM.

Conclusions: The number of people using CAM insurance benefits was substantial; the effect on insurance expenditures was modest. Because the long-term trajectory of CAM cost under third-party payment is unknown, utilization of these services should be followed.

From Lafferty WE et al: Insurance coverage and subsequent utilization of complementary and alternative medicine providers [abstract]. *Am J Manag Care* 12:397-404, 2006.

Good Stuff from the Government

NATIONAL INSTITUTES OF HEALTH

The National Institutes of Health provides a wealth of information about complementary and alternative medicine (CAM), including definitions, typical costs for treatment, and eligibility insurance reimbursement.

A health savings account (HSA) is a type of tax-exempt account. It is for people who participate in a high-deductible health plan (i.e., catastrophic health plan). In an HSA, you—not your employer—establish and maintain the account, although some employers make contributions. You can also invest your HSA funds to earn tax-deductible interest. Similar options include a flexible spending account (FSA) and a health reimbursement arrangement (HRA).

The Internal Revenue Service (IRS) has further information on these accounts. The IRS does not allow the same expenses to be reimbursed through an FSA or HSA and to be claimed as tax deductions. In tax year 2005, the IRS allowed taxpayers to deduct medical expenses for a limited number of CAM services and products, such as acupuncture and chiropractic care.

GovBenefits (http://www.govbenefits.gov/) and USA.gov (http://www.usa.gov/) are two Internet resources that explain federal health benefit programs. GovBenefits has a test you can take about qualifying for programs. State and local departments of health or social services also have financial assistance programs for eligible residents, and you can contact them directly to inquire.

The National Center for Complementary and Alternative Medicine (NCCAM) Clearinghouse provides information on CAM and NCCAM, including publications and searches of federal databases of scientific and medical literature. Two of its publications are *Selecting a CAM Practitioner* and *Are You Considering Using CAM?* The Clearinghouse does not provide medical advice, treatment recommendations, or referrals to practitioners.

PUBMED

A service of the National Library of Medicine (NLM), PubMed contains publication information and, in most cases, brief summaries of articles from scientific and medical journals. CAM on PubMed, developed jointly by NCCAM and NLM, is a subset of the PubMed system and focuses on the topic of CAM.

AGENCY FOR HEALTHCARE RESEARCH AND QUALITY

The Agency for Healthcare Research and Quality (AHRQ) conducts research on health care outcomes, quality, costs, use, and access. Publications for consumers include *Choosing and Using a Health Plan* and *Checkup on Health Insurance Choices*.

DEPARTMENT OF LABOR

The Department of Labor (DOL) has publications on federal health care laws, including the Health Insurance Portability and Accountability Act of 1996 (HIPAA) and Consolidated Omnibus Budget Reconciliation Act (COBRA), that apply to job seekers, workers, and retirees.

INTERNAL REVENUE SERVICE

The IRS is the nation's tax collection agency. Among its services are publications for consumers:

- Publication 969: *Health Savings Accounts and Other Tax-Favored Health Plans*
- Publication 502: *Medical and Dental Expenses*
  All links are available on the Evolve Web site.

HMO, HSA, or something else, each has appropriate codes and methods that must be used to achieve the desired results. Some therapists may prefer to outsource to an insurance biller to have the most effective insurance outcomes. The CPT codebook provides a concise and accurate description of codes a type of dictionary for insurance billing. However, the therapist needs to understand and use the codes accurately to be successful at this component of the business.

Bibliography

Collins SA: Billing for massage-specific CPT codes. Dynamic Chiropractic 24(14), 2006. Available at http://findarticles.com (August 20, 2008).

Council for Affordable Health Care: Resources and health insurance. Available at http://www.cahi.org/cahi_contents/resources/pdf/HealthInsuranceMandates2008.pdf (accessed January 12, 2009).

Denning E: Massage therapy medical codes for 2004. *Massage Bodywork* Feb-Mar, 2004.

Madison-Mahoney V: Coding for insurance billing and Medicare issues. *Massage Today* 6(2), 2006.

National Center for Complementary and Alternative Medicine (NCCAM): Consumer financial issues in complementary and alternative medicine. Available at http://nccam.nih.gov/health/financial/index.htm#15 (accessed May 16, 2006).

National Center for Complementary and Alternative Medicine: Home page. Available at http://nccam.nih.gov (accessed June 2009).

Onofrio J: Introduction to The Massage Insurance Billing Manual. LMP June 2004. Available at http://www.thebodyworker.com/guesteditorial (accessed September 2009).

United States Department of Health & Human Services Agency for Healthcare Research and Quality: Information about insurance. Available at http://www.ahrq.gov/consumer/insuranceqa/ (accessed June 2009).

Evolve Annotated Web Links

Academic Consortium for Complementary and Alternative Health Care (http://ihpc.info/accahc/accahc.shtml)

Agency for Healthcare Research and Quality (AHRQ) (http://www.ahrq.gov)

Bodyworker (thebodyworker.com) and Massage School Notes (www.thebodyworker.com)

Complementary and alternative medicine (CAM) on PubMed (http://www.nccam.nih.gov/camonpubmed/

Council for Affordable Health Care (http://www.cahi.org/cahi_contents/resources/pdf/HealthInsuranceMandates2008.pdf)

Definitions of health insurance terms (http://www.bls.gov/ncs/ebs/sp/healthterms.pdf)

Department of Health and Human Services, Centers for Medicare and Medicaid Services: (http://www.cms.hhs.gov/)

Department of Labor (DOL) (http://www.dol.gov/)

Department of Labor (DOL), Consumer Health Plans and Benefits Information (http://www.dol.gov/dol/topic/health-plans/index.htm)

Federal Trade Commission (http://www.ftc.gov/)

Integrated Healthcare Policy Consortium (http://ihpc.info/)

Internal Revenue Service (IRS) (http://www.irs.gov/)

Internal Revenue Service (IRS), Publication 502, Medical and Dental Expenses (http://www.irs.gov/pub/irs-pdf/p502.pdf)

Internal Revenue Service (IRS), Publication 969, Health Savings Accounts and Other Tax-Favored Health Plans (http://www.irs.gov/pub/irs-pdf/p969.pdf)

MedlinePlus, drugs, supplements, and herbal information (http://www.nlm.nih.gov/medlineplus/druginformation.html)

National Cancer Institute, search for clinical trials (http://www.cancer.gov/clinicaltrials/search)

National Center for Complementary and Alternative Medicine (NCCAM) Clearinghouse (nccam.nih.gov)

PubMed (http://www.ncbi.nlm.nih.gov/sites/entrez?db-pubmed)

U.S. Department of Health and Human Services, Agency for Healthcare Research and Quality, questions and answers about health insurance (http://www.ahrq.gov/consumer/insuranceqa/; http://www.cahi.org/cahi_contents/resources/pdf/HealthInsuranceMandates2008.pdf)

U.S. Food and Drug Administration (http://www.fda.gov/)

U.S. Food and Drug Administration, dietary supplements overview (www.fda.gov/Food/DietarySupplements/default.html)

U.S. Government official Web portal (http://www.usa.gov/)

Workbook

1. Identify the four parties affected by insurance benefits and the roles of each.

2. Identify the types of insurance benefits programs.

3. Explain a standard insurance claim form.

4. What are the differences between using a paper claim form and an electronic claim form?

_____

_____

_____

_____

_____

_____

_____

_____

5. Identify five actions that constitute benefits fraud.

_____

_____

_____

_____

_____

_____

_____

_____

6. Explain procedure codes.

_____

_____

_____

_____

_____

_____

_____

_____

ACCOUNTING CONCEPTS

KEY TERMS

Accounting	Balance	Nonsufficient funds (NSF) check
Accounts payable	Bookkeeping	Receipt
Accounts receivable	Credit balance	Statement
Adjustment	Credit bureau	

LEARNING OUTCOMES

Mastery of the content in this chapter will enable the reader to:

- Define key terms
- Define bookkeeping
- Define accounting
- Explain basic mathematical procedures
- Describe common bookkeeping systems in massage therapy
- Explain the function of a computerized accounts receivable program
- Describe the components of a pegboard bookkeeping system

- Explain the procedures used in a pegboard bookkeeping system
- Explain the common systems of statement production
- Identify common payment and credit policies
- Describe the various laws affecting credit policies and collection procedures
- Identify common problems in maintaining a credit policy
- Identify the functions of a credit bureau
- Explain the function of a collection agency
- Compose collection letters

e Guidelines for the Learning Activities and answers to the Workbook questions are located on Evolve at http://evolve.elsevier.com/Fritz/business.

Certain things are best left to the professionals. This means that a small business owner will need to hire an accountant at one time or another. If you are an employee, you will not be directly responsible for accounting and bookkeeping. It is important, however, to understand the demands of the accounting process. *Accounting*, which is the recording, classifying, and summarizing of financial and business records, usually is the job of an accountant. If self-employed (i.e., business owner), it is highly recommended that you have an accountant who audits the books and computes a variety of tax reports and financial statements. There are too many changes in tax law yearly to keep up with while you run your business.

Although this textbook gives you a brief introduction to business accounting, the intricate and ongoing changes of finances and taxes mandate an expert. You can, however, make the accountant's job much more efficient and more cost effective by keeping the bookkeeping process in order.

Bookkeeping, or the recording of financial transactions, typically is the responsibility of the business owner. This may be your employer or you if you own the business.

Just as with massage therapy, the best way to find an accountant is the recommendation of other satisfied business owners. Small business accounting is much the same for all types of business. Do not look only for tax preparation services. If the size of your business warrants, you should look for more than simple tax preparation from an accountant. The small business owner should contract with the accountant to provide advice in the areas of business structuring, record keeping, timing of expenses or payments, and reduction of tax liability.

FINANCIAL SYSTEMS

Because massage therapy is a business as well as a health profession, sound business practices must be integrated into the management of the massage business office. The two financial systems used in a massage business office are *accounts receivable* and *accounts payable*. If you are self-employed, you are responsible for both. If you are an employee, your paycheck is part of accounts payable, because you are receiving a paycheck from the business.

The accounts receivable system includes all production; data are entered for treatment rendered and payments received, and new balances are calculated. After all computations have been made, the current accounts receivable amount, or the amount of money owed to the massage therapist (i.e., incoming money), is determined. Accounts payable refers to all of the massage therapist's financial obligations, or money the massage therapist owes (i.e., outgoing money). This chapter discusses accounts receivable; Chapter 16 details accounts payable and other financial systems.

Records management is a primary business responsibility. Financial records are as important as clinical records but should be maintained separately. They provide (1) protection for both the massage therapist and the client, (2) information for tax purposes, and (3) data for a business analysis. Inaccurate records result in poor public relations and may create unnecessary litigation with the state or federal government.

UNDERSTANDING BASIC MATHEMATICAL COMPUTATIONS

Before you can become proficient at computing financial activity on various records, you must review some basic mathematical rules. Because computers are used to produce so many documents, it often is easy to forget how to perform basic calculations.

Although a computer with the appropriate software can make the necessary calculations, you are responsible for entering the data in the appropriate fields to ensure that the final figures are accurate. You often need to add and subtract figures with decimals and perform other business-related computations. Most people use manual or electronic calculators for these tasks; however, relying solely on technological devices without having an understanding of basic computation can result in embarrassment, client dissatisfaction, and possibly loss of cash flow when errors are detected. The following descriptions cover basic mathematical procedures used for routine bookkeeping entries.

Decimals

ADDING AND SUBTRACTING DECIMALS

Place the numbers to be added or subtracted in a vertical column, aligning the decimal points, before performing the addition or subtraction. To add columns of figures with decimals, add the numbers in each column, beginning with the column farthest to the right and working your way to the left:

$$
\begin{array}{r}
0.5 \\
2.8 \\
30.50 \\
67.945 \\
+\underline{750.000} \\
851.745
\end{array}
$$

To subtract, follow the same procedure. Place the numbers to be subtracted in a vertical column, aligning the decimal points. Each amount must have the same number of decimals, and it may be necessary to add zeros before performing this procedure. For example, to subtract 1.75 from 3.876, add one zero at the end of the 1.75:

$$
\begin{array}{r}
3.876 \\
-\underline{1.750} \\
2.126
\end{array}
$$

MULTIPLYING DECIMALS

To multiply decimals, perform the procedure as you would for all whole numbers, except the decimal point must be placed correctly in the answer. Count the number of digits to the right of the decimal point in the multiplicand and in the multiplier; then count the same number of places from right to left in the product and insert the decimal point:

600.75	2 decimals (multiplicand)
× .20	2 decimals (multiplier)
120.1500	2 + 2 = 4 decimals

or

$800.50	2 decimals
× .75	2 decimals
400250	
560350	
$ 600.3750	2 + 2 = 4 decimals

or

$800	0 decimals
×.75	2 decimals
$600.00	0 + 2 = 2 decimals

Percentages

Working with percentages is a common function of routine posting of accounts receivable data. To change a percent to a fraction, drop the percent sign, place the number over 100, and reduce the fraction to the lowest terms. If the numerator is a decimal, multiply both the numerator and denominator by an appropriate power of 10 to clear the decimal. For instance,

$$5\% = \frac{5}{100} = \frac{1}{20}$$

or

$$7.5\% = \frac{7.5}{100} = \frac{75}{1000} = \frac{3}{4}$$

To change a percent to a decimal, move the decimal point two places to the left and drop the percent sign.

$$15\% = 0.15$$
$$2\% = 0.02$$
$$110\% = 1.1$$

To find a certain percentage of a number, convert the percent amount to a decimal amount, and multiply by the number. The following computation shows how to calculate 80% of $670:

$$\begin{array}{r} \$670 \\ \times .80 \\ \hline \$536 \end{array}$$

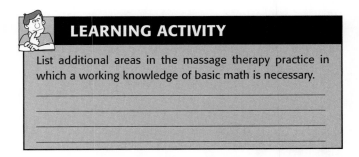

LEARNING ACTIVITY

List additional areas in the massage therapy practice in which a working knowledge of basic math is necessary.

_____

_____

_____

_____

BOOKKEEPING SYSTEMS

Types of Systems

Bookkeeping is the recording of financial transactions. If you are responsible for bookkeeping, you can select from a variety of bookkeeping systems, including the pegboard ("write it once") system, which, until the 1990s, was the system most often used in small business offices. With the pegboard system, one notation provided an entry on the daily journal sheet, the ledger card, the *receipt,* and in some cases, a statement. The current system of choice is a computer software program, which goes beyond the basic transactions of the pegboard system to provide all financial records, insurance claim forms (if applicable), future appointments, and recall management, and documents for practice analysis.

A computerized bookkeeping system can be integrated into total records management. In other words, you can make a clinical entry on a client's record that can then be transferred to a financial record. Using designated codes, you can transfer this information to a client's statement, and an insurance claim form can be generated from the original data entry. This type of system is more than a mechanism for bookkeeping. The CD that accompanies this book has a basic bookkeeping system.

Components of a Computerized Bookkeeping System

Chapter 5 described the use of massage office management software. One component of most of these systems is the accounts receivable program. By entering data for a client account it is also possible to generate myriad reports, forms, or other types of information.

To generate accounts receivable data, you follow specific steps outlined in the software package. The following description is an overview of some of the common steps in basic data entry on the CD at the back of the book. Table 15-1 presents some common commands used in a variety of accounts receivable programs.

OPENING THE PROGRAM

When you open the program, you commonly are required to enter your name or your user name and a password. When you enter a password, the characters are not displayed on the screen as you key them in. Most systems allow for reentry of your password in case you make an error, but after a specified number of erroneous entries, the program may abort.

TABLE 15-1	Common Commands in Accounts Receivable Software
COMMAND	**MEANING**
ADD	Enter additional data; create a new record
APPOINTMENT/ SCHEDULER	Enter data for a client appointment
DEL	Delete; to eliminate part or all of the data entry
EDIT	Alter or change data
ENTER	Insert data
ESC	Leave the screen
FILE	Open, close, print, or take action on files
INSURANCE	Make a data entry or obtain a hard copy of a claim form
LIST	Provides a screen view or hard copy of lists of clients, accounts, or other data
LOCATE	Find a client, an account, or other data
N	No
CLIENT	Enter a field of client records
POST	Enter data, financial or other
PRINT	Produce a hard copy of a document
RECALL	Enter data about a client for recall
REPORTS	Obtain some form of report programmed into the system
SYSTEM	Change the system setting, log in, or password
TRANSACTION	Reference to financial activity
VIEW	Changes the format of the screen view
WINDOW	Allows a different configuration of the screen
WORD PROCESSOR	Program that allows letter writing
Y	Yes

LOCATING ACCOUNT INFORMATION

When you make a selection, such as Clients, a box opens; you then find a list of your current clients. Click on the name of one client. The account information window opens (Fig. 15-1). If no account appears, one can be added by clicking on the NEW button and creating a new client record (Fig. 15-2). Certain basic account information is common to most systems, such as an identification (ID) number, massage therapist (the primary provider if an office has several massage therapists), user codes, name and address, personal data (e.g., telephone number or numbers, Social Security number, date of birth, gender, age), insurance, employment, and special notes, such as last update, last payment, date of admission, and insurance numbers.

EDITING ACCOUNT INFORMATION

Sometimes, you need to edit account information, such as when a client's name or address changes. To do this, you enter the client window and select Edit (which refers to the task of changing existing data).

ADDING OR DELETING A CLIENT

You may add clients to an account in the system shown by selecting the NEW command. This is commonly done to add a spouse or dependent to an account, but it also may be required in the case of marriage, divorce, or death or when older children are transferred to their own accounts. If your client has not visited in a given amount of time, you can simply move the account to the inactive tab rather than deleting it.

POSTING TRANSACTIONS

A common daily activity in bookkeeping is entering transaction data. From the transaction screen (Fig. 15-3), most systems are designed to allow you to enter clinical data about treatment, for which you may insert appropriate codes. When the data are entered, the program computes the financial activity and produces an account *balance*. Before these data are stored, fill out any necessary insurance claim forms or other activity (e.g., recall or appointment scheduling). A walk-out statement (Fig. 15-4) and an insurance claim form should be generated after these data entries are complete.

BACKING UP DATA

Maintaining all the practice data on a computer's hard drive is dangerous. Valuable information can be lost as the result of a power surge, computer crash, or misdirected ERASE or DEL command. For this reason, the hard drive must be backed up regularly. This can be done using a CD-ROM, DVD, or some other type of storage device. The office procedures manual must describe the backup procedure step by step, and a backup log must be maintained (Fig. 15-5).

SPECIAL PROBLEMS

A day would not be complete without some unusual activity that cannot be recorded using the procedure exactly as listed previously. Several such situations and their solutions are presented in the following discussion.

A *credit balance* often occurs when payment is made in advance, such as when a client buys a gift certificate for a massage or a massage package such as 10 massage sessions for the price of 9 sessions. A credit balance of $50, for example, can be noted in three ways: (1) with the amount preceded by *CR* (CR$50); (2) with the amount preceded by a minus sign (−$50) as shown in Figure 15-6; and (3) with the amount in color and enclosed in parentheses ($50).

When a gift certificate is redeemed or a massage is received, charges are made against the credit balance, reducing it. The credit balance represents what is owed to the client in services. The credit balance is also shown when a client pays on the account (Fig. 15-7).

Nonsufficient funds (NSF) checks, or checks returned to the office because of a lack of account funds, require some form of adjustment to the account. You may redeposit the check and not make an entry on the books. However, it may be necessary to charge the account with this returned check. Collection fees are paid to an agency for collecting a delinquent account, and these fees usually are deducted from the payment before it is sent to the massage therapist. For the returned check in Figure 15-8, an NSF notation has been made, and a service charge of $25 has been assessed to the account.

A courtesy discount is given when the massage therapist extends a professional courtesy to a client. The courtesy discount is entered in the adjustment column (Fig. 15-9).

PAYMENT POLICIES AND STATEMENTS

Many payment policies are used in massage business, but a few are common to all practices:

Cash only: The cash-only system is common and eliminates much paperwork in the business office, but it may place limitations on the massage practice.

Payment of statement in full: Unless other arrangements have been made with the office, the client is expected to pay in

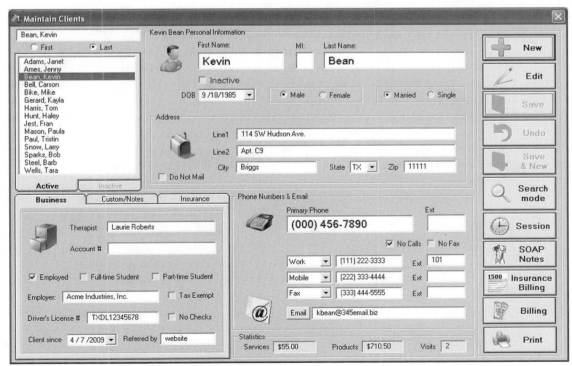

FIGURE 15-1. Account information screen. *(Courtesy of Island Software.)*

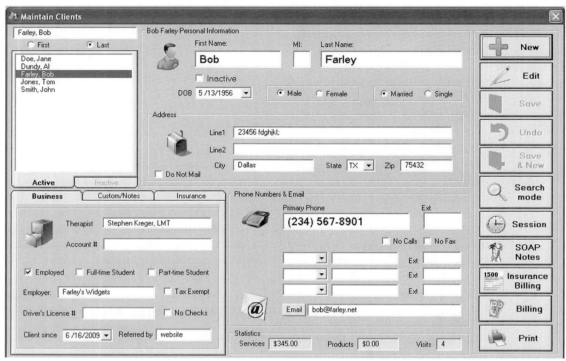

FIGURE 15-2. New client information screen. *(Courtesy of Island Software.)*

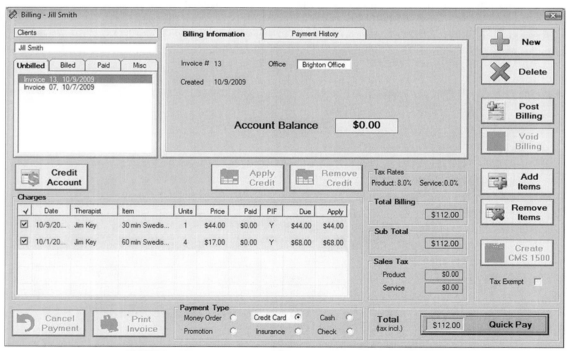

FIGURE 15-3. Transaction screen. *(Courtesy of Island Software.)*

full within 10 days of receipt of the statement. Some form of notice, such as appropriate signage or a written policy statement, must be presented to the client.

Extended payment: Regulation 2 of the Truth in Lending Act requires that an agreement exists between the massage therapist and the client if payment for services is to be made in more than four installments. Even if no finance charge is involved, the truth in lending form (Fig. 15-10) must be completed to verify that such a payment agreement has been reached.

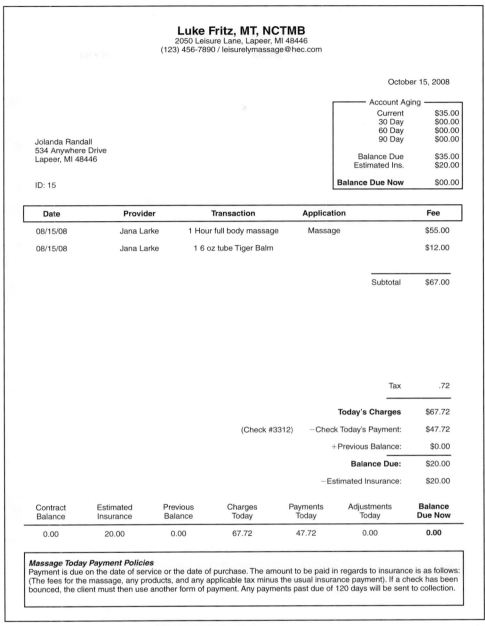

FIGURE 15-4. Walk-out statement.

A *statement* informs clients of their financial status with the massage therapist and indicates the charges, payments, and balances of their accounts for the month just concluded. The statement is also a request for payment. Monthly statements may be sent on day 1, 15, or 30 or on a staggered basis according to the alphabet. The important factor is consistency; be sure to send the statements at the same time each month.

A statement can be generated on the computer with an automated bookkeeping system. The itemized statement shows the dates of payments and the treatments for each member of the family during the month. With a computerized system, you can add special messages or aging columns to statements to enhance the collection process.

USING A CREDIT BUREAU

Perhaps the best way to define a *credit bureau* or *consumer reporting agency* (CRA) is to explain what it does not do. It does not lend money; it does not deny credit; and it is not a collection agency. A credit bureau reports specific information about a person's previous payment habits on deferred

BACKUP LOG

Date	Disk/Tape	Initials	Storage Location
____	_____	_____	_____
____	_____	_____	_____
____	_____	_____	_____
____	_____	_____	_____
____	_____	_____	_____
____	_____	_____	_____
____	_____	_____	_____
____	_____	_____	_____
____	_____	_____	_____
____	_____	_____	_____
____	_____	_____	_____
____	_____	_____	_____
____	_____	_____	_____
____	_____	_____	_____
____	_____	_____	_____
____	_____	_____	_____
____	_____	_____	_____
____	_____	_____	_____
____	_____	_____	_____
____	_____	_____	_____

FIGURE 15-5. Backup log. *(From Finkbeiner BL, Finkbeiner CA: Practice Management for the Dental Team, ed 6, St. Louis, 2006, Mosby.)*

payment plans. It reports on accounts placed for collection and provides information of public interest, such as that regarding bankruptcies, judgments, and lawsuits.

The Fair Credit Reporting Act (FCRA) was passed in 1992 to promote accuracy, fairness, and privacy of information in the files of all CRAs. Most CRAs are credit bureaus that gather and sell information about a person (e.g., whether a person pays bills on time or has filed bankruptcy) to creditors, employers, landlords, and other businesses. The full text of this legislation is available on the Federal Trade Commission (FTC) Web site. Consumers may have additional rights under state law, and a state or local consumer protection agency or a state attorney general can provide that information.

CRAs charge a nominal fee for supplying information. When seeking information from a credit bureau, complete data should be given about the prospective credit applicant. This information should include the following information about the individual:

- Full name, including first and middle names, is supplied. Accurate spelling is essential. The spouse's name should be used as a cross-reference for identification purposes only.
- Address or addresses for the past 3 years
- Place of employment for the past 3 years
- Names of stores and firms where credit has been established
- Name of bank or banks
- Social Security number

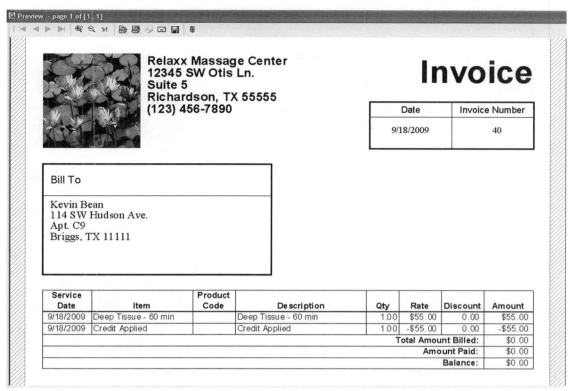

FIGURE 15-6. The current credit balance on the account is indicated by the amount preceded by a minus sign on the invoice. *(Courtesy of Island Software.)*

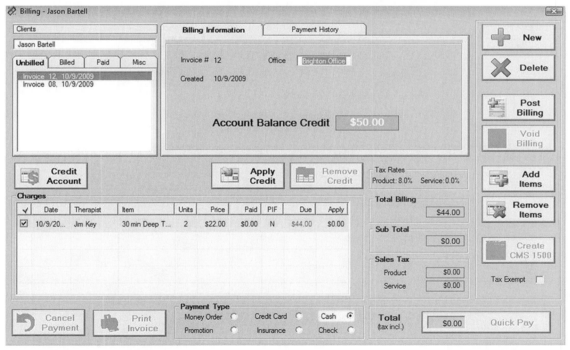

FIGURE 15-7. Credit is adjusted on receipt of a payment by the client. *(Courtesy of Island Software.)*

After this information has been given to the credit bureau, you will receive a credit report on the applicant. Care must be taken to record the information accurately. The Associated Credit Bureaus of America have designed a common language, which incorporates symbols, for reporting this information (Table 15-2). The symbols should mean the same things throughout the consumer credit industry, such as *O* for open, *R* for revolving, and *I* for installment.

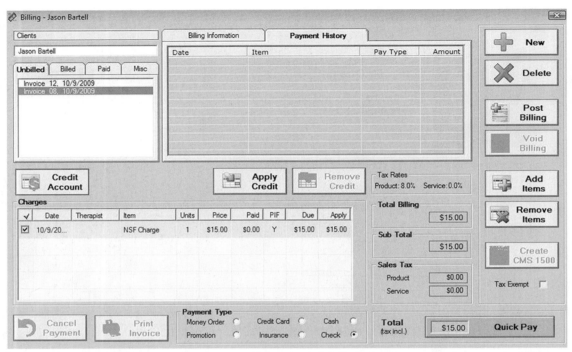

FIGURE 15-8. Account transaction screen indicates a nonsufficient funds (NSF) check with a service charge attached. *(Courtesy of Island Software.)*

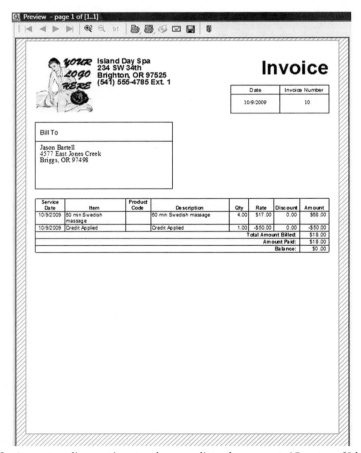

FIGURE 15-9. A courtesy discount is entered as a credit to the account. *(Courtesy of Island Software.)*

FIGURE 15-10. Truth in lending form. (*Courtesy of SYCOM, Madison, WI. In Finkbeiner BL, Finkbeiner CA:* Practice Management for the Dental Team, *ed 6, St. Louis, 2006, Mosby.*)

TABLE 15-2	Language Used in Consumer Credit Reports

USUAL MANNER OF PAYMENT	SYMBOL
Open account, 30-day account, 90-day account	0
Too new to rate; approved but not used	0-0
Pays (or paid) within 30 days of billing; pays 90-day accounts as agreed	0-1
Pays (or paid) in more than 30 days but not more than 60 days	0-2
Pays (or paid) in more than 60 days but not more than 90 days	0-3
Pays (or paid) in more than 90 days but not more than 120 days	0-4
Pays (or paid) in 120 days or more	0-5
Bad debt; placed for collection; suit; judgment; bankrupt; skip	0-9
Revolving or option account R or R $ _____ *	R*
Too new to rate; approved but not used	R-0
Pays (or paid) according to the terms agreed	R-1
Not paying (or paid) as agreed but not more than one payment past due	R-2
Not paying (or paid) as agreed and two payments past due	R-3
Not paying (or paid) as agreed and three payments past due	R-4
Bad debt; placed for collection; suit; judgment; bankrupt; skip	R-9
Installment account I or I $ _____ *	I*
Too new to rate; approved but not used	I-0
Pays (or paid) according to terms agreed	I-1
Not paying (or paid) as agreed but not more than one payment past due	I-2
Not paying (or paid) as agreed and two payments past due	I-3
Not paying (or paid) as agreed and three payments or more past due	I-4
Repossession	I-8
Bad debt; placed for collection; suit; judgment; bankrupt; skip	I-9

*When the monthly payment is known, it should be shown (e.g., R $20 or I $78).
Modified from the Associated Credit Bureau of America.

Extending credit to a client in the massage practice is not common but has the potential to increase. More people use massage on a regular basis and would prefer to pay a fixed amount each month. The massage therapist decides whether to extend credit to a client. If the client is denied credit, FCRA requires that the client be informed of the reason for denial of credit and the name of the bureau from which a credit report was obtained. It is not required to report the specific data obtained from the bureau; a client who wants this information should contact the bureau personally.

COLLECTING FEES

Collecting fees in the massage office can be easy or difficult. Collecting fees for a cash-only business is relatively easy. You can accept cash, credit or debit cards, or checks. Difficulties may include a client forgetting his checkbook or one who did not have enough cash. Another situation is NSF checks. Most clients pay when they receive their next massage, but not all do.

Experience has shown that clients pay health care bills last. People pay their rent for fear of eviction, their car payments for fear of repossession, utility bills for fear of losing service, and loans because banks usually adhere to stricter enforcement of collection procedures than the massage therapist does. Fortunately, only about 5% of clients become "uncollectable," but this 5% can be exasperating. A cash only policy prevents the need for collection.

SELF-REFLECTION

Have I ever been unable to pay all my bills? What was that like? What did I do? How did I respond when someone asked me for the money? Did I tell the truth and attempt to work out something? Did I avoid the collector or make excuses? What will I do when someone does not pay me for massage services? How will it feel to ask someone for the money? How will I ask to be paid? What will I do if I do not get paid?

Fair Debt Collection Practices Act

Collection procedures are regulated by the Fair Debt Collection Practices Act of 1996. This bill act was passed to protect the public from unethical collection procedures. The activities outlined in the law are listed in Box 15-1, and these regulations usually apply to collection agencies. When choosing a collection agency, it is important to verify debt collection regulations and ensure that the agents adhere to them. These same regulations should be considered when performing collection procedures in the office.

BOX 15-1 | Provisions of the Fair Debt Collection Practices Act

- Debtors may not be subjected to harassment, oppressive tactics, or abusive treatment. The law prohibits the collector from making any false statements to a debtor, such as claiming to be an attorney or a government agency.
- Debtors may not be called at work if the employer or the debtor objects and requests no calls.
- Debtors may not be called at inconvenient places or times, such as before 9 AM or after 9 PM.
- No one except the debtors themselves may be told they are behind on their bills.

Collection Letters

Letters may be sent at the discretion of the massage therapist. In offices that use a computer, a reminder notice can be included on the statement, and the first collection letter (Fig. 15-11) is automatically generated when an account becomes past due. You may use a series of computer-generated reminder notices automatically sent at specified intervals (e.g., 30, 60, and 90 days past due) before assigning an account to a collector. Be responsible, however, in reviewing the list of delinquent accounts. One of these accounts may be a client of long standing who, because of extenuating circumstances, was unable to pay the account. It is not wise to risk the loss of a well-established client relationship by adding a message or sending an account to a collector without first checking to see if a reason exists for the oversight.

The collection process should have four stages: reminder, inquiry or discussion, urgency, and ultimatum. The previous discussion concerned the first stage (reminder), which is accomplished through a notice on the statement. In the second stage (inquiry), you personally contact the client to determine the problem. The final two stages can be completed with letters. The letter of urgency must be persuasive (Fig. 15-12). An urgent phone call may be used as a follow-up as long as it does not result in harassment. In either situation, you should be courteous, considerate, and helpful but firm.

The final stage, the ultimatum, arrives when a client has failed to respond to all messages sent. You must confront the client with an ultimatum. Refrain from referring directly to lawsuits, attorneys, or collection agencies unless you intend to follow through. Send only one ultimatum letter with a deadline date (Fig. 15-13). Send this letter by certified mail with a return receipt requested to prove that the debtor has received the letter. If payment is not received by the designated date, the account must be turned over immediately to an attorney or a collection agency. The following rules can guide the composition of collection letters:

1. Keep the letter brief.
2. Make sure that data about the account are complete and accurate.

Luke Fritz, MT, NCTMB
2050 Leisure Lane, Lapeer, MI 48446
(123) 456-7890 / leisurelymassage@hec.com

October 20, 20xx

Serena Jarvez
321 Counting Lane
Your Town, State 00000

Dear Ms Jarvez:

Your account of $160.00 is over 90 days past due. If you are unable to pay this account in full, perhaps we can help you make arrangements for a payment plan.

Please contact us before November 15, 20xx, at 5:00 PM.

Sincerely,

Your signature

Luke Fritz, MT, NCTMB
Massage Therapist

FIGURE 15-11. First collection letter.

Luke Fritz, MT, NCTMB
2050 Leisure Lane, Lapeer, MI 48446
(123) 456-7890 / leisurelymassage@hec.com

November 20, 20xx

REGISTERED

Serena Jarvez
321 Counting Lane
Your Town, State 00000

Dear Ms Jarvez:

Since we have not heard from you regarding your account of $160.00 from June 1, 20xx, please be informed that it will be necessary to transfer this account to a collection agency.

The account must be paid in full by Friday, December 1, 20xx, to avoid such action.

Sincerely,

Your signature

Luke Fritz, MT, NCTMB
Massage Therapist

FIGURE 15-12. Urgent collection letter.

3. Use simple words and uncomplicated sentences.
4. Use phrases that will motivate the client, such as "cooperation" or "maintenance of a good credit rating."
5. Do not make statements that you do not intend to carry out. If you tell the client that the account will be sent to a collection agency in 10 days, give a specific date, and then follow through if necessary.
6. Set a specific date by which you expect payment, rather than saying "by the end of the month" or "in 10 days."
7. Be firm and polite.
8. Include a "thank you" in the letter closing because this, too, can be an important part of the collection procedure, and it is a valuable aid to public relations.

Telephone as a Collection Instrument

Many find it difficult to use the telephone in collecting delinquent accounts. The telephone allows a more personal contact with a client. When a client who normally pays the account on time becomes delinquent, a phone call seems less formal

Luke Fritz, MT, NCTMB
2050 Leisure Lane, Lapeer, MI 48446
(123) 456-7890 / leisurelymassage@hec.com

December 3, 20xx

REGISTERED

Serena Jarvez
321 Counting Lane
Your Town, State 00000

Dear Ms Jarvez:

Please be informed that your account of $160.00 from June 1, 20xx, has been transferred to the Dunhill Collection Agency for collection.

Sincerely,

Your signature

Luke Fritz, MT, NCTMB
Massage Therapist

FIGURE 15-13. Final collection letter.

than a letter and helps maintain a friendly relationship. Specific rules should be followed when using the telephone for collections:

1. Do not call before 9 AM or after 9 PM.
2. Verify that you are speaking to the person whose account is overdue. Ask, "Is this Mr. Johnson?"
3. Identify yourself.
4. Ask whether it is a convenient time to talk. If not, ask when you may call back, or find out when the client will be able to call you. Do not give details to a third party or leave detailed messages on an answering machine or voicemail.
5. State the purpose of your call. Be friendly and display a helping attitude.
6. Be positive. Do not say, "I'm sorry to call you." Act as though you know the client intends to pay and you are determining the arrangements for such a payment.
7. Have all of the information about the account in front of you.
8. Attempt to obtain a definite commitment, including the date and the amount of the payment. Follow up with written confirmation of the telephone discussion.
9. Make calls in a private area out of the hearing range of anyone in the reception room.
10. Do not threaten the client.
11. Follow up on the promises the client makes.
12. Do not discuss the account with anyone else.

Collection Agency

After every attempt has been made to collect an account, it may be necessary to engage the services of a collection agency. These services are required when the client fails to respond to a final collection letter or can no longer be located and becomes a "skip."

Delay in sending the account to a collection agency results in less chance of recovering a portion of the fee. Although the agency's fee reduces the portion recovered, continued unsuccessful attempts by the office are even less rewarding.

A collection agency should be selected that maintains high standards of professionalism. Investigate the agency thoroughly to determine its ethics and reliability:

- Check the ownership of the agency through a banker, the local Chamber of Commerce, or the Better Business Bureau.
- Contact the National Retail Credit Association or the Associated Credit Bureaus of America for information about the agency.
- Find out whether the agency has contacts out of town to aid in collection of accounts.
- Make sure the agency will not start legal action without the massage therapist's consent.
- Make sure the agency understands your needs and that you want reports on its activities.

After the business has sought the services of an agency, the office should use these services routinely. To allow action to be taken promptly, complete data about each case should be given to the agency, including the following:

- Debtor's full name
- Last known address and phone number
- Total amount of account
- Date of last entry on account (credit or debit)
- Debtor's occupation
- Business address and phone number
- Any other pertinent information

When an account is turned over to a collection agency, you no longer pursue collection procedures on it. However, the massage office staff must cooperate with the agency. The staff should do the following:

- Send no more statements
- Indicate the transfer to the collection agency on the ledger card, giving the date of transfer
- Refer the client to the agency if the person contacts the office
- Report the amount to the agency when payment is received in the office
- Rely on the agency staff members to do the job (i.e., do not pester them with calls of inquiry about the account)

Good Stuff from the Government

The U.S. Small Business Association offers many free online training courses. You can log on and complete courses in financing and accounting, including the following:
- Finance Primer: Guide to SBA's Loan Guaranty Programs (http://www.sba.gov/financialassistance)
- How to Prepare a Loan Package
- Assessing Financial Needs
- Introduction to Accounting
   Bean Counter (http://www.dwmbeancounter.com/) is an excellent nongovernment site that provides links to many Web sites, including government sites, and that offers free bookkeeping training.

SUMMARY

Unless the message therapist has studied accounting, she or he should probably hire an accountant to audit the books and compute a variety of tax reports and financial statements. The daily bookkeeping transactions remain the responsibility of the business owner. The two financial systems used are accounts payable and accounts receivable. A business owner who is not proficient in math can use the appropriate computer software to perform computations. However, basic mathematical procedures must be understood to detect errors.

Basic bookkeeping systems such as the pegboard system are being used less because of the many entries needed for basic transactions and the availability of software. The most popular system is a computerized bookkeeping system; from one entry, the system can produce an entry into a client's statement or insurance claim form and generated specific reports. This system also can generate accounts receivable and accounts payable summaries at the end of the day with a click of a button. The system can generate client statements to be mailed or given out to clients as they come in so they can keep payments up to date and keep track of the number of treatments. The reports generated can act as reminders that certain clients have payments due or have a birthday coming up.

A massage business requires common payment and credit policies, which can be printed on the client's statements. Common policies include when payments must be made, when payments are considered late, when unpaid bills will be turned over to collections, fees for missing appointments, and other rules. The laws must be adhered to and policies followed to support efficient work. If needed, a collection agency can be used for a fee.

Bibliography

Bean Counter: Home page. Available at http://www.dwmbeancounter.com/index.html (accessed June 2009).

Internal Revenue Service: Home page. Available at http://www.irs.gov/ (accessed June 2009).

U.S. Small Business Association: Online training courses, Available at http://www.sba.gov/training/index.html (accessed June 2009).

Evolve Annotated Web Links

http://evolve.elsevier.com/Fritz/business

Bean Counter (http://www.dwmbeancounter.com/index.html)

U.S. Small Business Association, online training courses (http://www.sba.gov/services/training/onlinecourses/index.html)

Workbook

1. Explain the differences between accounting and bookkeeping.

_____

_____

_____

_____

_____

_____

2. List the common types of bookkeeping systems used in massage therapy.

_____
_____
_____
_____
_____
_____

3. List and explain the function of the components of a pegboard system.

_____
_____
_____
_____
_____
_____

4. List and explain the function of the components of a computer bookkeeping system.

_____
_____
_____
_____
_____
_____

5. What are the advantages of an electronic bookkeeping system compared with a manual system?

_____
_____
_____
_____
_____
_____

6. Describe how monthly statements are prepared.

_____
_____
_____
_____
_____
_____

7. Identify the function of each of the following:
   a. Credit policy

   _____

   b. Credit bureau

   _____

   c. Collection agency

   _____

8. Explain the contents of an effective collection letter.

_____
_____
_____
_____
_____

MANAGING MONEY

KEY TERMS

American Bankers Association (ABA)
Automatic teller machine (ATM)
Bank card
Bank deposit
Bank draft
Bank statement
Budget
Cashier's check
Certified check
Check card
Checks

Credit card
Debit card
Employee's Withholding Allowance
  Certificate (Form W-4)
Employer identification number
Endorsement
Expenditures
Federal Insurance Contributions Act
  (FICA)
Form SS-4
Gross wages

Merchant account providers
Money order
Net pay
Petty cash
Revenue
Traveler's check
Voucher check
Wage and Tax Statement (Form W-2)
Withholding

---

e Guidelines for the Learning Activities and answers to the Workbook questions are located on Evolve at http://evolve.elsevier.com/Fritz/business.

LEARNING OUTCOMES

Mastery of the content in this chapter will enable the reader to:

- Explore his or her relationship with money
- Explain the function of a budget
- Explain the use of electronic banking
- Identify the parts of a check
- Write a check and determine the correct balance on a checkbook register
- Identify various types of checks
- Prepare checks for deposit with correct endorsements and complete a deposit slip
- Reconcile a bank statement
- Explain the purpose of a monthly expense sheet
- Explain the purpose of a yearly summary

- Identify the purpose of payroll records
- Explain the purpose of the employee's earnings record
- Calculate gross and net wages
- Explain how withheld income tax and Social Security taxes are deposited
- Explain how federal unemployment taxes are deposited
- Describe how to complete a Form W-2
- Explain the importance of retaining payroll records
- Explain the use of an automated payroll system
- Use the Internet as a resource for financial forms and instructions

All massage practices, regardless of size, have financial matters that need to be addressed by internal or external accounting procedures. You can expect to perform many tasks in addition to the accounts receivable activities highlighted in the previous chapter. These tasks may include receiving and organizing statements, paying for materials and supplies, processing payroll or tax forms, and recording and analyzing expenses.

In processing financial documents, accuracy is essential. Verification of data and attention to detail are necessary to ensure that the processed information is accurate. Incorrect data can mean improper cash flow analysis, inaccurate accounts receivable, erroneous claim form preparation, or inaccurate budget and expense figures. All of these effects can have serious repercussions for the entire business.

This chapter presents the major types of financial systems and the data that must be processed and managed in a modern massage practice. You will learn how technology is applied to the financial operations of a practice to make it more productive. Resources available through the Internet can guide you in procuring and filling out many of the financial forms needed by the practice. This chapter also addresses a more abstract relationship to business finances, sometimes described as *prosperity consciousness* or *abundance awareness*.

Much of this textbook teaches you very concrete activities, such as math or how to use a collection agency, as described in the previous chapter. However, a philosophy of success also has been advanced throughout the book. An important aspect of success is to understand how you measure success. Your relationship to money is part of that understanding. Value occurs in many ways, as does compensation for services rendered. Money is only one way to be compensated, but it is what keeps the business afloat. If you are uncomfortable asking for and receiving money, your attitude will interfere with your ability to manage money. Exploration of this topic is where we begin the chapter.

ABUNDANCE, ENOUGH, NOT ENOUGH: BALANCE

There are many definitions of abundance, enough, and scarcity (not enough). A few definitions are needed to develop an understanding of a money relationship.

Balance is as much as is needed (enough). If enough is just right, scarcity is not enough, and abundance is more than enough. Scarcity or not enough is easiest to understand. Most have experienced the sensation of not enough time. Some have experienced not enough food. When really hungry, we feel empty. However, not enough does not mean without. The thing we want is available, but not enough of it to feel satisfied. If there is enough, we are satisfied, but is there enough to share? If there is more than enough, we may save for a time when there may not be enough, or we may feel generous and distribute the excess. For example, if we have just enough to eat, we will be satisfied, but if we share, we will not be full. Will we share when resources are scarce—not quite enough but could be if everyone contributed a small amount?

How do we know when enough is enough? What happens when the pursuit of one thing in abundance—money or athletic performance for example—results in not enough time for friends, children, relaxing, or sleeping? This dilemma is often reflected in ancient health systems such as the balance of Yin and Yang. Most disease can be described in terms of too much in one area that results in not enough in another.

In massage, if you spend too much time working on the back, there is not enough time to adequately massage the rest of the body. It all becomes a management issues (i.e., practice of managing, handling, supervision, or control).

There is a difference between a need and a want. A need indicates that something is necessary for life, such as nutritious food, clean water, a specific medication, or shelter. A want is something we do not need, but it brings a sense of satisfaction. When truly hungry, we need and want food. We can meet the need with beans, rice, and spinach mixed together in a quantity that can fit in an individual's hands cupped together, or we can meet the need with something we want, such as a pint of ice cream, a huge steak, or a whole bag of candy. Many of the current diseases plaguing affluent societies come from meeting a need with a want. Too much of a good thing becomes a bad thing. Obesity and the resulting diabetes stem from overeating the wrong types of food. To counteract obesity caused by too much of the food we want and not enough exercise, we need to shift the balance. Reducing the food and creating scarcity on purpose and increasing the exercise so there is enough movement will result in a reduction of what we do not need: excess body fat. Easily said but sometimes very hard to do.

We do need some fat reserves, and in a similar manner, we do need money reserves. It is important to save appropriately so there is enough during times of scarcity. For example, there are natural slow times in the massage business. When the weather becomes nice in the spring or around holidays, people may get a massage less often. For a couple of weeks, business is slow, and income diminishes. Financial management anticipates the seasonal fluctuation in income, and money from periods of abundance is saved for times of relative scarcity. It is a balance.

Abundance is more than enough. Abundance can be wonderful or not. Abundance means that we have more than we need, but when we have more than we need, what do we do with it? Use it anyway? Save it? Hide it? Share it? A combination of all four options? Only you can answer this, and how you answer the question can provide insight into your relationship with money. Abundance is a worthwhile goal. Financial abundance is one aspect to consider. Financial abundance means that we can achieve some of our wants (e.g., ice cream for dessert along with the beans, rice and spinach), clean water pumped to the house instead of having to carry it from a distant well, and owning a house with a yard instead of living in the car or shelter. Abundance means that we can set aside resources to sustain ourselves when there are times of scarcity. Saving money is like preserving food during the abundance of the fall harvest to feed ourselves during the winter.

We all need to consider our future needs and wants, as well as the needs of those who depend on us, such as our children. It is important to regularly save from the current abundance in some sort of investment retirement plan. Investments grow and produce income. Investments can include savings accounts that earn a small amount of interest and purchasing property that will increase in value. Investment means that we are doing something productive with our abundance when the resources are more than enough. We can hide abundance, but hiding is a secret. People may hide income so that they do not have to pay taxes. That money cannot grow because it cannot be seen. If you are paying taxes, it means that you have earned an abundance in income. Those who make an income below a certain level (i.e., barely enough) do not have to pay very much in income taxes, whereas those who have more than enough income pay on the abundance. Some of the tax money is used to help those who do not have enough (e.g., social programs such as WIC, which provides federal grants to states for supplemental foods, health care referrals, and nutrition education for low-income pregnant, breastfeeding, and nonbreastfeeding postpartum women and to infants and children up to age 5 years who are found to be at nutritional risk.) Taxes can be seen as a form of sharing abundance. The tax laws are convoluted and not always fair, but the concept is sound. If you are paying taxes, you are making at least enough money to meet survival needs (Box 16-1).

BOX 16-1   Income Considered To Be Barely Enough, Not Enough, Enough, and Abundance

Collection financial standards are used to help determine a taxpayer's ability to pay a delinquent tax liability. Allowable living expenses include those expenses that meet the necessary expense test. The necessary expense test is defined as expenses that are necessary to provide for a taxpayer's (and his or her family's) health and welfare and production of income. The actual tables are on the Evolve Web site (http://evolve.elsevier.com/Fritz/business).

Examples are given for a single person who is 30 years old. All amounts are averages and estimates.

■ Just barely enough, no monetary abundance: meets needs only

Monthly expenses:
   Food, clothing, and other items: $500
   Transportation (monthly loan or lease payments, monthly operating costs): $700
   Housing and utilities: $1,100
   Health care (insurance and out of pocket): $200
Total monthly expenses: $2,500
Total yearly expenses: 30,000

■ Poverty level annual income: $8,900 (approximately one third of barely enough)
■ Enough $36,000 (approximately one-third more than barely enough)*
■ Abundance: $50,000 (almost double enough)

*These figures are estimated net incomes, provided to illustrate the concepts of scarcity and abundance.
Figures are adapted from the Internal Revenue Service. (http://www.irs.gov/individuals/article/0,,id=96543,00.html)

Abundance in all things—faith, hope, love, material resources, beauty, joy, and courage—allows us to rise higher on Maslow's hierarchy of needs (see Chapter 3), from survival and security needs to function at the social level of caring for others. Meaning does exist beyond survival with abundance. There is enough to share, but abundance does not mean that there will only be good times. Life is a balance. We cannot appreciate light without knowing the dark, love without understanding loss, more without feeling compassion for those with less. The saying "no rain, no rainbows" summarizes this concept (Box 16-2).

It is good business to strive for abundance if you maintain balance in all aspects of your life. This is hard to do if you are planning on career development as a business owner. Starting a business requires a balance of energy. The business is a baby and needs constant care, but it will mature and be able to stand alone in time. You will need the understanding and support of those around you during this time. They are investing in you, and in time, you will be able to repay the investment. During the process, seek balance, and do not overlook those things that are most important.

Wise use of abundance requires a plan. A financial plan begins with a budget.

SELF-REFLECTION

What is most abundant in my life? Is there a balance? What will I do with the abundance from my massage career? Am I afraid of money? Is money my friend? Is money my tool?

BOX 16-2	Perspective

"The least of things with a meaning is worth more in life than the greatest of things without it."—*Carl Jung*

"You must give some time to your fellow men. Even if it's a little thing, do something for others, something for which you get no pay but the privilege of doing it."—*Albert Schweitzer*, Nobel Peace Prize winner

"Money can't buy happiness, but neither can poverty."—*Leo Rosten*, U.S. (Polish-born) author

"Abundance is, in large part, an attitude."—*Sue Patton Thoele*, U.S. author

"Though I am grateful for the blessings of wealth, it hasn't changed who I am. My feet are still on the ground. I'm just wearing better shoes."—*Oprah Winfrey*, U.S. actress and television talk show host

"Making a living and having a life are not the same thing. Making a living and making a life that's worthwhile are not the same thing. Living the good life and living a good life are not the same thing. A job title doesn't even come close to answering the question 'What do you do?'"— *Robert Fulghum*, U.S. author

DETERMINING A BUDGET

A *budget* is a massage practice's financial plan of operation for a given period, usually 1 year. The purpose of the budget is to establish the practice's financial goals. To achieve an acceptable level of profit, *expenditures*, the amount of money spent to operate the practice, must be kept in balance with *revenue*, the amount of income received by the practice. Massage therapists can use spreadsheet software to develop a budget so that they can plan more thoroughly and in less time than with paper and pencil methods. Spreadsheets allow planners to see how a change in one calculation affects all the related calculations. A template of a business budget modified for a massage practice is shown in Figure 16-1. A template of a personal budget and a personal finance statement is shown in Figure 16-2.

LEARNING ACTIVITY

Analyze your current financial status; include income and expenses. Develop a personal budget based on your income and expenditures. Analyze the budget for areas that can be improved.

BANK ACCOUNTS

One of the daily routine functions of the massage office is control of the *cash flow,* or the amounts of money received and the amounts disbursed. A good understanding of banking technology and procedures is necessary. Banking responsibilities include managing debit and credit cards, check writing, accepting checks from clients for payment of services, endorsing and depositing checks, keeping an accurate bank balance, and reconciling the bank statement.

Electronic Banking

For many massage offices, electronic banking means 24-hour access to cash through an *automated teller machine* (ATM) or direct deposit of paychecks and accounts receivable into a checking or savings account. Electronic banking now involves many different types of transactions.

Electronic banking, also known as *electronic funds transfer* (EFT), uses a computer and electronic technology as a substitute for checks and other paper transactions. EFTs are initiated through devices such as cards or codes that let the massage therapist or those authorized by the massage therapist access an account. Many financial institutions use ATMs or debit cards and personal identification numbers (PINs) for this purpose. Other institutions use devices such as debit cards or a signature or scan to access to an account. The federal Electronic Fund Transfer Act (http://www.fdic.gov/

MASSAGE BUDGET

Month/Year:

SUMMARY	ACTUAL	BUDGETED	OVER BUDGET	UNDER BUDGET	
Total income					
Total expenses					
Income less expenses:					

INCOME DETAILS	ACTUAL	BUDGETED	OVER BUDGET	UNDER BUDGET	NOTES
Fees					
Interest earned					
Rent					
Royalties					
Other					
Total income:					

EXPENSE DETAILS	ACTUAL	BUDGETED	OVER BUDGET	UNDER BUDGET	NOTES
Accounting					
Contributions					
Equipment purchases					
Insurance					
Legal					
Loans					
Office supplies					
Postage					
Professional Dues					
Rent & maintenance					
Salaries and wages					
Employee benefits					
Payroll taxes					
Telephone					
Travel					
Utilities					
Other					
Total expenses:					

FIGURE 16-1. Business budget for a massage practice.

regulations/laws/rules/6500-1350.html) covers some electronic consumer transactions.

ATMs, which provide 24-hour service, are electronic terminals that allow banking at almost any time. To withdraw money, make deposits, or transfer funds between accounts, an ATM card is inserted and a PIN number is entered. ATMs must indicate if a fee is charged and give the amount on or at the terminal screen before the transaction is completed.

Direct deposit enables a person to make a deposit to the account on a regular basis. In this system, the massage therapist may preauthorize recurring bills, such as insurance premiums, mortgages, and utility bills, to be paid automatically.

Pay by phone systems allow a person to call the financial institution with instructions to pay certain bills or to transfer funds between accounts. An agreement must exist between the institution and the company being paid that allows these funds to be transferred.

Personal computer banking allows the account to be accessed from a remote location, such as a personal computer. The account holder can view the account balance, request transfers between accounts, and pay bills electronically.

The use of electronic transfers should be monitored carefully. The massage therapist and any other person responsible for electronic banking must read the documents received from the financial institution that issued the access device. No one should know the PIN except the responsible person

Cost-of-living budget

Regular or fixed monthly payments*

Mortgage or rent	$
Automobile payment	$
Automobile insurance	$
Appliances	$
Loan	$
Health insurance	$
Personal property insurance	$
Telephone	$
Utilities (gas or electric)	$
Water	$
Other non-emergency expenses	$

Discretionary or variable payments

Clothing, laundry, cleaning	$
Medicine	$
Doctor and dentist	$
Education	$
Dues	$
Gifts and donations	$
Travel	$
Subscriptions	$
Automobile maintenance and gas	$
Spending money and entertainment	$

Food expenses

Food—at home	$
Food—away from home	$

Taxes

Federal and state income tax	$
Property	$
Other taxes	$

Other

Other	$

Total monthly payments	$

Sample recommended budget expenditures

Shelter (rent or mortgage)	20%
Food	25%
Clothing	12%
Transportation	12%
Medical and dental	6%
Dues and charities	9%
Education and entertainment	10%
Savings	6%*

*Financial advisors recommend that savings should cover expenses for at least 3 months.

A

Personal financial statement

Assets

Cash	$
Securities (stocks, bonds, CDs)	$
Real estate	$
Automobile	$
Furniture	$
Receivables (money owed to you)	$
Other	$

Value should be determined by the amount that could be obtained from a "quick" sale.

Total owned	$

Debts

Household bills unpaid	$
Installment payments:	
Automobile	$
Appliances	$
Loans	$
Real estate payments	$
Other	$
Insurance:	
Automobile	$
Personal property	$
Health	$
Other	$
Taxes	$
Other debts	$

Total owed	$

Total owned minus total owed = Total worth	$

B

FIGURE 16-2. Personal budget (**A**) and financial statement (**B**). *(From Gerdin J: Health Careers Today, ed 4, St. Louis, 2007, Mosby.)*

or persons. Before any electronic transfer system is used, the institution must provide the following information, which you should keep filed:

- A summary of the practice's liability for unauthorized transfers
- The telephone number and address of the person to be notified if an unauthorized transfer has been or may have been made, a statement of the institution's business days, and the number of days you have to report suspected unauthorized transfers
- The type of transfers that can be made, the fees for transfers, and any limits on the frequency and amount of transfers
- A summary of the right to receive documentation of transfers and to stop payment on a preauthorized transfer, as well as the procedures for stopping payment
- A summary of the institution's liability
- Privacy assurance

If problems arise in the use of the EFT, a complaint can be filed through the Web site for the state member banks of the Federal Reserve System (http://www.federalreserve.gov/).

Credit and Debit Card Payment

Being able to accept credit cards for massage service payment makes the business more attractive to customers. Some massage therapy business owners are intimidated by the process of accepting credit and debit cards or are worried about the associated fees. Accepting credit cards is not difficult, and the increased volume and other benefits almost always outweigh the fees that business owners have to pay for this capability.

There is a process for accepting credit and debit cards. You need a merchant account, which is where credit card payments will be deposited. *Merchant account providers* give businesses the ability to accept credit and debit cards.

A *credit card* is a method of payment. The issuer of the card (i.e., Visa, Discover) grants a line of credit to the consumer. The consumer is borrowing money for payment. When a purchase is made, the credit card user agrees to pay the card issuer. The cardholder indicates his or her consent to pay by signing a receipt with a record of the card details and indicating the amount to be paid. The card needs to be verified to ensure the card is valid and the credit card customer has sufficient credit to cover the purchase. Verification is performed using a credit card payment terminal, which is a device used to swipe or key in required credit card information and to transmit data to the merchant service provider. Data from the card are obtained from a magnetic stripe or chip on the card.

A *debit card* (i.e., bank card or check card) provides an alternative payment method to cash when making purchases. Functionally, it can be called an electronic check, because the funds are withdrawn directly from the bank account.

To get a merchant account, you can use a bank, a third-party provider such as PayPal, or an independent sales organization. Most massage business owners are best suited by working with an independent sales organization. Many merchant account providers have special packages for small businesses, so take the time to shop around for the best deal. They also have access to the equipment you will need to process the payment. There are hundreds of merchant account providers. Contact your Better Business Bureau (http://www.bbb.org/) for listings. Take the time to shop around, and be sure that you understand all the associated fees and compare deals until you find the one that is best for your specific needs.

Security and fraud are important issues when accepting these types of payments. Examine each credit card closely to make sure it is valid. Be aware of possible counterfeit, stolen, or fraudulently used credit cards. Do not allow clients' financial information to be observed. Identity theft is the fastest growing crime, and business owners need to protect their clients. One of the most common ways that information is snatched is through lost credit cards.

Establishing a Checking Account

As a rule, the checking account for the business was opened before you began working. In opening the account, the massage therapist decides what type of account to use and signs a signature card (Fig. 16-3) that permits him or her to write checks against the account. If another person is permitted to write checks against the account, that person's signature must also appear on a signature card for the account or on the same signature card that the massage therapist signed.

CHECKS

Checks are a means of ordering the bank to pay cash from the customer's bank account. In the past, checks accounted for more than 90% of all financial transactions in the United States; however, the current use of checks is below 60%, and the rate will continue to decline because of the move to a paperless financial culture. Checks are still used, however, and you need to understand how they work.

Many parts of a check are self-explanatory; however, some parts need additional explanation. In Figure 16-4, part 3 is the *American Bankers Association* (ABA) bank identification number. Under this coding system, every bank is given its own number, which constitutes a numeric name for the bank. This number aids the sorting of checks for distribution to their proper destination. The ABA number is a fraction and usually is printed in the upper right corner of the check or slightly to the left of the check number. Part 4 of the check is the *payee*, the individual or company that will receive the money. Part 7, the *drawee*, is the bank that pays the check. Parts 8 and 9 are magnetic ink character recognition (MICR) numbers. These are encoded on all checks to facilitate high-speed handling by machine. The first number is the bank

FIGURE 16-3. Signature card. *(From Finkbeiner BL, Finkbeiner CA:* Practice Management for the Dental Team, *ed 6, St. Louis, 2006, Mosby.)*

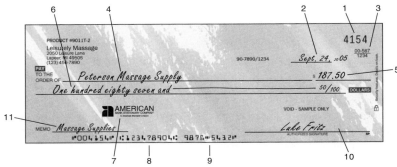

FIGURE 16-4. Parts of a check. 1, Check number. 2, Date of check. 3, American Bankers Association (ABA) bank identification number. 4, Payee, the person or company to be paid. 5, Amount of check (in numerals). 6, Amount of check (in words). 7, Drawee, the bank on which the check is drawn. 8, Bank identification number magnetically printed for electronic processing. 9, Customer account number magnetically printed for electronic processing. 10, Signature of drawer. 11, Reason the check was written. *(Courtesy of SYCOM, Madison, WI. Modified from Finkbeiner BL, Finkbeiner CA:* Practice Management for the Dental Team, *ed 6, St. Louis, 2006, Mosby.)*

identification number (also found in the ABA identification number). The second number is the check writer's checking account number. These numbers can easily be read by people or by machine. Part 10 of the check is the signature of the *drawer* or check writer, the person who orders the bank to pay cash from the account.

WRITING CHECKS

Check writing can be done manually or with the help of a computer system. The check stub or checkbook register should be completed before the check is written or printed. The stub or register provides a record of (1) the check number, (2) the date, (3) the payee, (4) the amount of the check, (5) the purpose of the check, and (6) the new balance brought forward after the amount of the check has been subtracted, or it provides the new balance if a deposit is to be added to the previous balance, as shown in the manual system (Fig. 16-5).

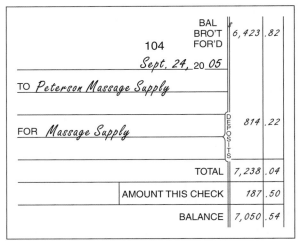

FIGURE 16-5. Check stub. *(Modified from Finkbeiner BL, Finkbeiner CA:* Practice Management for the Dental Team, *ed 6, St. Louis, 2006, Mosby.)*

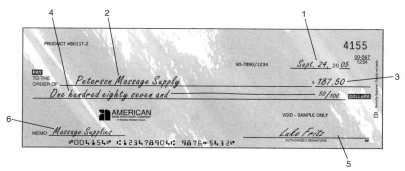

FIGURE 16-6. How to write a check. 1, Date the check. 2, Key or write the name of the person or firm to whom the check will be payable. 3, Enter the amount of the check (in figures) opposite the dollar sign. 4, Write the amount of the check (in words) under the "Pay to the order of" line. Start as far to the left margin as possible. 5, The name on the signature line should be signed as it appears on the bank signature card. 6, On the memo line, record the purpose of the payment. *(Courtesy of SYCOM, Madison, WI. Modified from Finkbeiner BL, Finkbeiner CA:* Practice Management for the Dental Team, *ed 6, St. Louis, 2006, Mosby.)*

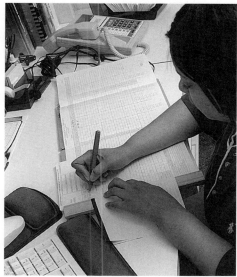

FIGURE 16-7. Pegboard check system. *(From Young AP:* Kinn's the Administrative Medical Assistant, *ed 5, St. Louis, 2003, WB Saunders.)*

Figure 16-6 presents a step-by-step procedure for writing a check. A similar procedure is followed for entering checks in the one-step system (Fig. 16-7) or for entering check information in a computerized bookkeeping system.

TYPES OF CHECKS

The following list describes a few of the types of checks that you may receive:

Certified check: A certified check is a guarantee that funds have been set aside to cover the amount of the check. The person goes to the bank and writes a personal check for the proper amount. The bank sets aside that amount from the customer's account, placing it in a special account, and then stamps *Certified* across the face of the check. Usually, a nominal fee is charged for certifying a check.

Cashier's check: A cashier's check is the bank's order to make payment out of the bank's funds. When a cashier's check is purchased, the person specifies to whom the bank makes the check payable and receives a carbon or stub of the check as a record. A fee is usually charged for this type of check.

Money order: A money order is a means of transferring money without using cash or a personal check. People who do not maintain a personal checking account often use money orders to pay their creditors. The money order may be purchased in the form of a bank money order, a postal money order, or an express money order. The money order shows the name of the purchaser and the person who is to receive the payment (i.e., payee). A fee is charged for this service.

Traveler's check: Even though the *traveler's check* is designed as a payment device for a person who is away from home, it is not uncommon to receive a traveler's check in payment for massage services. Traveler's checks are purchased through a bank, American Express, or Railway Express Agency. The checks are preprinted in various denominations, usually $10, $20, $50, and $100. A small fee, determined by the amount purchased, is charged. When the checks are purchased, the individual signs his or her name in a designated place on each check. When the checks are used for payment or are cashed, they are *countersigned;* that is, the purchaser signs them again in the presence of the individual who cashes the check or accepts it for payment.

Bank draft: A bank draft is a check drawn by the cashier of one bank on another bank where the first bank has available funds on deposit or credit. A bank draft is used if a person or company wants to send a sum of money and a personal check is not acceptable.

Voucher check: A voucher check provides a detachable stub, which serves as an excellent accounting record for itemizing payment of invoices or any other type of itemization the payer would like as a reference.

ACCEPTING AND CASHING CHECKS

Many different types of checks may be used as payment for services. When you accept a check, make sure that it is (1) legibly written in ink or typewritten, (2) currently dated, (3) signed by the check writer, (4) drawn on a U.S. bank, (5) made payable in a certain sum of money (the amount in figures and the amount in words should agree), and (6) made payable to a payee or bearer.

Sometimes, you may be asked to accept a check for more than the charges. This may present a problem. For example, if the individual owes $50 and wants to pay $50 but writes a check for $100 and asks for $50 to be returned, a question may arise at a later date if the client tries to use the canceled check as a receipt for full payment of the account. Another problem that may be encountered is the acceptance of payment for more than the balance and the return of the difference in cash to the client. If the bank returns the client's check for insufficient funds, you have paid cash out from the business, and the client has the cash. To avoid problems of this nature, it is better to establish a firm policy of not accepting checks for more than the amount owed.

Cash

Because some clients pay their accounts with cash, some cash must be kept in the office. However, large amounts of cash should not be routinely kept in the office, because it may end up being counted as part of the total cash receipts for the day. A separate cash balance can be maintained for petty cash (discussed later).

SELF-REFLECTION

How do I pay my bills? Do I use checks, debit cards, credit cards, cash, money orders, or electronic transfers? Do I pay off the credit card each month or accumulate a balance? What do I do if I overdraw an account and spend money I do not have? Can I have cash in my wallet and discipline myself to not spend it? Do I spend money on impulse, or do I think about purchases a while before buying?

Deposits

MAKING A DEPOSIT

Depositing money into the practice's checking account is usually a daily routine. A bank deposit represents the accumulation of money received for a single day or possibly for a longer period. The bank provides checking account deposit slips, which have the massage practice's name and account number imprinted on them. Follow the step-by-step procedure presented in Figure 16-8 when completing the deposit

DEPOSIT TICKET

PRODUCT 419

CHECKS AND OTHER ITEMS ARE RECEIVED FOR DEPOSIT SUBJECT TO THE TERMS AND CONDITIONS OF THIS BANK'S COLLECTION DEPARTMENT. PLEASE LIST EACH CHECK SEPARATELY.

PRODUCT #419-4
Leisurely Massage
2050 Leisure Lane
Lapeer, MI 49505
(123) 456-7890

YOUR BANK NAME HERE
321 MAIN STREET
CITY, STATE AND ZIP

Date		DOLLARS	CENTS
CURRENCY			
COIN			
1	11-82	225	00
2	12-416	75	00
3	2-412	80	00
4	16-308	55	00
5	10-012	135	00
6	MONEY ORDER	40	00
7	MASTER CHG.	140	00
8	AM.EXP.TRAV.CH.	50	00
9			
10			
11			
12			
13			
14			
15			
16			
17			
18			
19			
20			
21			
22			
23			
24			
LESS CASH RETURNED			
TOTAL ITEMS	TOTAL DEPOSIT	800	00

FIGURE 16-8. Deposit slip. 1, Write or type the date on the front side. 2, List currency and coins to be deposited. 3, Identify checks to be deposited individually; if there are more than three, use the back side of the deposit slip. Checks should be listed on the deposit slip by the American Bankers Association (ABA) numbers. However, you may prefer to list checks with the client's name and number. If it is a money order, traveler's check, or MasterCard or VISA charge receipt, the total amount of money and the name of the item are listed. 4, Enter the total from the back on the front side of the deposit slip. 5, Total the entire deposit (net deposit). 6, Optional: some deposit slips provide a line in case the depositor wants part of the deposit back in cash. The amount desired is entered on this line and subtracted from the total line above; the net deposit then is entered as in 5. (*Modified from Finkbeiner BL, Finkbeiner CA:* Practice Management for the Dental Team, *ed 6, St. Louis, 2006, Mosby.*)

form. A duplicate copy of the deposit form may be retained for office use to verify with the check register and bank statement at the end of the month.

Another type of bank deposit slip may be used. In the era of computers, software is available for the massage practice,

October 24, 2009 at 3:05p   Page 1

                              DEPOSIT SLIP
                                PRACTICE
                    Dates Included: 10/24/09 to 10/24/09

Leisurely Massage
2050 Leisure Lane
Lapeer, MI 49505
(123) 456-7890

Account Number:

Code	Bank No.	Check No.	Amount	Reference (ID, Name)
3	87/44323	634	150.00	(7301) Gable, Catherine M
3	55/980	978	80.00	(12202) Page, Michael W
3	90/4532	709	50.00	(26901) Glass, Steven
3	77/345-0	4793	150.00	(48201) Nair, Ernest
3	445/0983	345	50.00	(50101) O'Brien, Armando
3	12-9855	746	125.00	(234101) Jackewitz, Jerry

TOTAL

        6 Checks   Total   605.00

        Total Cash   211.00

        Total Deposit   816.00

FIGURE 16-9. Computer-generated deposit slip. (*Modified from Finkbeiner BL, Finkbeiner CA:* Practice Management for the Dental Team, *ed 6, St. Louis, 2006, Mosby.*)

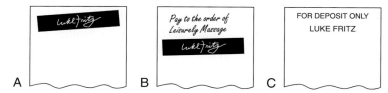

FIGURE 16-10. Check endorsements. **A,** Blank endorsement, which is an endorsement that consists of the signature of the payee. A blank endorsement makes the check payable to any holder. **B,** Endorsement in full, which is an endorsement that states to whom the check is to be paid and the signature of the payee. This endorsement specifies that the check can be cashed or transferred only on the order of the person, bank, or company named in the endorsement. **C,** Restrictive endorsement, which is an endorsement that includes special conditions or that limits the receiver of the check in the uses that can be made of it; this type of endorsement commonly is used when checks are prepared for deposit. (*Modified from Finkbeiner BL, Finkbeiner CA:* Practice Management for the Dental Team, *ed 6, St. Louis, 2006, Mosby.*)

and frequently, the massage management software is written by a massage therapist. A common application on the computer is the management of the daily cash flow. At the end of the day, the bank deposit slip is generated from funds entered into the accounts receivable program (Fig. 16-9).

DEPOSITS BY MAIL

Making deposits of the day's receipts by mail saves time for you. Mail deposit slips and envelopes are provided by the bank. Each check should be carefully endorsed on the back with a restrictive *endorsement* and the signature or stamp of the payee and then placed in the envelope with the deposit slip. The three most common types of endorsements are explained in Figure 16-10. Currency and coins should not be sent through the mail unless sent by registered mail. On receipt of the deposit, the bank sends the customer a receipt of the deposit and another mail deposit slip and envelope. Mail deposits are rapidly being replaced with electronic transfers.

NIGHT DEPOSITORY

Sometimes, the practice receives large amounts of money after banking hours. The night depository is a means of depositing money in the bank vault when the bank is closed. Usually, the deposit is completed the next business day by a bank teller; the depositor must go to the bank to pick up the deposit bag and receipt. However, if the depositor prefers, the deposit bag can remain locked until the person arrives at the bank to make the deposit personally.

BOX 16-3	Important Points to Remember When Using an Automatic Teller Machine

- Never use an ATM to deposit cash or other items that can be used by unauthorized personnel.
- You receive only receipts of deposit; no copies of deposit slips are given.
- Use an ATM only to deposit checks with restrictive endorsements.
- Notify the bank immediately of any discrepancies between its records and transactions on the office bank statement.
- Notify the bank immediately if your office ATM access card is lost or stolen.

FIGURE 16-11. Bank statement. (*Modified from Finkbeiner BL, Finkbeiner CA:* Practice Management for the Dental Team, *ed 6, St. Louis, 2006, Mosby.*)

AUTOMATIC TELLER MACHINE

In conjunction with the checking account, financial institutions offer special access cards that can be used to perform banking transactions 24 hours per day, 7 days per week. The cards can be used at ATMs, which are computer workstations that electronically prompt the user through most routine banking activities. Deposits or withdrawals can be made, or funds can be transferred between accounts. However, some precautions must be taken when using an ATM (Box 16-3).

Reconciling the Bank Statement

Although procedures may differ, most banks send a *bank statement* (Fig. 16-11) to the depositor each month. The bank may return the *canceled checks* (i.e., checks that have been paid) along with the bank statement showing the balance of the account at the beginning of the month, deposits made during the month, checks drawn against the account, corrections or charges against the account (e.g., service charge, stop payment charges), and the bank balance at the end of the month. To maintain an accurate record of the checking account, you should reconcile the bank statement as soon as the records are received from the bank.

You should use the following procedure to reconcile the bank statement.

1. Verify the amount of the canceled checks with the amounts on the bank statement. The canceled checks are usually returned in the order listed on the statement.
2. Arrange the canceled checks numerically.
3. Compare the amounts on the canceled checks and the deposits with the amounts written in the checkbook register. Check-off all canceled checks and deposits in the checkbook register.
4. List the *outstanding checks* (i.e., checks not yet returned to the bank), including the check number and the amount.

5. Total the outstanding checks. If a deposit has been made but does not appear on the bank statement, the deposit must be added to the bank statement balance before the outstanding checks are subtracted.
6. Look for charges other than checks that have been deducted from the account, such as service charges (SC), debit memos (DM), and overdrafts (OD). These charges must be subtracted from the checkbook register.

In Figure 16-12, a reconciliation of the bank statement has been prepared for the practice of Massage Associates, PC (see Fig. 16-11 for end of the month figures to determine how these computations were made).

PETTY CASH

Although the cash receipts are deposited in the bank and invoices and miscellaneous items are paid by check, a small amount of cash should be kept in the office. This should be established as a *petty cash* fund and controlled with the same accuracy as the checking account.

When it has been determined how much cash will be placed in the petty cash account, a check is written against the business account and cashed, and the cash is returned to the office and kept in a separate fund. To help eliminate errors in disbursements from the fund, one person in the

Leisurely Massage
Bank Reconciliation
July 25, 2009

Balance per Bank Statement		$7,790.47	Balance per checkbook		$7,743.26
+ Deposit of 07-20- not on statement		400.00	Subtract		
		$8,190.47	Debit memo	$5.00	
			Service charge	8.40	13.40
Less Outstanding Checks					
No. 1102 -	$50.00				
No. 1106 -	150.61				
No. 1110 -	75.00				
No. 1111 -	66.40				
No. 1112 -	118.60				
Total Outstanding checks		460.61			
Adjusted Bank Balance		$7,729.86	Adjusted Checkbook Balance		$7,729.86

FIGURE 16-12. Bank reconciliation. *(Modified from Finkbeiner BL, Finkbeiner CA:* Practice Management for the Dental Team, *ed 6, St. Louis, 2006, Mosby.)*

Petty Cash Voucher

No.________ Date________

Paid to ______________________ Amount

For ______________________ ________

Charge to ______________________

________________ Approved by ________________ Payment received

FIGURE 16-13. Petty cash voucher. *(From Finkbeiner BL, Finkbeiner CA:* Practice Management for the Dental Team, *ed 6, St. Louis, 2006, Mosby.)*

office should have control over the petty cash. A voucher is completed each time money is taken from the fund. The voucher shows the date, voucher number, amount of payment, what the payment was for, to whom the payment was made, and the name of the person approving the payment (Fig. 16-13).

After the voucher is completed, it is placed in the drawer as a reminder of the amount of cash taken from the fund. The vouchers and cash together should equal the original balance of petty cash.

A formal record of petty cash disbursements may be used. This record shows all the disbursements in chronologic order, the voucher number, and special columns for each expense item disbursed from the fund. It also provides a complete summary of how the money was disbursed. At the end of the month, the fund must be replenished. This involves writing another check for cash purposes and charging the various expense accounts for the amount used from the petty cash.

RECORDING BUSINESS EXPENSES

As invoices are processed, the expenditures represented on them need to be analyzed and verified for payment. A check is then made out to each supplier for payment of these statements. You then record each item in an expense category. A monthly income and expense register provides a list of all the expenditures for the month, including the date of payment, the company to which the payment was made, the category of deduction, and the amount of payment. These totals are transferred to the annual summary. This combination checkbook and expense record provides space for deposit entries and checkbook balances, as well as itemization of each expenditure into specific categories. A software alternative allows expenses to be recorded and checks printed using a computer system. Either of these systems can keep a running total of expenses or provide monthly and yearly totals.

MAINTAINING PAYROLL RECORDS

Various federal and state laws require that most businesses keep records to provide information about wages paid and to help in the preparation of required tax reports. You must have a good working knowledge of payroll and tax records.

Initial Payroll Procedures

As an employer, the massage therapist must apply for an *employer identification number,* a nine-digit number assigned to sole proprietors or corporations for filing and reporting payroll information. The application, *Form SS-4,* is available from the Internal Revenue Service (IRS). Some states also require a state employer identification number. Any forms you may need can be found online (http://www.irs.gov) and can be printed, downloaded, or even obtained by fax.

EMPLOYEE'S EARNINGS RECORD

Exemptions _____ Name _____
Date of Birth _____ Address _____
Date Employed _____ _____
Phone _____ Soc. Sec. No. _____
In Emergency Notify _____

REMARKS	DATE	CHECK NO.	GROSS SALARY	FEDERAL W.H. TAX	F.I.C.A.	STATE W.H. TAX	OTHER	OTHER	NET CHECK
THIRD QUARTER									
FOURTH QUARTER									
YEAR'S TOTALS									

FIGURE 16-14. Employee's earnings record. *(Courtesy SYCOM, Madison, WI.)*

The employer is required to have every employee complete an *Employee's Withholding Allowance Certificate (Form W-4)*. This form is needed to determine the status of each employee for income tax deductions from wages. Employees are required to complete a new Form W-4 when they change the number of withholding exemptions claimed.

Employee Earnings Record

The employer must maintain employees' earnings records, including a summary of information for each employee. If the record has been properly designed, it provides the information needed for quarterly and annual reports. The employee's earnings record should contain the following information, which is used for various state and federal reports (Fig. 16-14).

1. Name, address, Social Security number, rate of pay, withholding exemptions claimed, marital status, and special deductions (e.g., credit union account, bonds, United Fund contribution)
2. The number of pay periods in a quarter and the date on which each pay period ends
3. Columns for regular earnings, overtime earnings, and total earnings (earnings records are available that provide

columns for rate of pay and hours or days worked in a pay period)

4. A column for each deduction and for total deductions
5. A column for entering the net amount (net pay) received (i.e., difference between total earnings and deductions)
6. A column for recording accumulated taxable earnings, which provides the employer with information on taxable earnings, *Federal Insurance Contributions Act* (FICA) deductions (discussed later), and taxable wages for unemployment taxes
7. Columns for quarterly and annual totals

Determining Employee Wages

The employer and employees must reach an agreement on an acceptable wage. This may be determined as an hourly rate, a weekly rate, or a monthly amount. After this rate has been established, the procedure must be decided for determining net pay.

1. The hourly wage is $20 per hour.
2. If the workweek is based on 40 hours per week, the *gross wages* (amount earned before deductions) are $800 (40 hours × $20 per hour = $800).
3. Deductions are made from wages, as in the example that follows:

   a. *FICA deduction (Social Security and Medicare taxes):* The amount to be withheld is determined by calculating at the combined 2000 rate (7.65% [or 0.0765] × $800 = $61.20). This tax rate is divided into two parts: the Social Security part, which is 6.2% on the first $76,200 earned in 2000, and the second part, for Medicare, which is 1.45% on all earnings, no ceiling. These tax rates are subject to change by Congress. The employer must keep track of such changes and make deductions according to the current rate. The *Employer's Tax Guide—Circular E,* available from the IRS, can be used to check the current tax rates.

   b. *Withholding (income tax deductions):* The amount withheld depends on the number of exemptions indicated on Form W-4. The tax amount withheld is determined from a table in the *Employer's Tax Guide—Circular E.* The withholding tax on $800 for a married person claiming one exemption is $94.

   c. *Local income tax:* Some cities and states have personal income taxes that must be deducted. The employer must be familiar with the state and local laws regarding these taxes.

   d. *Other deductions:* In addition to the standard deductions, you may have a weekly deduction of $60 for the credit union (noted on the earnings record).

4. The *net pay* (take-home pay), the amount for which the paycheck is written, is $584.80.

Gross Wages	Minus Deductions	Total Deductions	Net Pay
$800.00	FICA: $61.20 Withholding tax: $94 Credit union: $60	$215.20	$584.80

The net pay for each member of the business staff must be calculated. After the amounts have been determined, the paychecks are written, the information is entered on each employee's earnings record, and a record is made on the expense sheet.

A pegboard system similar to the one described earlier, which uses a write-it-once method, can be a great time saver. With this type of system, the employee's earnings are recorded on the earnings record and the monthly expense disbursement sheets when the check stubs are written. The columns on the check stubs, earnings records, and monthly expense disbursement sheet coincide. These systems have proved very popular with employers who have a number of employees.

Depositing Withheld Income Tax and Social Security Taxes

The employer must deposit withheld income tax, Social Security, and Medicare taxes in an authorized commercial bank or a Federal Reserve Bank. Since January 1, 2000, new coupon forms have been used for depositing taxes. The IRS sends the employer a Federal Tax Deposit (FTD) Coupon Book (Form 8109) containing 15 coupons for depositing all types of taxes. FTD forms are no longer mailed out periodically. If additional forms are needed, the FTD Reorder Form (Form 8109A) provided in the coupon book is used. If you do not have a coupon book, you may request one from the IRS district office.

The amount of taxes determines the frequency of deposits. These taxes are owed when the employer pays the wages (or makes the payments from which the taxes are withheld), not when the payroll period ends. To determine when the taxes are due and the amount on which they are based, you should check the instructions on the reverse side of the Employer's Quarterly Federal Tax Return (Form 941).

Although the employer probably will make monthly deposits for the withholding taxes and FICA deductions, he or she must file a quarterly return on Form 941. The returns and tax payments are due on the following dates:

Quarter	Quarter Ending	Date Due
January to March	March 31	April 30
April to June	June 30	July 31
July to September	September 30	October 31
October to December	December 31	January 31

The employer completes Form 941 by entering the summarized payroll data for the quarter. Information about total wages and taxable FICA wages is obtained from the employee's earnings record. Further instructions are available in the IRS pamphlet instructions for Form 941.

Federal Unemployment Tax

The employer is subject to a federal unemployment tax under the provisions of the Federal Unemployment Tax Act (FUTA). This tax is 6.2% of wages paid and applies to the first $7000 of wages paid during the calendar year. A credit may be taken against the federal unemployment tax for contributions to be paid into state unemployment funds. The federal unemployment tax is imposed on employers and must not be deducted from employees' wages. On or before January 31, the employer must file an unemployment tax return (i.e., Employers' Annual Federal Unemployment [FUTA] Tax Return [Form 940]) and deposit or pay the balance of the tax in full. For deposit purposes, the employer must compute the federal unemployment tax on a quarterly basis. The deposit must be made on or before the last day of the first month after the close of the quarter.

To determine whether your employer must make a deposit for any of the first three quarters in a year, compute the total tax as follows:

1. Multiply the first $7000 of each employee's annual wages paid during the quarter by 0.008.
2. If the amount subject to deposit (plus the amount subject to deposit but not deposited for any prior quarter) is more than $100, a deposit should be made during the first month after the quarter.

Wage and Tax Statement: Form W-2

A federal Wage and Tax Statement (Form W-2) for a calendar year must be provided for each employee no later than January 31 of the following year. Form W-2 is prepared in six parts and distributed in the following manner: one copy for IRS use; one copy to state, city, or local tax

LEARNING ACTIVITY

Look at different payroll checks, and identify the deductions. Describe the difference between government deductions and other deductions. List the various types of other deductions that may be taken from gross wages by the employer.

_____

_____

_____

Describe how self-employed individuals pay income and payroll taxes.

_____

departments; three copies to the employee (i.e., one for filing federal tax returns, one for state or local tax purposes, and one for the employee's files); and one copy retained by the employer. Form W-2 includes the following information:

- Employer's identification number, name, and address
- Employee's Social Security number, name, and address
- Federal income tax withheld
- Total sum of wages paid to the employee
- Total FICA employee tax withheld (Social Security and Medicare)
- Total wages paid that are subject to FICA
- State and local taxes withheld when applicable

To correct a Form W-2 after one has been issued to an employee, a corrected statement must be issued. The corrected statement must completely replace the original statement and be clearly marked as "CORRECTED RETURN" in capital letters directly above the title, Wage and Tax Statement. If a Form W-2 is lost or destroyed, the substitute copy issued to the employee is marked as "REISSUED RETURN."

REPORT OF WITHHELD INCOME TAX

On or before February 28, copy A of all Form W-2s issued for the year and Form W-3, Transmittal of Wage and Tax Statements, must be sent to the IRS.

RETENTION OF PAYROLL AND TAX RECORDS

The employer must keep all records pertaining to employment taxes available for inspection by the IRS. Although no form has been devised for such records, the employer must be able to supply the following information:
- Amounts and dates of all wages paid
- Names, addresses, and occupations of employees
- Periods of employees' employment

SELF-REFLECTION

Did I realize how payroll is calculated? Have I ever challenged how payroll deductions were made when I thought there was a mistake? How do I feel about the difference between gross and net pay in my paycheck? If I am going to employ massage therapists, how do I feel about paying a portion of their taxes?

- Periods for which employees were paid while absent because of sickness
- Employees' Social Security numbers
- Employees' income tax withholding allowance certificates
- Employer's identification number
- Duplicate copies of returns filed and the dates and amounts of deposits made

These tax records should be kept for at least 4 years after the date the taxes to which they apply become due.

Employer's Responsibility for Tax Information

The *Employer's Tax Guide—Circular E* summarizes the employer's responsibilities for withholding, depositing, paying, and reporting federal income tax, Social Security taxes, and federal unemployment tax. The circular is available to all employers and may be obtained from a local IRS office. Because tax rates often increase, it is wise to check with the IRS to ensure that current forms and percentages are used for tax calculations. Additional information and help are available at the American Payroll Association Web site (http://www.apa.com/).

ACCOUNTS PAYABLE SOFTWARE

Most massage office software packages do not provide a mechanism for writing checks and maintaining payroll records; therefore, the massage therapist must rely on some form of commercial software to accomplish this task. QuickBooks Financial Software gives small business owners the power to run their businesses more effectively. For small businesses with 1 to 20 employees, QuickBooks helps to save time and increase productivity because it offers improvements to commonly used features and provides better help and learning tools to increase the user's knowledge and confidence. The software is available in a variety of editions, and you should review the needs of the office before making a selection. The package has several benefits:

- Pay bills
- Print checks
- Create invoices and purchase orders
- Track business payments and expenses
- Manage payroll processing
- Direct deposit paychecks
- Create state and federal forms
- Track workers' compensation payments and easily calculate bonuses

 Explore the tutorial on the accounting capabilities of the practice management software. Based on the inventory management you already established, pretend you need to order a certain supply and fill out the various screens involved in this process.

Good Stuff from the Government

A number of government and private organizations have information about various aspects of identity theft and fraud: how it can occur, what you can do about it, and how to guard your privacy. To help you learn more about the problem and its solutions, the U.S. Department of Justice Web site lists other Web sites on identity theft and related topics. Links to the information provided here also can be found on the Evolve Web site.

THE UNITED STATES SECRET SERVICE

The United States Secret Service Web site (http://www.secret-service.gov) provides information on the following topics:

How can I detect counterfeit currency?

How can I protect myself against credit card fraud?

What should I do if I think I have been victimized by credit card fraud or identity theft?

How do I report a case of advance fee fraud (also known as "4-1-9 fraud")?

How can I protect myself against check fraud?

How can I protect myself against telemarketing fraud?

How can I protect my privacy?

FREE ANNUAL CREDIT REPORT

According to the Fair and Accurate Credit Transactions Act of 2003 (http://www.whitehouse.gov/news/releases/2003/12/20031204-3.html), U.S. residents are entitled to one free credit report a year from AnnualCreditReport.com (https://www.annualcreditreport.com/; phone number: 877-322-8228). Experts suggest ordering one from a different agency every 4 months. Check the number of open accounts on the report to make sure that the total agrees with what you would expect. You are also entitled to a free credit report when you have reason to suspect identity fraud.

THE INTERNAL REVENUE SERVICE

There is much valuable information on the IRS Web site (http://www.irs.gov/businesses/small). A few of the highlights are presented here, and a more complete list is available on the Evolve Web site. You can find answers to many questions about being self-employed individuals or independent contractors.

(Continued)

Good Stuff from the Government—cont'd

Who is self-employed? If you are in business for yourself or carry on a trade or business as a sole proprietor or an independent contractor, you can consider yourself a self-employed individual. You are an independent contractor if the person for whom you perform services has only the right to control or direct the result of your work, not what will be done or how it will be done.

Do I need an identification number? You must have a taxpayer identification number to operate your business. This usually is your social security number or an individual taxpayer number. However, if you have employees and in some other circumstances, you will need an employer identification number.

Useful forms and publications: A collection of relevant forms and publications related to understanding and fulfilling your filing requirements.

Operating a business: Learn about the various responsibilities associated with operating your own business. You will find many topics, such as types of business taxes that may apply, how to structure retirement plans for your employees, deducting the cost of running your business, and much more.

Closing a business: There is more involved in closing your business than just locking the doors. This section provides procedures for getting out of business, including what forms to file and how to handle additional revenue received or expenses that you may incur.

Tax trails: Quick and interactive, answer a few yes or no questions, and you have insight into your deductions, credits, and more.

RECORDKEEPING

Good records can help you monitor the progress of your business, prepare your financial statements, identify source of receipts, keep track of deductible expenses, prepare your tax returns, and support items reported on tax returns. Log on to the IRS Web site to find information on the following topics:

Why should I keep records?

What kinds of records should I keep?

How long should I keep records?

How long should I keep employment tax records?

How should I record my business transactions?

What is the burden of proof?

SUMMARY

Money has monetary value and emotional value. One person's sense of financial security may be completely different from another's.

A business is an operation that needs to make money to stay in business, and the use of a budget is essential. You must calculate the total expenditures and revenue and then determine how much each expenditure should be allowed. This calculation should include the funds needed when revenue is below average and the bills still need to be paid.

Just as you need to know the parts of a check you write, you should be able to identify those areas on the checks you receive to make sure they provide the necessary information to obtain payment. There are many payment methods that you may want to provide your client, but when offering credit payment, there are additional expenses. The most secure forms of payment are cash, certified check, cashier check, money order, traveler's check, and debit card. At the end of the day, these checks need to be entered on a deposit slip or printed if you are of a computer software program and then stamped with the account number on the back of the check. Monthly, all deposits and expenditures of the business need to be reconciled with the bank statement.

Bibliography

Department of the Treasury: *Internal Revenue Service: Employer's Tax Guide*, publication no, 15, circular E *(revised)*. Washington, DC, 2005, Internal Revenue Service.

Fulton PJ: *General Office Procedures for Colleges*, ed 12, Cincinnati, OH, 2003, South-Western.

Hall J: *Consumers Now Favor Credit and Debit over Cash and Checks*, Washington, DC, December 2003, American Banking Association.

Evolve Annotated Web Links

http://evolve.elsevier.com/Fritz/business

American Bank Association (http://americanbankassociation.com)

American Bank Association (www.apa.com)

Annual Credit Report (https://www.annualcreditreport.com/cra/index.jsp)

Better Business Bureau (www.bbb.org)

Federal Deposit Insurance Corporation (http://fdic.gov)

Federal Electronic Fund Transfer Act (EFT) (http://www.fdic.gov/regulations/laws/rules/6500-1350.html)

Federal Reserve (www.federalreserve.gov)

Federal Trade Commission (www.ftc.gov)

Internal Revenue Service, publications online (http://www.irs.gov/publications)

Internal Revenue Service, tax information for businesses (http://www.irs.gov/businesses/)

Intuit, QuickBooks (http://www.quickbooks.com/support)

United States Department of Justice: Where can I find out more about identity theft and fraud? (http://www.usdoj.gov/criminal/fraud/websites/idtheft.html)

United States Secret Service, FAQ: How do I protect myself against credit card fraud? (http://www.secretservice.gov/faq.shtml#faq11)

1. Name and define the parts of a check.

_____
_____
_____
_____
_____

2. List the necessary steps in writing a check.

_____
_____
_____
_____
_____

3. Explain the differences between a certified check and a cashier's check.

_____
_____
_____
_____

4. Describe the procedure for making a bank deposit.

_____
_____
_____
_____
_____

5. Define the following:
   a. Blank endorsement

_____
_____
_____

   b. Endorsement in full

_____
_____
_____

   c. Restrictive endorsement

_____
_____
_____
_____

6. Describe the procedures for reconciling a bank statement.

_____
_____
_____
_____

7. Explain the function of a monthly expense sheet.

_____
_____
_____

8. Explain the function of a yearly summary.

_____
_____
_____
_____
_____

9. Why is it necessary to maintain accurate payroll records?

_____
_____
_____
_____
_____

10. What is the purpose of an employee's earnings record?

_____
_____
_____
_____
_____

11. Explain the difference between gross and net wages.

_____
_____
_____
_____
_____

12. What is the purpose of Form 941, and when is the form prepared?

_____
_____
_____
_____
_____

13. On what amount of the employee's wages must the employer pay unemployment taxes?

_____
_____
_____
_____
_____

14. What information is included on Form W-2?

_____
_____
_____
_____
_____

15. Explain the importance of payroll and tax record retention.

_____
_____
_____
_____
_____

MAINTAINING A SAFE WORK ENVIRONMENT

KEY TERMS

Acquired immunodeficiency syndrome
(AIDS)
Asepsis
Autogenous infection
Barrier techniques
Blood-borne pathogens
Centers for Disease Control and
Prevention (CDC)
Communicable disease
Cross-contamination

Disease transmission
Disinfectants
Disinfection
Environmental Protection Agency
(EPA)
Hazard
Hazardous waste
Hepatitis B virus (HBV)
Human immunodeficiency virus (HIV)
Infection

Infectious waste
Occupational Safety and Health
Administration (OSHA)
Personal protective equipment (PPE)
Risk
Sanitization
Sexual harassment
Sharps containers
Sterilization
Standard precautions

e Guidelines for the Learning Activities and answers to the Workbook questions are located on Evolve at http://evolve.elsevier.com/Fritz/business.

LEARNING OUTCOMES

Mastery of the content in this chapter will enable the reader to:

- Define key terms
- Identify the importance of an understanding of disease transmission
- Identify the routes of disease transmission
- Describe basic infection control procedures
- Identify regulatory agencies that may affect the massage therapy office

- Identify the records required by the Occupational Safety and Health Administration that are maintained in the business office of health care professionals
- Explain routine procedures to maintain quality assurance in the office
- Institute the necessary procedures and protocols for dealing with harassment in the workplace

A fundamental principle of massage therapy practice is safe and secure care. Attending to this process begins before the client enters the door. Is the entrance to the massage office safe and secure? Is the area well lighted and maintained in inclement weather. In the massage theory and practice segment of your education, you learned specific information about infection control and safety procedures. It may seem odd that this topic occurs in a book about career development, but all aspects of the business environment must be maintained in a safe and sanitary manner. The reception area, business equipment, and other features of the business are used by many people and therefore can become a route for infection transmission and provide a *hazard* for an accident, such as a fall or burn.

Unfortunately, there is potential in any work environment, including massage therapy, for harassment and various forms of workplace violence. These concepts are in opposition to the compassionate, nurturing environment of massage, and it may be inconceivable that such situations could occur. Although uncommon, they do unfortunately happen, and you have to know how to protect yourself and others if necessary. This chapter describes these important safety aspects of business operations.

SELF-REFLECTION

How safe do I feel when I go to school, shopping, work, the doctor, or home? What steps do I take to maintain a safe personal environment? Does the topic scare me? What can I do to be safer in my environment?

SANITATION IN THE HEALTH CARE BUSINESS OFFICE

Sanitation procedures entail more than keeping the environment neat and clean. Specific procedures are used in the business setting to protect the health and safety of employees and clients. If you are working in a health care environment

such as a pain management clinic, you must follow stringent sanitation requirements as set up by the *Occupational Safety and Health Administration* (OSHA). There are also very specific sanitation requirements for any location, such as a spa, where the public may use hydrotherapy equipment.

Several responsibilities must be attended to as part of business operations; the number of responsibilities depends on the environment. Because you may not know where you will be working, it is necessary to understand how infection control is maintained (Table 17-1).

Disease Transmission

Unlike treatment in the setting of nursing or dentistry, which involves several sources by which infectious diseases can be transmitted, including blood, saliva, and nasal discharge, massage therapists typically do not come in contact with body fluids. However, some instances of *disease transmission* may occur, as in the case of an unexpected nosebleed or a client with some degree of incontinence. Massage therapists routinely come in contact with the client's skin, hair, and clothing. When someone sneezes, mucus droplets are sprayed in the environment. Any of these events can transmit a microbial *infection*. Table 17-2 lists several *communicable diseases* and their routes of transfer.

Types of Infections

Infections can be divided into two categories: autogenous infections and cross-infections. *Autogenous infections* are infections that result from a person's own microflora. For example, a client who undergoes dental procedures may subsequently develop endocarditis; this condition can result from the spread of virulent organisms (e.g., staphylococci, pneumococci) that live in the mouth and that can be introduced into the bloodstream. *Cross-infections* are transferred from one person to another. For example, when a child has an infection and coughs or sneezes, the caregiver may contract the infection through airborne or droplet transmission.

Routes of Infection Transmission

Microbial transmission through secretions and exudates occurs by three routes: (1) direct contact with a lesion, organisms, or debris; (2) indirect contact through contaminated surfaces, supplies, equipment, or records; and (3) inhalation of microorganisms aerosolized from a client's saliva during coughing and sneezing.

INFECTION CONTROL IN THE MASSAGE THERAPY OFFICE

Because client care begins in the business office, it is important to maintain infection control in all areas of the business environment. Every health care worker, including the massage the therapist, is responsible for breaking the cycle of disease transmission (Fig. 17-1). Safe practice is based on the following principles:

■ A complete and accurate client history must be obtained.
■ Aseptic techniques must be observed, using *personal protective equipment* (PPE) if necessary.
■ Health care workers must strictly adhere to acceptable *disinfection* and *sterilization* procedures.
■ Equipment and supplies must be maintained in a sanitary manner.

The first step in safe practice is obtaining complete and detailed information about the client. The records discussed in Chapter 7 must be completed, dated, signed, and reviewed thoroughly. You must make sure that protocols are followed and the necessary barrier materials are available for use. You must ensure that the records used during the treatment procedure are transferred safely from the massage area to the business office without *cross-contamination.*

Table 17-3 presents several situations that massage therapists may encounter in attempting to maintain safe practice in the office. You must be able to distinguish between right actions and wrong actions and must understand the consequences of a wrong action in infection control.

Health Protection Program for the Massage Therapy Staff

Whether you are a therapist working in a health care environment, spa, or your own business, there is a role for an infection control coordinator, and you should be familiar with the aspects of this process. The office's personnel policy must include a health service program for the staff that covers the following:

■ Education and training
■ Immunizations
■ Exposure prevention and postexposure management

SELF-REFLECTION

If you can agree with each of the following statements, you probably can perform your duties safely and free of potential risks. If you cannot agree with one of these statements, you may jeopardize your own health and the safety of others with whom you have contact.

1. I completely understand the Occupational Safety and Health Administration (OSHA) concepts and the need to perform my duties safely.
2. I am sure that the pencils, pens, and records with which I come in contact regularly are free of contamination.
3. I am never in contact with exposed surfaces, body fluids, or contaminated areas or involved with sterilization processes.
4. I will never be required to provide emergency care to clients or others without protective personal barriers.
5. I never come in contact with infectious waste.
6. I never assume that the client is not potentially contagious because he or she is a family member or personal friend.

I understand that if I answered no to any of the preceding points, I must proceed only if I strictly adhere to the appropriate barriers and protocols provided by the *Centers for Disease Control and Prevention* (CDC) and OSHA.

■ Medical conditions, work-related illness, and work restrictions
■ Allergies or sensitivities to work-related materials, such as latex
■ Records maintenance, data management, and confidentiality issues
■ A referral arrangement with a medical physician who is available to treat staff members for emergencies and perform medical evaluation and treatment quickly and appropriately
■ Confidential, up-to-date medical records for all workers

Government Regulations

All health professionals are expected to comply with current guidelines and regulations governing infection control, hazard communication, and medical waste disposal. Several agencies are responsible for providing the regulations affecting each of these areas. The employer is primarily responsible for maintaining current copies of all state and federal regulations. These guidelines must be reviewed, and their implementation in the office must be documented.

In 1986, OSHA established guidelines to protect workers from occupational exposure to blood-borne diseases. In 1988, employees in direct contact with blood or infectious

TABLE 17-1	Management of Occupational Exposures to Blood-Borne Pathogens	
MASSAGE THERAPY WORKER	**EMPLOYER OR INFECTION CONTROL COORDINATOR**	**QUALIFIED HEALTH CARE PROVIDER**
Before an Exposure Occurs Receives training in risks of occupational exposures, immediate reporting of injuries or exposures, and massage therapy office reporting procedures	Establishes referral arrangements and protocol for employees to follow in the event of exposures to blood or saliva by puncture injury, mucous membrane, or nonintact skin or other potentially infectious materials Trains occupationally exposed employees in postexposure protocols Makes available and pays for hepatitis B vaccine for workers at occupational risk	Contracts with employer to provide medical evaluation, counseling, follow-up care to employees exposed to blood within the practice setting Keeps current on public health guidelines for managing occupational exposure incidents and is aware of evaluating health care provider's responsibilities ethically and by law
When an Exposure Occurs 1. Performs first aid 2. Reports injury to employer 3. Reports to the designated health care professional for evaluation and follow-up care, as indicated 4. Receives copy of Written Opinion.	1. Documents events in the office setting 2. Immediately directs employee to evaluating health care professional 3. Sends to evaluating health care professional: • copy of standard job description of employee • exposure report • source client's identity and bloodborne infection status (if known) • employee's HBV status and other relevant medical information • copy of the Occupational Safety and Health administration (OSHA) Bloodbourne Pathogen Standard 4. Arranges for source client testing, if the source client is known and has consented 5. Pays for postexposure evaluation and, if indicated, prophylaxis 6. Receives Written Opinion from evaluating health care professional • files copy of Written Opinion in employee's confidential medical record (if maintained by employer) • provides copy of Written Opinion to exposed employee	1. Evaluates exposure incident, worker, and source client for HBV, HCV, and HIV, maintaining confidentiality • arranges for collection and testing (with consent) of exposed worker and source client as soon as feasible (if serostatus is not already known) • in the event that consent is not obtained for HIV testing, arranges for blood sample to be preserved for up to 90 days (to allow time for the exposed worker to consent to HIV testing) • arranges for additional collection and testing as recommended by the U.S. Public Health Service/CDC • notifies worker of results of all testing and of the need for strict confidentiality with regard to source client results • provides counseling • provides postexposure prophylaxis, if medically indicated 2. Assesses reported illnesses/side effects 3. Within 15 days of evaluation, sends to the employer a Written Opinion, which contains (only):* • documentation that the employee was informed of evaluation results and the need for any further follow-up • whether HBV vaccine was indicated and if it was received

*All other findings or diagnoses remain confidential and are not included in the written report.
Modified from http://www.cdc.gov/mmwr/

materials and substances were required to use *standard precautions*; that is, all clients must be treated as if they are potentially infected with the *human immunodeficiency virus* (HIV, the cause of *acquired immunodeficiency syndrome* [AIDS]), the *hepatitis B virus* (HBV), or other infectious organisms. Some massage therapists may have additional massage contracts outside the main massage practice, and because the

massage practice is becoming common in the health care industry, an overview of the latest required OSHA standards is presented in Box 17-1.

When standard precautions are used, additional procedures are not necessary for treating a client known to have an infectious disease. Under standard precautions, each workplace must

TABLE 17-2 Transmission of Communicable Diseases

DISEASE	MEDIUM OF TRANSMISSION	ROUTE OF TRANSMISSION
Acquired immunodeficiency syndrome (AIDS)	Blood, semen, or other body fluids, including breast milk	Inoculation by use of contaminated needles or by direct contact so that infected body fluids can enter the body
Gonococcal disease	Lesions, discharge from infected mucous membranes	Direct contact, as in sexual intercourse; towels, bathtubs, toilets; hands of infected individuals soiled with their own discharges; through breaks in hands of attendant
Hepatitis B (viral)	Blood and serum-derived fluids, including semen body fluids	Contact with blood and vaginal fluids
Measles (rubella)	Discharges from nose and throat	Direct contact, hands of health care worker, articles used by and about client
Mumps	Discharges from infected glands	Direct contact with person affected
Pneumonia	Sputum and discharges from nose and throat	Direct contact, hands of health care worker, articles used by and about the client
Rubeola	Secretions from nose and throat	Through mouth and nose
Streptococcal sore throat	Discharges from nose and throat, skin lesions	Through mouth and nose
Syphilis	Infected tissues, lesions, blood	Direct contact, kissing, or sexual intercourse; transfer though placenta to fetus; contaminated needles and syringes
Tuberculosis	Saliva, lesions, feces	Direct contact, droplet infection from a person coughing with mouth uncovered, saliva transferred from mouth to fingers and then to food and other articles

Modified from http://www.cdc.gov/mmwr/

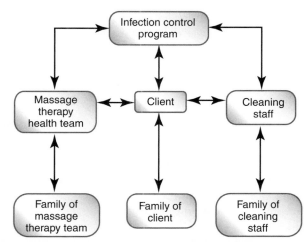

FIGURE 17-1. Cycle of disease transmission. *(Modified from Finkbeiner BL, Finkbeiner CA: Practice Management for the Dental Team, ed 6, St. Louis, 2006, Mosby.)*

- Be hazard free
- Provide personal protective clothing and equipment
- Display poster no. 2203, a guide to OSHA regulations, in a prominent location

The *Environmental Protection Agency* (EPA), a federal regulatory agency, developed a program for overseeing the handling, tracking, transportation, and disposal of medical waste. The CDC, a division of the U.S. Public Health Service, also provides recommendations for health care workers. It is responsible for investigating and controlling various diseases, such as hepatitis and tuberculosis (the incidence of which is increasing).

Maintaining Regulatory Records

Employers are responsible for the job of maintaining the myriad records required to meet the various standards and regulations. A control form can help to ensure that all records are kept as required. Examples of all records should be included in the office procedures manual or the *Regulatory Compliance Manual*. These records should be kept confidential and should include the following:

- Exposure determination forms, which describe the office infection control program and procedures
- Employee medical records
- Employee training records, which describe hepatitis B vaccination availability, requirements, and implementation
- Informed refusal for hepatitis B vaccination
- Postexposure evaluation and follow-up training

TABLE 17-3	Recognizing Right and Wrong Infection Control Patterns	
WRONG	**EFFECT**	**RIGHT**
Shaking hands while wearing gloves	Disease transmission may occur through cross-contamination.	Remove gloves and wash hands before leaving.
Pulling mask on and off	Contact with the face with contaminated gloves can expose unprotected tissues to disease. If mask is contaminated, contact with gloved or ungloved hands can allow disease transmission.	Nod and speak greetings to the individual.
Wearing the same mask for more than one client	Masks become moist fields, allowing penetration of particles through the mask.	Always change masks between clients, and use more than one mask if treatment procedure is lengthy.
Reusing gloves for different clients	Most gloves have microscopic openings, allowing penetration of microbes. Washing gloves increases the potential for disease transmission.	Gloves are always changed between clients; gloves may need to be changed during a treatment procedure that is lengthy.
Placing client records in treatment room	Records may become exposed to aerosols or through handling; these records are transferred to the business office after treatment, exposing the business personnel to the potential for disease.	Records other than radiographs should be kept outside the treatment room to avoid contamination. If the records must be in the treatment room, they should be kept out of the reach of aerosols and handled with clean hands or with overgloves rather than examination gloves.
Eating in a contaminated site	Surfaces can become contaminated from instruments or materials exposed to client aerosols or handling.	A staff lounge or eating area must be available in a site away from potentially contaminated materials.
Wearing a V-neck laboratory coat	Garments under laboratory coat can become contaminated. If wearing a V-neck shirt underneath, skin will be exposed.	Always wear high-neck laboratory coat when working with clients or in a laboratory.
Wearing dangling earrings, piercings, necklaces, bracelets	Items can become contaminated. They may hang near the client's face or catch on something.	Minimize jewelry to only wearing wedding bands and small post earrings.

Modified from http://www.cdc.gov/mmwr/

- Employee informed refusal of postexposure medical evaluation
- Incident report of exposure to occupational illness

Hazard Communication Program

OSHA's hazard communication standards require all health professionals to develop and implement a program involving employee training, compile a list of hazardous chemicals, maintain material safety data sheets (MSDSs), and label all chemicals in the office. This program must apply to all activities in which an individual may be exposed to hazardous chemicals under normal working conditions. The hazardous chemicals most likely to be encountered by a massage therapist are cleaning and sanitizing chemicals.

One individual in the office is designated the hazard communication program coordinator. A sole business practitioner automatically becomes the coordinator. This person is responsible for the following:

- Disseminating information about the program
- Recognizing the hazardous properties of chemicals found in the workplace
- Keeping up to date on procedures for safe handling of chemicals
- Implementing measures for protecting the office staff from hazardous chemicals

MATERIAL SAFETY DATA SHEETS

If you are assigned the job of hazard communication program coordinator, you should make and maintain an updated list of all products in the office that contain hazardous chemicals. For the massage therapy business, these chemicals are typically cleaning supplies, but essential oils in large volume can also be hazardous, and those that contain

| BOX 17-1 | Overview of Standards Established by the Occupational Safety and Health Administration (OSHA) |

IMPORTANT SANITATION AND SAFETY TOPICS

■ Acquiring a thorough understanding of the routes of disease transmission
■ Maintaining an adequate inventory of acceptable disinfectants, sterilants, and barrier covers
■ Maintaining records verifying compliance with the requirements of the Occupational Safety and Health Administration (OSHA)
■ Attending training sessions
■ Verifying employee compliance with OSHA
■ Maintaining employee records
■ Scheduling continuing education courses for the staff
■ Verifying quality assurance
■ Maintaining all Material Safety Data Sheets (MSDSs)
■ Arranging for the disposal of hazardous waste
■ Providing infection control training for new employees as designated by the employer
■ Interacting with outside agencies

RESPONSIBILITIES OF EMPLOYERS AND EMPLOYEES

■ Employers must identify and train workers "reasonably anticipated" to be at risk of exposure. They also must reduce or eliminate exposure and offer medical care and counseling if exposure occurs.
■ Employers must have written exposure control plans identifying workers with occupational exposure to blood and other infectious materials and specifying ways to protect and train those workers.
■ Employers must have a plan that includes protocols for barrier techniques, sterilization, disinfection, hepatitis B vaccination, and the handling of office accidents, including exposure to infectious materials. They must also have plans to protect and train employees; these plans must be reviewed and updated annually and must be available to employees at all times.
■ Employers must provide laundering of protective clothing. Laundering of protective clothing at home is prohibited.
■ Workers must wear gowns and gloves when a risk exists of exposure to or skin contact with blood, body fluids, or saliva. General work clothes are not considered protection against exposure to blood, body fluids, or saliva.
■ Employers must provide personal protective equipment to be worn by all employees (i.e., gowns, gloves, masks, and eyewear) at no expense to employees.
■ Sharps containers must be labeled and easily accessible to areas where sharps are used.
■ Hepatitis B vaccinations must be offered to employees at no cost after training is completed but within 10 days of placement in a position that involves occupational exposure. If a worker declines the hepatitis B vaccination, access is still required if the employee has a change of mind.
■ Employers must provide a training program during working hours for all employees in occupational exposure positions by June 4, 1992, and annually in subsequent years.
■ Training records must be kept for 3 years after the training sessions.
■ The following must be handled as infectious waste (i.e., placed in special, labeled containers): pathologic waste sharps; blood and body fluid items that release blood, body fluid, or saliva when compressed; and items caked with dried blood, body fluid, or saliva if such contaminants can be released from the materials during handling.

A variety of diseases can be transmitted when receiving or giving massage. The Centers for Disease Control (CDC) Web site (http://www.cdc.gov) is an ongoing source of up-to-date information and should be visited regularly. On this site are recommendations for (1) educating and protecting health care personnel; (2) preventing the transmission of blood-borne pathogens; (3) hand hygiene; (4) personal protective equipment; (5) contact dermatitis and latex hypersensitivity; (6) sterilization and disinfection of client care items; and (7) environmental infection control.

There are no specific recommendations for massage; however, it would be prudent to follow the recommendations of similar health care providers, such as physical therapists.

Modified from U.S. Department of Labor; Occupational Safety and Health Administration: CP2-2.69; Exposure procedures for occupational exposure to bloodborne pathogens.

clove and cinnamon are very caustic. Hydrotherapy procedures that use a hot tub require hazardous chemicals to maintain water quality.

MSDSs, which are government-approved, or equivalent forms that provide specific information about chemicals purchased for use in a workplace, are an important part of the records. MSDSs for all products with hazardous potential are compiled and kept updated in a master list available to all individuals. An MSDS should include the manufacturer's name and address, the product name, the generic name (if applicable), potential routes of entry, the organs affected by the chemical, and means of protecting against or reducing the effects of chemical exposure (e.g., eyewash).

LABELING OF HAZARDOUS MATERIALS

The hazard communication program coordinator is responsible for properly labeling hazardous chemicals and substances. Many products purchased from supply companies arrive with permanently affixed information about hazardous chemicals. When items are purchased in bulk and then transferred to smaller containers, hazard communication labels must be put on the secondary containers. The label must show that the MSDS was obtained and must designate the chemical's hazard class, the routes of entry into the body, and the organs affected. Labeling kits and informational materials are available from a variety of companies.

EQUIPMENT FOR HAZARDOUS SITUATIONS

The massage therapist may be responsible for ordering equipment and training office staff members in the use of a variety of materials during a hazardous situation. Although you may not work directly with hazardous materials, it is your responsibility to ensure that safe practice is implemented, to understand how to prevent accidents, and to know how to react in the event of an accident.

The following equipment should be readily available for use in preventing or dealing with a hazardous spill:

- Fire extinguisher
- Eyewash stations
- Masks approved by the National Institute for Occupational Safety and Health (NIOSH)
- Protective clothing (e.g., long sleeves, high neck, fluid-impervious fabric)
- Kitty litter, broom, and dustpan
- Protective nitrile gloves and glasses
- Bags in which to seal spilled materials and contaminated objects
- Well-ventilated areas for work (which allow the ventilation to be turned off if an accident occurs)

Infection Control Techniques

In the course of massage therapy treatment, some contamination of equipment, surfaces, instruments, and other devices occurs. The goal of any infection control program must be to maintain sanitation and to prevent cross-infection through aseptic technique.

ASEPTIC TECHNIQUE

The term *aseptic technique,* or *asepsis,* refers to procedures that break the circle of infection and ideally eliminate cross-contamination. With cross-contamination, a previously noncontaminated environment is exposed to harmful agents.

Several procedures are used to maintain asepsis and prevent cross-contamination:

- Barrier coverings are used on surfaces that cannot be sterilized.

- Exposed surfaces are cleaned and disinfected.
- Sterile disposable items are used whenever possible.
- All contaminated reusable items are cleaned and sterilized.
- Contaminated gloved hands are not allowed to touch protective eyewear, masks, or the hair.
- The hands are washed regularly throughout the day with an antimicrobial cleanser, such as before and after lunch and just before and immediately after the treatment of each client.
- A complete and comprehensive health history is obtained for every client.

Under OSHA standards, employees are allowed access to a client's health history information. This is especially important if an employee is exposed to *blood-borne pathogens* in the massage therapy office. Such information is maintained as part of a confidential medical record for employees. OSHA requires that these records be kept for all employees at risk for blood-borne pathogen transmission in an occupational setting.

All clients should be treated in the same manner, as potentially infected with HBV, HIV, or other blood-borne pathogens or as having an infectious disease. Consistent adherence to these standard precautions is a primary professional standard of care and reduces the guesswork of determining a client's infection status (Box 17-2). The following sections describe techniques that can be used to minimize contamination during treatment procedures.

PERSONAL PROTECTION

Personal protection involves two basic considerations: immunologic protection (i.e., immunization) and barrier protection.

Immunization

Immunization is the process by which resistance to an infectious disease is induced or augmented. The human body can produce immunity to particular diseases or conditions. When no natural immunity exists for a disease, immunization may be provided through certain vaccinations. There may be an individual preference to avoid immunizations. If this is the case, it is important to understand the process of immunization.

Immunization to prevent and control cross-infection is an important aspect of health care for massage therapy professionals, especially as massage has moved into the medical environment. The HBV vaccine, for example, is effective and widely available. However, several other diseases may pose a threat to the health and well-being of massage therapy personnel and clients.

The occupational risks for hepatitis B, measles, rubella, influenza, and certain other microbial infections can be minimized considerably by stimulation of artificial active immunity. Common childhood immunizations may be given for several diseases, including diphtheria, tetanus, pertussis, polio, and rubella. Other vaccinations help prevent rubella, mumps, and influenza. The tuberculin Mantoux test can determine whether an individual has been exposed to or has

BOX 17-2	Examples of Sanitation Requirements

(a) Each massage establishment shall be maintained in accordance with applicable state and local sanitary or health code(s) and regulations.

(b) A massage establishment and all fixed equipment shall be thoroughly cleaned on a routine basis and shall be rendered free from harmful organisms by the application of an accepted bactericidal agent.

(c) Each massage establishment must maintain its facilities cleanliness, sanitation, and repair at all times.

(d) Toilet facilities shall be kept clean and sanitary without offensive odor and in working order at all times. Restrooms shall not be used as storage rooms.

(e) Each massage establishment shall provide hand washing facilities, including hot and cold running water, located near or adjacent to the toilet room or rooms. Hot air blowers or suitable holders for sanitary towels and dispensers for soap shall be provided, and be adequately supplied at all times.

(f) All trash containers must be emptied daily and kept clean by washing or using plastic liners.

(g) Disposable sheets, towels or protectors that cannot be disinfected will be disposed of in a waste receptacle immediately after use.

(h) Furniture, equipment, or other fixtures shall be of a washable material and kept clean and in good repair. Electrical equipment shall be kept sanitary and safe at all times.

(i) Clean sheets shall be used on each client.

(j) Oiled sheets are to be discarded. After a sheet has been used once, it shall be deposited in a partially closed receptacle, container, or basket, and shall not be used again until properly laundered and disinfected.

(k) Used towels shall be laundered in chlorinated hot water by regular commercial laundering or by a noncommercial laundering process.

(l) Oil must be kept in closed containers.

(m) Each massage establishment must have adequate ventilation.

From §141.52 Sanitation Requirements for Massage Establishments, Texas, http://www.dshs.state.tx.us/massage/mt_rules.pdf (accessed June 2009).

tuberculosis. This test is important, because the incidence of tuberculosis, once thought to be almost nonexistent in North America, is increasing.

Although the topic of immunization can be somewhat controversial, it is an important consideration for massage therapists. Global interaction has led to increased exposure to infectious agents that were previously almost eradicated in many countries. A generation of people may not be immunized completely and are now susceptible to once-controlled diseased such as polio. The decision about whether to receive immunizations is a personal matter, but it does need to be made from an informed position.

Barrier Protection

Although vaccines are effective at minimizing the transmission of certain infections, they are not sufficient protection against the wide variety of potential pathogens encountered during client interaction in the business office or while receiving massage. Physical barriers are a fundamental component of an infection control program. Gloves, gowns, and disposable linens or sanitized linens are examples of barrier protection.

SELF-REFLECTION

What would I do if exposed to a contagious disease? How do I feel about being immunized against various conditions? What would I do if I was working with an individual with a condition such as hepatitis? How do I respond to this statement?

We are no longer a relatively isolated population. Global interaction has led to increased exposure to infectious agents that were almost eradicated in many developed countries. A generation of people has not been immunized completely and is now susceptible to once rare and controlled diseases, such as polio.

Disposables

Disposable items are manufactured and identified for single use only. Disposables are becoming more widely available as manufacturers, distributors, and office personnel recognize their usefulness. There is a conflict in using disposables and maintaining an environmentally sound business practice. Multiple-use products that can be sanitized in an acceptable manner need to be carefully considered even though the cleaning process may require more work. Linens are the primary example. When disposables such as paper cups are used, buy the most environmentally friendly products possible and recycle responsibly.

EDUCATING CLIENTS ABOUT INFECTION CONTROL PROGRAMS

Effective infection control must become a routine component of professional activity. The use of standard precautions in the treatment of all clients greatly minimizes occupational exposure to microbial pathogens, because it addresses the reality that most potentially infectious individuals are asymptomatic and therefore undiagnosed.

Procedures aimed at preventing the spread of infectious disease are constantly evaluated by the profession and by consumer agencies. The best course of action is to educate the staff and clients about the importance of safe practice and the use of standard precautions for all clients. Massage therapists should be willing to freely discuss infection control with clients, using valid data. The two best ways to avoid potential litigation and OSHA inspections are prevention and good documentation. It is important for massage therapy professionals to keep up with developments and incorporate new technology into their practices as it becomes available.

INFECTIOUS WASTE DISPOSAL IN THE MASSAGE THERAPY OFFICE

According to OSHA, *infectious waste* means blood and blood products, contaminated sharps, pathologic wastes, and microbiologic wastes. All infectious waste destined for disposal should be placed in closable, leak-proof containers or bags that are color coded or labeled appropriately.

Warning labels should be affixed to containers of infectious waste, to refrigerators and freezers containing blood, to other containers used to store or transport blood or other potentially infectious materials, and to any potentially infectious materials. The labels required by OSHA should be used in the office. These labels should be fluorescent orange or orange-red or predominantly so and should have lettering or symbols in a contrasting color.

LEARNING ACTIVITY

Develop a checklist for evaluating the sanitation of a location based on the information in this chapter. Choose an environment such as the student clinic at school, a classroom, or a government office building, and use the checklist to do an inspection. If violations are identified, develop corrective action plans to support improvement.

_____

_____

_____

_____

All infectious material should be disposed of in accordance with federal, state, and local regulations. A medical waste tracking form is completed for medical waste disposal, and a shipment log is used to verify the mode of transport and other vital information.

WORKPLACE SAFETY

For any individual to perform well and work productively, a relaxed, congenial work environment must ensure physical safety and help to maintain mental balance. Workplace safety is emerging as one of the key risk management and regulatory compliance focus areas. Because therapeutic massage promotes a sense of safety, relaxation, comfort, and support, it is necessary to make sure that the environment provides these elements. For example, burning candles can be relaxing, but the danger of a fire or of someone being burned and exposure to the chemical scent are health and safety hazards. Burning candles in the massage environment is not worth the risk. Any type of throw rug in the environment can be a tripping hazard even if it is part of a beautiful decorating scheme. Plants in the environment are beautiful and can positively affect air quality, but some are very poisonous, and people may be allergic to the pollen. Ensuring the safety of the massage environment requires regular assessment of potential hazards. Consider what could possibly happen, and then do what you can to eliminate or reduce the risk.

Workplace safety is a category of management responsibility in most places of employment. It includes the health and safety of any individuals in that environment. Different businesses may have different types of physical hazards, but none is entirely injury proof. Maintaining a safe environment in the massage therapy business involves attending to areas of parking and entrance to the office, the reception area, business office, all hallways, restrooms, and treatment rooms.

Identifying Health and Safety Hazards

A *hazard* is something that may cause harm or injury. A *risk* refers to the likelihood that a hazard will cause specific harm or injury to persons or may damage property. A health hazard is any agent, situation, or condition that can cause an occupational illness, also referred to as occupational hazards. A safety hazard is anything that may cause an injury. Safety hazards cause harm when workplace safety controls are not adequate. Health hazards include the following:

- Chemical substances such as cleaning supplies
- Biologic agents such as bacteria, viruses, dusts, and molds
- Physical agents or energy sources that are strong enough to harm the body, such as electric currents, heat, light, vibration, and noise
- Work design, also referred to as ergonomic hazards, that are associated with musculoskeletal injury
- Injuries or illnesses that may be caused by forceful exertions, constrained poor postures, and long-duration or continuous work
- Harassment, violence, or working alone

  Safety hazards include the following:

- Slipping and tripping hazards, such as injury caused by electrical cords across floors
- Fire and explosion hazards
- Safety and stability of the massage table and other massage specific equipment
- Moving parts of machinery, tools, and equipment (i.e., pinch and nip points)

- Pressure and heat systems and other equipment (e.g., stream heat, hydrotherapy equipment)
- Lifting and other manual handling operations
- Materials falling from height, rolling, shifting, or caving-in
- Potential for violent action (e.g., working alone at night)

Safety Measures

Risk management is a process by which the management assesses the risks, determines the control measures, and takes appropriate measures or actions to reduce such risks. Risk assessment is an important activity to reduce risk in the workplace. Effective workplace safety and health programs and measures have reduced injuries and illnesses in the workplace.

An effective policy that adheres to effective workplace safety must satisfy the following criteria:

- Working in a safe and healthy way is a condition of employment.
- Safety and health is everyone's responsibility; employers and employees are both accountable.
- Safety is given as much importance as productivity, quality, or cost control.
- All hazards are identified and controlled.
- Safety and health education needs to be consistent and ongoing.
- All accidents and near accidents are reported and investigated.

Several areas need to be addressed to ensure health and safety in the workplace (Boxes 17-3 and 17-4):

- Emergency action plan is reviewed and revised periodically.
- Emergency escape procedures and routes have been developed and communicated to all.
- An alarm emergency warning system is recognizable and perceptible above ambient conditions and is properly maintained and tested regularly.
- All workers know their responsibilities for reporting emergencies, responding to emergency warnings, performing rescue, and providing first aid.
- All work areas are clean and orderly.
- Walking surfaces are dry or slip-resistant.
- Spilled materials or liquids are cleaned up immediately.
- Combustible scrap, debris, and other wastes are safely contained and removed promptly.
- The appropriate number of toilets and washing facilities are provided, and toilets and washing facilities are sanitary.
- Areas are adequately lighted.
- All exits are marked with an exit sign and illuminated by a reliable light source if used in darkness.
- Directions to exits are marked with visible signs if the exits are not immediately apparent.

- Doors, passageways, or stairways that are neither exits nor access to exits and that could be mistaken for exits are marked NOT AN EXIT, TO BASEMENT, STOREROOM, or otherwise clearly designated.
- Exit signs are provided with the word EXIT in lettering at least 6 inches high, and the lettering is at least 0.75-inch wide.
- Exit doors are side-hinged.
- All exits are kept free of obstructions and unlocked.
- There are sufficient exits to permit prompt escape in emergencies.
- The number of exits from each floor of a building and the number of exits from the building itself are appropriate for the building occupancy load.
- When workers must exit through glass doors or storm doors, the doors are fully tempered and meet the safety requirements for human impact.
- There is a written fire prevention plan that describes the types of fire protection equipment and systems that are available and established practices and procedures to control potential fire hazards and ignition sources.
- The workplace has a fire alarm system that is it tested at least annually.
- Metal guards protect sprinkler heads where they could be physically damaged, and proper clearance is maintained below the sprinkler heads.
- Portable fire extinguishers are provided in adequate numbers and type, mounted in readily accessible locations, recharged regularly, and have dates noted on the inspection tags, and individuals are trained to use the fire extinguisher.
- Workers are trained and rehearsed on how to immediately evacuate the building in a fire emergency. They are familiar with the emergency rescue plan of the building, are able to recognize the fire alarms installed in the building, know to crawl (not walk) to find ways to escape, avoid elevators completely, and stay calm.
- All equipment is maintained in safe working order through inspection and preventative maintenance programs.
- Workers are trained to switch off equipment at the power point before pulling out the plug and to not overload circuits and fuses by using too many appliances from the one power point.
- Electrical cords are kept off the floor to reduce the risk of damage from drag or contact with sharp objects. A damaged electrical cord can cause a fatal electric shock.
- All equipment is used according to the instruction booklets.
- Management employs only licensed electrical workers to perform electrical work. This includes new electrical installations and alterations and repairs to existing installations. An unqualified person should not be employed to undertake electrical work.
- Supplies are stored so that they do not create a hazard or block lights, fire extinguishers, sprinklers, aisles, exits, or electrical-control panels.

BOX 17-3	Example of Office Safety Guidelines

TEN PRINCIPLES OF SAFETY

The following 10 points sum up how a Captial Projects Office feels about safety and forms the policies to ensure safe workplaces.

1. We believe that preventing all injuries and occupational illnesses is a realistic goal and not just a theory.
2. We are all directly responsible for preventing injuries and illness with each level accountable to the one above and responsible for the level below.
3. Safety is as important as production, quality, and cost control.
4. Safety awareness does not come naturally. Management must establish procedures and safety performance standards for each job or function.
5. We must audit performance in the work place to assess the effectiveness of facilities and programs and to detect areas for improvement.
6. All deficiencies must be corrected promptly, such as bettering employees' training and disciplining constructively and consistently.
7. It is essential to investigate all unsafe practices and incidents with injury potential, as well as injuries.
8. Serious illnesses and injuries involve tremendous cost directly or indirectly.
9. Safety off the job is just as important as safety on the job. (See related information on home safety.)
10. People are the most critical element in the success of a safety and health program. Management responsibilities must be complemented by individuals' suggestions and their active involvement in keeping work places clean.
    Keeping our workplace clean and neat is a big contribution that everyone can make toward creating a safe workplace.

Housekeeping not only improves the appearance of a workplace, it also helps prevent injuries. A tidy work environment helps to make our work go faster and more efficiently. Seven steps are the keys to good housekeeping:

1. Remove all unnecessary items.
2. Arrange necessary items properly so that they can easily be picked up for use.
3. Clean your workplace periodically to ensure cleanliness.
4. Maintain a high standard of housekeeping and workplace organization at all times.
5. Ensure ample leg room.
6. Maintain a minimum space of 3 feet wide wherever people need to walk.
7. Keep perishable goods or samples in proper storage conditions.

CREATING A SAFE WORKPLACE

Remember the following four points. They summarize nearly all you need to know to play your part in creating a safe workplace.

1. Removing the causes of accidents is the first step in preventing them. Our workplaces should be made hazard free and accident proof.
2. Unsafe actions by staff members cause the largest number of office injuries. Staff members can prevent accidents by changing their behavior.
3. Slips, trips, and falls cause most of the serious injuries in offices. Hazards that might cause falls should not be allowed to exist.
4. Fingers and hands suffer the most frequent office injuries, which occur while employees are handling everyday materials such as paper. Employees should take special care to avoid injury to their hands.

POTENTIAL HAZARDS

If you see any of these common office hazards, take action to solve the problem.

Furniture

Protruding keys left in a file cabinet lock: A passer-by may bump into them and get a painful poke. Remove keys after using a filing cabinet.

Jaws drawers: Filing cabinet and desk drawers are known to "bite" fingers. Avoid being bitten by drawers by using the handles.

Open drawers: There is always someone who has a fatal attraction for open drawers and will bump into them when you least expect it, and opening several file drawers at a time can tip over a cabinet. Keep drawers closed when not in use. Open only one file drawer at a time.

Obstacle courses: When furniture is badly arranged, it can form an obstacle course for people trying to move about the office. Arrange furniture to allow people to move around freely and easily.

Passageways and Storage

Blockages: Large objects or groups of people standing around blocking doorways and passageways increase the likelihood of bumps and knocks, because vision is blocked and space is tight. Keep doorways and passageways clear at all times, especially emergency exits. Make sure that any area where people walk is at least 3 feet wide. *Do not* place objects close to fire extinguishers, fire hydrants, and fire alarms.

Climbing: Reaching for high objects while standing on a stack of boxes or a chair with wheels is dangerous. Always use a suitable ladder or step stool.

Heavy objects: These objects are dangerous if they fall. Store heavy objects near floor level.

Toxic chemicals: Do not store toxic chemicals in or near the office.

Swing doors and corners: You cannot guess when someone may be approaching the other side of a closed door or around a corner. Do not open doors suddenly. When working behind a closed door, lock it. Approach corners and doors cautiously.

Running: This should be strictly a lunchtime or after-work activity for keeping fit. It has no place in an office, where it can cause close encounters of an embarrassing or even painful kind. Walk; do not run. Better to arrive late than without your two front teeth!

BOX 17-3	Example of Office Safety Guidelines—cont'd

Floors

Extension cords and other wires snaking loosely across the floor: These items can cause injury but and the abrupt shutting down of electrical equipment such as computers. (You will not be happy if you did not save your document!) Clamp electric wires securely to the floor.

Litter: Small items left lying on the floor have caused some dreadful accidents. Although somebody slipping on a banana peel may be funny in a comedy film, tripping on a pencil in the office may not seem so humorous. Food dropped on the floor is unhygienic as well as hazardous, and it should be disposed of in kitchen area garbage cans only. Anything dropped on the floor should be removed immediately.

Work Methods and Tools

Using the wrong tools: Fingers are not suitable tools for jobs such as removing staples. Use the right tools for the job.

Not using safety glasses: Eyesight is precious. Always wear safety glasses when working with hand tools.

Sharp and pointed objects: Even paper has sharp edges, as many office workers know to their cost. Scissors, knives, pencils, letter openers, and paper cutters are common sharp objects in the office. Use and store sharp objects carefully. Sheath them before storing in a drawer. Point them away from you on your desk. Do not use razor blades as cutters.

Unreported injuries. Reporting injuries reduces the chances of the same injury happening to someone else in future. Report accidents to help make the office safer for others.

Kitchen Area

Clean up your spills: Dispose of food waste in the proper container.

Microwave oven: Cover food in the oven to prevent spattering. Do not put metal containers, paper objects or Styrofoam inside the oven. Keep all flammable objects clear of it.

Hot objects: Use a cloth or mittens to handle hot objects.

Kitchen area housekeeping: Do not stack glasses too high. Store knives and can openers in the right place. Wrap broken glass in paper labeled *broken glass* and place in the kitchen garbage can. All waste food must be thrown only in the kitchen garbage cans. Keep the floor dry to prevent slips.

Equipment and Tools

Using tools wrongly can be hazardous. It can be dangerous to use tools that are not properly maintained.

Offices use a lot of electrical equipment. When using it, we should watch out for any obvious signs that something is wrong, such as loose wires, faulty connections, excessive heat, smoke, or sparks.

Never tamper with any electrical equipment. If repair is needed, always seek help from the qualified personnel in our office services department.

Computers, printers, and other electrical equipment should be switched off at the socket.

Do not overload the socket outlet. If uncertain, check with your manager.

Use proper adapters for two-pin plugs.

Safety glasses are to be worn while using certain hand tools. Never fail to use them.

From Ron Fouty, Capital Projects Office (CPO), CPO Office Safety Guidelines, University of Washington (http://www.cpo.washington.edu/Safety-Office-Guidelines.htm).

■ Stored items are stacked, blocked, or interlocked so that they are stable, secure, and will not collapse.

■ Storage areas do not have tripping, fire, or explosion hazards.

■ Hazardous materials are stored separately from other materials and identified with appropriate warning signs. Special care is taken with items that may be dangerous, such as liquids and toner.

■ Materials and supplies are stored so that they are easy to find, get to, and put back.

■ Heavy objects, such as boxes of documents, are placed on shelves low enough to be safe, although not so low that back strain occurs when lifting them.

■ People use steps or a ladder to reach high objects, and never stand on chairs or stacked boxes.

■ Do not allow top-heavy filing cabinets. Place heavier items in lower drawers, and do not pull out more than one filing drawer at a time.

■ Do not put objects on top of high furniture.

■ Objects such as boxes, cartons, bins, and furniture must not be left placed in areas where people are moving around.

■ All floors are slip-resistant and are regularly cleaned to maintain a safe surface.

■ Photocopiers are located in well-ventilated rooms or work areas and are properly maintained to reduce the hazards of emissions, heat, noise, and toner dust.

■ Adequate ventilation is maintained throughout the office environment to provide fresh air.

■ First-aid supplies are available in a clearly marked container that protects them from damage, deterioration, or contamination.

■ Workers are trained in basic first aid procedures.

■ Emergency numbers with the address of the business location are clearly posted near all phones.

BOX 17-4 | Sample List for Monitoring Office Safety

OFFICE FURNITURE AND EQUIPMENT
- Office lighting adequate

Aisles well lit

Walkways and stairways well lighted

Storage areas well lighted
- Lighting fixtures intact
- Ventilation

All work spaces ventilated through supply air outlets or operable windows

Photocopy machines located in ventilated spaces or large open areas
- Adequate wall and telephone outlets
- Desks and file drawers not opened into aisles or walkways
- Desk and file drawers not left open
- File cabinets: heavy items in bottom drawers
- No more than one file drawer opened at any time
- File cabinets and shelving units bolted together or to the floor or wall
- Faulty or broken desks, chairs, or other office equipment not in use
- Only authorized persons permitted to operate office equipment
- Maintenance and repairs done by designated, trained personnel

WALKWAYS
- Aisle widths adequate for two-way traffic and unobstructed
- No tripping hazards in aisles
- Floors kept clear of pencils, bottles, and other loose objects
- Floors even and slip resistant
- Carpeting not torn, badly worn, or with curled edges
- No throw rugs or other tripping hazards
- Posted caution signs for doors that open onto stairways

- Stairways provided with suitable handrails, and free of worn stair treads
- Running on stairs, corridors, or elsewhere is prohibited

ELECTRICAL EQUIPMENT
- All electric fans protected with guards of not over half-inch mesh
- Worn electrical cords or plugs and loose outlet plates or connections absent
- Exposed metal parts of electrical office machines or appliances electrically grounded
- Light fixtures or fixture parts securely hung
- Extension cords not run over radiators, by steam pipes, through doorways, under rugs, or across walkways

MISCELLANEOUS
- No smoking in the workplace
- Windows easy to open
- Stable ladders readily available for reaching materials on high shelves and kept in safe, serviceable condition
- Materials not stacked to unstable heights
- Heavy materials stored at waist height or lower; all materials stored safely and without crowding on shelves
- No materials hanging over edges of shelves
- Employees instructed in safe lifting procedures
- Only nontoxic cleaning materials used
- Fire and emergency evacuation plans posted in appropriate areas
- Employees aware of nearest emergency exit
- Employees know the fire and ambulance phone numbers

SELF-REFLECTION

Am I aware of potential safety hazards, and do I ignore them? Do I regularly do safety inspections in my work and living environment? How does my school measure up to safety requirements and infection control? What can I do to be safer in my surroundings?

Workplace Violence

Massage therapy is based on safe, respectful, compassionate, professional human touch and interaction. Workplace violence is absolutely contrary to the principles of massage ethics, but as massage moves into a broader public arena, the massage professional is more likely to encounter individuals who do not live by the same standards of behavior. No textbook on the professional practice of massage therapy can ignore this subject.

Workplace violence can be any act of physical violence, threat of physical violence, harassment, intimidation, or other threatening, disruptive behavior that occurs at the worksite. Workplace violence can affect or involve employees and others (e.g., clients) in the environment.

Several events in the work environment can trigger workplace violence. It may even be the result of non–work-related situations such as domestic violence or road rage that has carried over into the workplace. Workplace violence can be inflicted by an abusive employee, a manager, supervisor, coworker, client, family member, or stranger. Whatever the cause or whoever the perpetrator, workplace violence cannot be accepted or tolerated.

There is no sure way to predict human behavior, and although there may be warning signs, there is no specific profile of a potentially dangerous individual. The best prevention comes from identifying any problems early and dealing with them (Fig. 17-2). The following are warning indicators of potential workplace violence:

- Intimidating, harassing, bullying, belligerent, or other inappropriate and aggressive behavior
- Numerous conflicts with customers or clients, coworkers, or supervisors

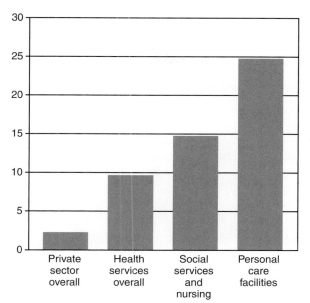

FIGURE 17-2. Incidence rates for nonfatal assaults and violent acts by industry in 2000. *(From U.S. Department of Labor, Bureau of Labor Statistics. Survey of Occupational Injuries and Illnesses, 2000. Washington, DC, U.S. Department of Labor, 2001.)*

- Bringing a weapon to the workplace (unless necessary for the job), making inappropriate references to guns, or making idle threats about using a weapon to harm someone
- Statements showing fascination with incidents of workplace violence, statements indicating approval of the use of violence to resolve a problem, or statements indicating identification with perpetrators of workplace homicides
- Statements indicating desperation (over family, financial, and other personal problems) to the point of contemplating suicide
- Direct or veiled threats of harm
- Substance abuse
- Extreme changes in normal behaviors

After you have noticed any signs of these indicators, you should take the following steps:

- If you are a coworker, you should notify management immediately about your observations.
- If it is a customer or client, notify management immediately.
- If you are management (business owner), you should evaluate the situation by considering what may be causing the employee's problems and investigating the situation.
- If it is your supervisor, notify that person's manager.
- If it is the owner or manager, there will be no avenues to pursue within the business, making this a very difficult situation. Possible avenues include a group intervention with the owner or notifying one of the owner's trusted peers. However, be aware of spreading rumors that are unfounded.

It is important to respond appropriately; do not overreact, but do not ignore a situation. Sometimes, the correct approach may be difficult to determine. Managers should discuss the situation with an expert resource to get help in determining how best to handle the situation.

Unacceptable behavior includes the following:

- Excessive noise
- Malicious allegations
- Offensive gestures
- General verbal abuse
- Racial and sexual abuse
- Drug and alcohol abuse
- Damage
- Theft
- Threats
- Violence

ADMINISTRATIVE AND WORK PRACTICE CONTROLS

Guidelines and procedures should be established to prevent violence and ensure safety (Box 17-5):

- State clearly to clients and employees that violence is not permitted or tolerated.
- Establish a liaison with local police and state prosecutors, and report all incidents of violence. Provide physical layouts of facilities to expedite investigations.
- Require employees to report all assaults or threats. Keep logbooks and reports of such incidents.
- Advise and assist assaulted employees requesting police assistance.
- Institute a sign-in procedure for everyone, with additional passes for visitors.
- Prohibit employees from working alone.
- Discourage employees from wearing necklaces to prevent possible strangulation.
- Provide staff with identification badges.

BOX 17-5	Risks for Workplace Assault

- Poorly lit parking areas
- Exchange of money
- Delivery of passengers, goods, or services
- Having a mobile workplace
- Working with unstable or volatile persons
- Working alone or in small numbers
- Working late at night or during early-morning hours
- Working in high-crime areas
- Guarding valuable property or possessions
- Working in community-based settings
- Lack of training to deal with assault

From National Institutes for Occupational Safety and Health (NIOSH), Current Intelligence Bulletin 57, DHHS (NIOSH) Publication No. 96-100, Violence in the Workplace, Risk Factors, and Prevention Strategies, 1996. http://www.cdc.gov/niosh/violrisk.html.

- Provide staff members with security escorts to parking areas.
- Use the buddy system, especially when personal safety may be threatened.
- Invite local police to visit and make recommendations for a safer workplace.

WHEN VIOLENCE OCCURS

After a violent incident, individuals experience three stages of crisis reactions to some degree:

Stage One: Emotional reactions are characterized by shock, disbelief, denial, or numbness. Also common is a fight-or-flight survival reaction, in which the heart rate increases, perceptual senses become heightened or distorted, and adrenaline levels increase to meet a real or perceived threat.

Stage Two: The impact stage involves a variety of intense emotions, including anger, rage, fear, terror, grief, sorrow, confusion, helplessness, guilt, depression, and withdrawal. This stage may last a few days, a few weeks, or a few months.

Stage Three: In the reconciliation stage, victims attempt to make sense of the event, understand its impact, and through trial and error, reach closure. This stage may be a long-term process.

Although it is difficult to predict how an incident will affect a given individual, several factors influence the intensity of trauma. These factors include the duration of the event, the amount of terror or horror the victim experienced, the sense of personal control (or lack thereof) the individual had during the incident, and the amount of injury or loss the victim experienced (e.g., loss of property, self-esteem, physical well-being). Other variables include the person's previous victimization experiences, recent losses (e.g., death of a family member), and other intense stresses (see Box 17-5).

SEXUAL HARASSMENT

Sexual harassment is a form of sex discrimination that violates Title VII of the Civil Rights Act of 1964 (http://www.eeoc.gov/policy/vii.html). Sexual harassment is any unwelcome sexual advances, requests for sexual favors, and other verbal or physical conduct of a sexual nature. According to the federal Equal Employment Opportunity Commission (EEOC) guidelines, sexual harassment is defined as "unwelcome sexual advances, requests for sexual favors, and other verbal or physical conduct of a sexual nature" when the following occurs:

- Submission to such conduct is made explicitly or implicitly a term or condition of employment.
- Submission to or rejection of such conduct by an individual is used as the basis for employment decisions affecting the individual.

- Such conduct has the purpose or effect of unreasonably interfering with an individual's work performance or creating an intimidating, hostile, or offensive working environment.

Sexual harassment can include the following:

- Verbal abuse (e.g., propositions, lewd comments, sexual insults)
- Visual abuse (e.g., leering or display of pornographic material designed to embarrass or intimidate an employee)
- Physical abuse (e.g., touching, pinching, cornering)
- Rape

Prevention

Prevention is the best tool to eliminate sexual harassment in the workplace. Employers are encouraged to take steps necessary to prevent sexual harassment from occurring. They should clearly communicate to employees, customers, clients, and anyone who enters the environment that sexual harassment is not tolerated. They can do so by prominent, highly visible posting of the business policy against sexual harassment, establishing an effective complaint or grievance process, and taking immediate and appropriate action when an employee complains.

Vulnerability to Sexual Harassment

Massage therapists may be the victim of sexual harassment by clients because there still exists confusion about the nature of touch in our society. Other health professionals also experience sexual harassment. Nurses, for example, often must deal with inappropriate behavior by patients. If sexual harassment occurs, do the following:

- Say *stop* immediately.
- Document the incident.
- Get witnesses' support.
- Directly inform the harasser that the conduct is unwelcome and must stop. Make a report using any employer complaint mechanism or grievance system available.
- Object! Make it clear to the harasser that his or her behavior is unwelcome. You may prefer to object verbally in the beginning, but if the harassment continues, object in writing, and keep a copy of the letter. Be specific about what behavior you find objectionable.
- Keep a log or diary of incidents, including the date, time, place, behavior, what was said, and names of witnesses. Keep the log in a safe place at home, not at work.
- Do not suffer in silence! The harasser is counting on you to keep it a secret.
- Do not blame yourself. Do not assume that you are doing something to provoke the harassment. Sexual harassment usually is about power rather than sex.

- Talk to friends and family. Let people who care about you offer their support.
- Talk to coworkers. Because harassers tend to be repeaters, you may learn of other victims of the same harasser. Your coworkers may provide support and some protection and, if alerted, may be able to corroborate incidents of harassment.

Take formal action and insist that the proposed "solution" does not adversely affect you. For example, the employer may propose transferring you away from the harasser. If the new job is in an inconvenient location or would adversely affect your seniority rights or promotional opportunities, you are within your rights to insist that the harasser—not you—be inconvenienced.

Because litigation can be expensive, time consuming, and traumatic for the sexual harassment victim, every effort should be made to deal with the problem at the workplace. If the problem cannot be so resolved, do the following:

- File a complaint with the state Fair Employment Practices (FEP) Agency or the federal EEOC. When investigating allegations of sexual harassment, EEOC looks at the whole record: the circumstances, such as the nature of the sexual advances, and the context in which the alleged incidents occurred. A determination on the allegations is made from the facts on a case-by-case basis (see Good Stuff from the Government section near the end of this chapter).
- Consult an attorney experienced in sexual harassment cases.
- If the harasser's behavior included assault and battery or rape, file criminal charges with the police.

The number of sexual harassment incidents in the massage business setting can be decreased by the following measures:

- Draft, publicize, and proximately post an anti–sexual harassment policy. The zero tolerance policy should be posted at the reception desk and in all treatment rooms.
- Implement a procedure for employees to follow if they feel they have been the victim of sexual harassment.
- Conduct organization-wide sexual harassment prevention training.
- Have all clients sign an agreement to be incompliance with the business zero tolerance policy to sexual harassment.

Important facts about sexual harassment include the following:

- The victim and the harasser may be a woman or a man. The victim does not have to be of the opposite sex.
- The harasser can be the victim's supervisor, an agent of the employer, a supervisor in another area, a coworker, or a client.
- The victim does not have to be the person harassed but may be anyone affected by the offensive conduct.
- The harasser's conduct must be unwelcome.

- Sexual harassment can occur off business premises if the activity is related to employment (e.g., company picnic, dinner).

Fraudulent Accusations of Sexual Harassment

The rights of sexual harassment victims are clear and protected. The rights of those accused of sexual harassment are less well defined. After millions of dollars in lawsuits filed by victims over the past 10 years, it is much less risky for employers to quickly err on the side of the accuser, even if this means that there is an increased risk of someone being accused unjustly.

There are many reasons why someone may make false accusations. For most, it is the potential for a monetary settlement. False accusations also occur as a form of retribution. For example, a female client attempts to engage a male massage therapist in a personal relationship but is told that it is not possible. The female client may then attempt to get back at him by claiming misconduct on the part of the massage therapist. A female massage therapist may be envious of the retention business success of another female massage therapist working in the same location. One way to remove the more successful massage therapist is though allegations of sexual harassment. Although it is not common for someone to falsely accuse another of this type of behavior, it does occur, and it most often is directed against men. Male massage therapists must be extremely cautious about their behavior and continuously assess their actions to prevent career-ending allegations.

Individuals accused of sexual harassment have privacy rights that prohibit other persons from divulging information concerning the complaint, except as part of the sexual harassment complaint resolution process. The accused is informed of the allegations, the identity of the complainant, and the facts surrounding the allegation. Individuals accused of sexual harassment have due process rights that prohibit such individuals from being disciplined without adequate notice and an opportunity to be heard.

The U.S. Equal Employment Opportunity Commission receives more than 12,000 sexual harassment charges per year. One half of them may be settled for "no reasonable cause." A percentage of those settle because it is emotionally, physically, and financially draining to sustain a legal action to prove innocence.

If unjustly accused, you need to get an attorney, and make sure the attorney contacts everyone who currently works or has worked with you to establish a pattern that you are not in the habit of sexually harassing anyone. If a client accuses you of sexual misconduct, the same process applies. The attorney should also investigate the accuser to see if he or she has a history of suing and may be able to find prior lawsuits filed by the accuser.

Do not speak to the accuser at all—not by phone, e-mail, or with any other contact whatsoever. *Absolutely do not talk* about the accuser or the sexual harassment incident with anyone unless it is your attorney or a government agency representative who is investigating the alleged incident.

It is difficult to prove sexual harassment if there is no proof, because it is his or her word against yours. This is why actual victims of sexual harassment have such a difficult time receiving help and why the laws and rules are more favorable for the victim. If, however, there is any prior conduct with others or if you have been accused before, this history can be considered as proof of a pattern of sexual harassment behavior.

You must protect yourself from accusations that are unfounded, and you must constantly be aware of how your conduct can be interpreted as sexual harassment. It is advantageous to take sexual harassment training courses to learn how to prevent sexual harassment behavior. Document that you have taken these classes. Most importantly, always be professional, and think before speaking or acting. Do not put yourself in situations in which you could be accused.

SPECIFICALLY FOR MALE MASSAGE THERAPISTS

Men must be more careful than women. Although this is unjust, it is the reality. For example, a male massage therapist should never go to the home of a female client alone; never work alone in the office with a female client; never lock the door of the treatment room while giving a massage; always have another female (e.g., another massage therapist or receptionist) in the office within hearing range; never work on the breast area of a female client (even if the work is justified for scar tissue management); never massage into the upper thigh region of a female client (always refer female clients to female massage therapist for this type of work); always meet female coworkers or employees only in a public area; and never invite female clients, coworkers, or employees to his home if he is alone.

Men must be careful about how they treat female coworkers and clients. Do not call them "honey," "babe," or other offensive terms of endearment. Do not make sexist comments, even if kidding. Do not allow anyone else to speak this way. No massage professional should allow anyone to hang sexist and offensive jokes, comics, cartoons, calendars, or anything else that depicts anything sexual in nature.

Install a window with blinds in a private office or treatment room, and never have the blinds closed when you are alone in your office or massage area with a female. Never lock the door. Inform the client that the blinds will be closed while they prepare to get on the massage table and then they will be opened. The door remains unlocked for their protection and yours to make sure nothing inappropriate occurs. Assure the client that meticulous draping procedures will provide privacy.

APPROPRIATE BEHAVIOR FOR ALL MASSAGE THERAPISTS

Always inform new clients that sexualizing the massage in any way by the client or the massage therapist is inappropriate. Inform the client of reporting procedures if she or he feels that the massage therapist behaved inappropriately. Inform the client that you will end the session immediately if you consider any behavior to be inappropriate. You will leave the massage session and report the behavior immediately to your supervisor. Taking this sort of action is more difficult if you are self-employed, and one of the advantages of working with others is protection in these instances. It may be advantageous for the receptionist or some other individual other than the massage therapist to discuss all office policies with new clients and coworkers to indicate that there is unified agreement about what constitutes appropriate and inappropriate behavior.

Be aware of behavior that others may consider offensive, even if you do not. Before acting or speaking, ask yourself the following questions:

- Would I do or say this if I knew it was going to be shown on TV?
- Am I stepping on this individual's personal boundaries?
- Would I want anyone to say or do this to my parent, spouse, or child?
- In what ways may this behavior or conversation be misinterpreted?

LEARNING ACTIVITY

Develop a checklist of appropriate and inappropriate professional behavior based on this section in the chapter. Use the checklist to assess your professional behavior. Develop a corrective action plan based on the results. (Do not think that you have no areas that need improvement. No one is perfect. We can all do better. Return to the list, and be more honest with yourself.)

_____

_____

_____

_____

ACCIDENTS HAPPEN, BUT BE CAREFUL

If an incident occurs and there may be a misunderstanding about the intent of the action, immediately acknowledge the error (e.g., slipped draping, unfortunate comment), apologize, and inform the client that you are required to document and report all accidents of this type to management.

If you are the management, the documentation should be placed in the client's file. This will let someone who is looking to falsely accuse know that the incident was already reported to the proper personnel. It is unfortunate that we have to be so cautious, but litigation is common, and it is important that you protect yourself.

Be careful but not fearful. A confident demeanor combined with professional etiquette will prevent most misunderstandings and provide communication channels to resolve unfortunate and unintentional issues. Remember that there is no excuse for unprofessional behavior. Your actions affect the entire massage therapy profession.

(CD) During a massage for one of your clients, the fire alarm in the facility went off. The building was evacuated. There was no injuries or damage. Using the practice management software, document this event in your client's record.

SUMMARY

Understanding the key terms in this chapter is important for the safety of you and your clients. The sanitary procedures that you follow on a daily basis can protect you and your clients from transmittal of many diseases. Understanding the OSHA concepts and keeping in compliance with them can assist you with these tasks.

The first step in safe practice is obtaining detailed health information from the client and then implementing the necessary protocols and barriers. Compliance with the safety protocols should be followed in regard to infection control techniques. The most important sanitation protocols for the massage therapist are to follow hand-washing techniques to the fullest every time and to follow standard precautionary measures when doing massage. In the office, standard precautionary measures, rules about health hazards, and safety guidelines must be followed in the reception area, hallways, restrooms, and parking lot. Make sure emergency exits are clearly defined and evacuation plans are posted. Keep fire extinguishers fully charged.

Harassment and violence in the massage environment can be minimized or prevented. Massage therapists should take classes about harassment and violence in the work area. A zero tolerance policy should be posted at the reception desk. If inappropriate behaviors happen, immediately report the incident, and follow the massage policy protocols.

Bibliography

Centers for Disease Control and Prevention (CDC): Guidelines for infection control in massage therapy health-care settings. MMWR Morb Mortal Wkly Rep 52(RR-17), 2003.

Molinari JA: Infection control: its evolution to the current standard (formerly universal) precautions, *J Am Dent Assoc* 134(5):569–574, 2003.

Occupational Safety and Health Administration (OSHA): State plans. Available at http://www.osha.gov/fso/osp/index.html (accessed June 2009).

Tommey AM: Guide to Nursing Management and Leadership, ed 8, St. Louis, Mosby, 2008.

Evolve Annotated Web Links

http://evolve.elsevier.com/Fritz/business

Find all links from this chapter plus additional information on the Evolve Web site.

Centers for Disease Control and prevention (CDC): Home page (http://www.cdc.gov/niosh/homepage.html)

Occupational Safety and Health Administration (OSHA): Home page (http://www.osha.gov)

U.S. Equal Employment Opporturnity Comission (EEOC): Home page (http://www.eeoc.gov/)

1. Explain why it is important that each member of the massage therapy team understand the concepts of infection control.

_____
_____
_____
_____
_____

2. Identify common barrier materials and explain their use.

_____
_____
_____
_____
_____

3. Explain the term *standard* (formerly universal) *precautions.*

_____
_____
_____
_____
_____

4. Describe the role you play in infection control.

_____
_____
_____
_____
_____

5. Using a sample form provided or from the office of employment, complete an accident report for the following situation. The massage therapist, Ray F. Thompson, experienced exposure to saliva and digestive fluids when Mr. Frank Oliver was receiving a massage and suddenly vomited. The massage therapist's address is 4001 Kinect Drive, Cutlerville, MI 49545, SS# 000-00-2111, date of birth 4/17/1981. The accident occurred at XYZ spa and golf resort. The massage therapist physician, Gerry Murphy, MD, was contacted for follow-up, but no hospitalization was necessary.

SAMPLE ACCIDENT REPORT

Employee(s) name(s): _____

Time and date of accident/incident: _____

Job title(s) and department(s): _____

Supervisor/lead person:_____

Witnesses: _____

Brief description of the accident or incident: _____
_____

Indicate body part affected: _____

Did the injured employee(s) see a doctor? ( )Yes ( ) No

If yes, did you file an employer's portion of a worker's compensation form? () Yes () No

Did the injured employee(s) go home during his or her work shift? () Yes () No

If yes, list the date and time injured employee(s) left job(s): _____

Supervisor's Comments:

_____

_____

What could have been done to prevent this accident/incident? _____

_____

_____

Have the unsafe conditions been corrected? () Yes () No

If yes, what has been done? _____

_____

If no, what needs to be done?

_____

_____

Employer or Supervisor's signature: _____

Date: _____

Additional comments/notes:_____

_____

_____

_____

6. Review various office situations and identify incidents that might require special attention to prevent the transmission of disease-causing organisms from the massage treatment room or business office.

_____

_____

_____

_____

_____

_____

_____

_____

_____

_____

7. Develop a sample fire safety plan.

_____

_____

_____

_____

_____

_____

_____

_____

_____

_____

8. Develop a no tolerance harassment and workplace violence policy.

_____

_____

_____

_____

_____

_____

_____

_____

18

PLANNING AND MANAGING YOUR CAREER PATH

OUTLINE

Employee or Self-Employed
Seeking Employment
    Self-Assessment: Identifying Assets and Liabilities
    Marketing Your Skills
    Career Priorities and Philosophy
    Determining Your Worth
Employment Opportunities
    School Placement
    Newspaper Advertisements
    Employment Agencies
    Professional Organizations and Journals
    Internet and World Wide Web
    Personal Networks
Getting the Job
    Preparing a Letter of Application

    Contacting an Office by Telephone
    Creating a Resume
    Completing the Job Application Form
    The Interview
Keeping the Job
    Professional Etiquette
    Asking for a Raise
Job Termination
    Resignation
    Being Fired
    Being Laid Off
Starting and Maintaining Your Own Business
    The Business Plan
    The Business Structure
Summary

KEY TERMS

Job application
Letter of application

Portfolio
Resume

LEARNING OUTCOMES

Mastery of the content in this chapter will enable the reader to:

- Determine career goals
- Identify personal assets and liabilities for a job
- Identify legal considerations in hiring
- Explain the use of pre-employment testing
- Describe new employee orientation
- Determine desirable characteristics for a job you may seek

- Determine methods of marketing your skills
- Identify personal priorities for a potential job
- Develop a philosophy for massage therapy
- Identify factors to consider in salary negotiations
- Identify potential areas of employment
- Prepare data for job applications and interviews
- Identify potential interview questions

Guidelines for the Learning Activities and answers to the Workbook questions are located on Evolve at http://evolve.elsevier.com/Fritz/business.

LEARNING OUTCOMES—Cont'd

- List suggestions for a successful interview
- Prepare an interview follow-up letter
- Explain how to advance on the job
- List hints for success in a job on the massage team

- Describe how to terminate a job
- Determine if you have the personality and skills to be self-employed
- Develop a business plan

A review is in order. The key ideas are summarized for each of the previous 17 chapters in the following paragraphs.

Chapter 1, The Business of Massage Therapy, emphasizes that business is business is business. There are overlapping themes in service businesses. For example, work in a dental office provides an excellent model, because the profession has systematically built a service concept based on prevention and regular maintenance care. Much can be learned by looking at this and other models for health service professions, but there is also something unique about massage. The business of massage has its own interesting and challenging business concepts. Chapter 1 introduced the idea of federal resources for business development and support.

Chapter 2, Being a Professional, dealt with the big picture and the small details. Inspiration, intention, and intuition were linked to the business process. The ideas of perception and gestalt can be abstract, such as a pattern of belief, or can be concrete, such as developing a logo that demands attention. Various approaches were used to describe massage therapy professional behavior.

Chapter 3, Focus on the Client, explained that a service business is client focused. It is about relationships. Relationships among people are complex and challenging. Communication is an art and science.

Chapter 4, Legal and Ethical Issues in the Massage Professional Practice, highlighted the roles for law, legislation, and ethics in dealing with clients and coworkers. Practice acts that regulate various professionals, including massage therapists, in most jurisdictions are in place to protect the public from harm and, in theory, support competent care. Legal matters are fairly concrete, and although open to interpretation, legislation is quite specific about what is acceptable and what is not. Ethical behavior is about relationships with yourself, peers or coworkers, other professionals, and clients. The code of ethics is based on principles of behavior. It is much harder to isolate ethical from unethical behavior than it is to differentiate legal and illegal behaviors.

Chapter 5, Technology in the Massage Practice, described how the massage therapist offers balance in the low-tech delivery of massage. Massage is slow, rhythmic, and nurturing, and it focuses on outcomes. There is a softness to massage, but there also is a technologic side that demands improvement of skills to make routine jobs much easier and more efficient. It is necessary to be at least minimally technologically competent. Advances are making it easier to incorporate the time-saving advantages that technology can offer in the business environment.

Chapter 6, Massage Business Office Design, described how ergonomics and aesthetic facility design soften the hardness of the high-tech business environment. Personality takes the lead in designing the office, but the clients' preferences also must be considered. If you love red walls with purple dots and sitting on a pillow on the floor, you can use this design to decorate your office, but you should expect that some potential clients may go elsewhere. However, it is likely that you will attract clients with similar preferences for red, purple, and pillows. Professional offices usually have a simple design because a generic plan is most comfortable for most people.

Chapter 7, Documentation, addressed record keeping. Many massage therapists neglect the entire process of creating and maintaining efficient and effective record keeping systems. Unfortunately, if business problems occur, these charts, contracts, receipts, and client files will be required to solve the problems. Regardless of personal feelings and skills, this is an area that requires diligence.

Chapter 8, Storage of Business Records, described the necessity of archiving records in a way that permits easy retrieval. After the paperwork is generated, it must be safely stored.

Chapter 9, Written Communication, described the fundamentals of writing messages and letters. Written communications are important in business, and technology is increasing the need for proficiency in writing clear messages. E-mail has replaced much snail mail, and text messaging has become a major way to communicate. To avoid miscommunication, shortcuts and abbreviations should be eschewed in favor of proper spelling, grammar, and punctuation.

Chapter 10, Telecommunications, continued the theme of communication. The telephone remains the single most important communication device in the business office. Modern phone systems are smart. They can do almost everything from e-mailing and text messaging to taking pictures and videos. Smartpones support the concept of a virtual office, which is excellent for a massage therapist who is a sole practitioner and must do it all.

Chapter 11, Appointment Management Systems, addressed the need to accurately schedule clients because massage professionals are not able to double-book or dovetail clients. A cosmetologist, for example, can do several tasks within the same time frame by moving from one client to the next during the wait times for services. While the color sits on the hair of one client, another can be under the dryer, and the stylist can be cutting hair. Massage therapists cannot multitask; each client requires total attention. Because of this, managing the appointment schedule is critical.

Chapter 12, Marketing the Massage Therapy Business, focused on getting and retaining clients. Marketing is about determining the needs of potential clients and then communicating how your massage skills are of value to them. Marketing, including advertising, is about informing, educating, and delivering services to clients. This requires understanding of how people perceive their world and their place in it and what you can do to make their lives better.

A successful business requires retention, retention, retention. Regular clients on a regular schedule are the hallmark of success, especially for self-employed massage therapists. One way to boost retention is to keep in contact with the client between appointments and to use incentives and persuasive methods that are compassionate and ethical to keep the clients coming for appointments. Clients who receive massage every week at the same time usually fall into the habit and schedule around their massage appointments. The remaining clients with appointments every 2 weeks, once each month, or on a random or as-needed basis need reminders and encouragement, which requires a recall system. Clients with irregular massage appointments need reminder calls, mailed notes, or e-mails.

Chapter 13, Inventory Systems and Supply Ordering, addressed the basic inventory of a massage business office. Running out of disinfectant or fresh linens is not good business. An inventory system can prevent this from happening.

Chapter 14, Insurance Reimbursement for Massage Therapy Services, delved into the details of money and where your business is going to get it. Money is an emotional and logical issue. The reason for being in business is to make money. If making money does not interest you, perhaps you should consider volunteer service. Money in return for massage services can be obtained through various forms of insurance. This can be profitable but complicated. Cash for services rendered is the simplest way to do business, but as massage therapy branches out into medical environments, it will be necessary to understand the insurance reimbursement process. Often, you will work for health professionals such as a chiropractor or physician, and the professional's office will handle the insurance billing, but you still need to maintain records in a way that supports the reimbursement process.

Chapter 15, Accounting Concepts, described procedures for business accounting. Typically, you will use a specialist such as an accountant or bookkeeper to help with these obligations, but you need to know how accounting is done to ensure a good job is done. Accounts receivable (money you get), accounts payable (money your give), and what is left (profit) are the basis of accounting. If you are employed, your wages are part of the accounts payable. If you are the business owner, the profit is your paycheck.

Chapter 16, Managing Money, described relationships with money. Abundance, enough, not enough, and balance are fundamental principles of success. We want our massage careers to be abundant. Money is one factor in that abundance. There are many more indicators of abundance, such as the pleasure in watching someone relax after a bad day or a new parent learning how to massage her baby or comforting the elderly with compassionate touch. It is difficult to place a monetary value on these types of abundance. In Maslow's hierarchy of needs, survival needs can be based on having barely enough for ourselves, let alone anyone else. We have to be successful to help others. We can best share and serve from a position high on the hierarchy's triangle. Individual success achieved through ethical business practices and skilled massage delivery is the vehicle for having more than enough, and it can give us the opportunity to share that abundance with others.

Money is transferred from one place to another by cash exchange, credit exchange, third parties, such as a bank, and checks or debits. Massage therapists must understand these transfer methods and which forms to use for paying bills and employees.

Chapter 17, Maintaining a Safe Work Environment, was about being safe. Feeling safe is a parasympathetic process. Massage professionals must feel safe enough to provide a gentle, relaxing, and healing environment. There are specific government regulations to ensure public safety. Like good health, safety comes from being proactive.

By the time you read this chapter, you are probably close to completing a formal educational program or course of study for therapeutic massage and you might have passed your certification examination or other credentialing examination. Your thoughts are turning to career development. This chapter emphasizes the tasks necessary to market your skills as an educated and credentialed massage therapist. You may feel nervous about the prospect of taking a credentialing examination, finding a job, or beginning a private practice in massage. However, cultivating positive attitudes and taking time to reflect on career goals can help you get on track. This is the time when you can reflect on all the skills you have acquired and allow intention, intuition, and inspiration to guide you toward success.

EMPLOYEE OR SELF-EMPLOYED

You have a major decision to make at the beginning of your massage therapy career. Will you begin as an employee or be self-employed? The following information may help you determine the best starting point.

How old are you? Those younger than 25 years may be well served by first seeking employment, gaining experience, and settling into the career track. After 2 or 3 years of experience, you will have a foundation to become a business owner.

How organized are you? If you struggle with details, paperwork, and much of the information provided in this textbook and do not want to be responsible for business operations, it is better to be employed.

How financially stable are you? Employment offers reliable income, whereas beginning a business requires money for startup costs and time to develop a client base.

What are your family obligations? Employment may provide a more structured work schedule. When self-employed, you can make your own schedule to some extent, but you will work more hours because you must provide massage sessions and all business operations.

How confident are you about your massage skills? It takes time for all the information learned in school to settle into confidence while giving a massage. It takes about 5000 massage sessions before the skills become natural. That is 3 to 5 years of giving massage full time, which is about how long it takes for most people in any career to be good at what they are doing. Employment may offer an environment in which clients' expectations will this development to occur. The same case can be made for self-employment. Whatever path you choose to achieve excellence, you must do lots of massage sessions.

As an experienced massage therapist and educator, I suggest employment for those just graduating. The second option is a secure position as an independent contractor. Why? Because it is a solid place to start to build experience and confidence. Starting your own business is a good option if you have access to a network of referrals, such as your uncle who manages a golf resort; you have been a nanny and know lots of nannies and families who would like to have massage in their homes; or your Grandma's exercise group wants to add massage to their wellness plan. However you choose to start your career, the most important thing is that you begin. To be a massage therapist, you must do massage.

In this chapter, various aspects of being an employee are described, followed by exploration of the process of starting your own business. Many of the activities, such as developing a resume, are just as important for those who are planning on being self-employed as for those seeking employment. Employees must understand, support, and respect the many business obligations of employers.

SEEKING EMPLOYMENT

When you apply for various positions, your prospective employers will assume that you have completed your studies and obtained your credentials as a certified or licensed massage therapist. If you are self-employed and starting your

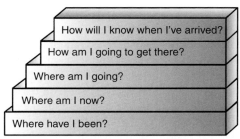

FIGURE 18-1. Job preparation ladder: questions to ask yourself when preparing for a job search. *(From Finkbeiner BL, Finkbeiner CA:* Practice Management for the Dental Team, *ed 6, St. Louis, 2006, Mosby.)*

own business, each client will have the same expectations. Employers and clients want certain skills in employees:

- Interpersonal skills
- Teamwork skills
- Verbal communication skills
- Critical thinking skills
- Technical skills
- Computer skills
- Written communications skills
- Leadership skills

These skills can be learned and are therefore called hard skills. In addition to hard skills, you need to develop soft skills, such as value clarification, self-discipline, ethical behavior, positive attitudes, creativity, and anger and stress management. As you reflect on your hard and soft skills, you should analyze what they mean to your career path.

Before you venture into the job market as a massage therapist, you must identify your career goals. A career path is based on careful planning and preparation, but it can be altered by unexpected opportunities and luck. To begin preparation, you should ask yourself the series of questions shown in the job preparation ladder (Fig. 18-1). Prospective employers will put your resume on the top of the job application pile if you spend some time reflecting on each of these questions: Where have I been? Where am I now? Where am I going? How am I going to get there? How will I know when I have arrived? Before going to any job interviews, you should share your thoughts about these questions with peers or spend some time alone reflecting on them. Sharing and introspection can help you build confidence in your plans and goals for a career.

Where have I been? This question helps you to review your past and identify some of the reasons you arrived where you are now. It forms the foundation of your preparation ladder. Some individuals may find looking at the past depressing, whereas others may yearn for the comfort of the past. Regardless of the impact of your past, reflection is worthwhile. Some personal information is confidential, and certain types of questions may not be asked during a job interview; however, it is wise to be prepared for questions about your past employment. For instance, if you have worked at several jobs in the past, you may be asked about your reasons for having changed jobs frequently. You should explain your job history honestly.

Where am I now? You need to reassure yourself about where you are in your career path. Where are you right now—completing a course of study in massage therapy, secure or insecure in a personal or family relationship, looking forward beginning your massage career soon, or waiting to begin your career sometime in the future? Knowing where you are at the present time enables you to continue on the career path.

Where am I going? This is a goal-oriented question that requires you to identify what you want to do. As you progress up the preparation ladder, you must stop to think about what you want in the near and the distant future. For some individuals, getting a job or beginning their business and gaining independence are their primary goals. For others, the job may be the means to a future goal. Obtaining a job now, gaining experience, and continuing with one's education may be several short-range goals that are needed to reach the ultimate goal, such as teaching or owning a massage clinic and spa. Regardless of your goals, you must realize that they may change; remaining flexible in your goals enables you to accept challenges along the way.

How am I going to get there? This question identifies the steps that must be taken to achieve your goals. For some, a job means independence or a sense of security and self-worth. For others who are pursuing additional education, a short-term job supports a return to school for advanced training in massage or cross-training in disciplines such as cosmetology or nursing.

How will I know when I have arrived? This is the top rung of the ladder. To answer this question, you must define what success means to you. For some people, the definition of success is always changing. Money, material goods, or a feeling of security and satisfaction can represent success. For others, the knowledge of service to others is the primary indicator of success. No one answer is correct for this question, and your response will likely be a combination of both ideas.

Taking time to prepare for your future career can influence a job interview. When an employer or office manager asks you to describe yourself, your background, and your career goals, you will be prepared. Simply saying, "Oh, I don't know. There isn't much to tell," indicates that you have not given your career much thought, and a potential employer may think you feel the same about employment (Box 18-1).

BOX 18-1   Preparing for the Future

If you watch future reports on television or read *Trend Letter*, *The Futurist* (The World Society publication), or current books (e.g., *The World is Flat: a Brief History of the Twenty-First Century* by Thomas L. Friedman), you will find comparable themes about the future. The following forecasts will affect massage therapy; it is possible to ask the "what if" questions with each:

- Knowledge will change dramatically, requiring that we all be dedicated learners.
- Knowledge will evolve from the intensity of the current information growth so that we will access content with meaning and applicability for our work.
- A power shift will occur toward health care because of the intensity of the developing knowledge and its use in making cost-effective decisions about care.
- The health care system must change to remain financially viable, and as employers limit health care coverage and genetics allow us to know more about how an individual would respond to treatment, a shift toward eliminating the current disparities is more likely to occur.
- The world will be seen increasingly as a continuum without borders that prevent trade and the exchange of inventions, including those related to health care.
- Technology will continue to revolutionize health care.
- Increasing diversity will result in more people who are older, more people moving to different parts of the country or the world, and a greater need for speaking two or three languages.
- People no longer will be satisfied with service; they will want an experience.
- There will be increased violence and, simultaneously, an increased expectation for civility.
- Stores will be very small or huge.
- Macromarketing (i.e., targeting masses) will be out; micromarketing (i.e., targeting specific populations) will be in.
- Job security will be out; career options will be in.
- Competition will be out; cooperation will be in.
- Work will be sporadic.
- More people will be living with chronic diseases.
- More people will be overweight and consequently experience related diseases.
- Bioengineering will make possible interventions that currently do not exist.
- Emphasis on prevention will redirect care efforts.
- Work will be accomplished by teams.
- Everyone will need to be a leader.

Modified from Yoder-Wise PS: *Leading and Managing in Nursing*, ed 4, St. Louis, 2006, Mosby.

Self-Assessment: Identifying Assets and Liabilities

As you embark on your career path ask yourself what skills and characteristics you can bring to a client and to a prospective employer. Take time to write down your skills, strengths, and weaknesses with a prospective job in mind.

BOX 18-2	Desirable Characteristics for a Massage Therapist

- Promptness
- Initiative
- Dependability
- Creativity
- Flexibility
- Self-motivation
- Enthusiasm
- Honesty
- Sense of humor
- Good general health
- Willingness to accept change
- Good listener
- Willingness to work with a team
- Effective organizational skills
- Knowledge of automated equipment
- Use of proper language skills in verbal and written communications
- Attention to detail

As you begin this exercise, you may find that you seem to concentrate on your weaknesses; this is not uncommon. Parents, teachers, and associates share criticism willingly, thinking it improves a person, but sincere praise may not be given as freely. Criticism may be so common that when praise is offered, it may be difficult to accept. Learn to accept praise, identify your positive characteristics, and develop your assets.

How do you begin? Identify your positive characteristics and your skills, and then identify your liabilities, but analyze how these weaknesses can be overcome. For instance, if you are prompt and seldom absent and you pay attention to details, you have characteristics that employers seek in an employee (Box 18-2). You may find it difficult to use a specific type of computer software, or you may have a problem remembering a specific massage method, but these skill deficiencies can be improved with experience. If a prospective employer asks about any weaknesses, you could explain that although you have had difficulty using a specific type of software used for client records, you would like to improve this skill and are willing to spend some extra time on your own to do so. This is a positive attitude that shows an interest in improving yourself, rather than an attitude of not caring.

Marketing Your Skills

A well-educated, experienced massage therapist with the appropriate credentials has valuable bargaining power for obtaining a job or potential client who requires these skills and provides adequate compensation. Stating that you are a graduate of a massage education program is a credible assertion; however, supporting this claim with valid data that demonstrates the positive effect you can have is likely to win you the job or the client even though you are just beginning your career.

You need a caring, positive attitude about your professional abilities and should present yourself in a positive manner. It is your responsibility, however, to live up to the claims you make. Your skills, knowledge, investment in your education, and credentials are tools that can be used to achieve compensation similar to that of other allied health or business professionals with similar backgrounds and responsibilities. Most states require licensing to be able to practice massage. Obtaining licensing is a mandated requirement to be able to practice massage, but certification that is voluntary and measures skills beyond the minimum basic requirements is a valuable way to demonstrate to potential employers how dedicated you are to your massage career.

Career Priorities and Philosophy

Everyone dreams about the ideal job. However, many people are so excited to be given an interview that they take the first job offer without considering their goals, needs, and priorities. Before applying for a job or preparing for a job interview, decide what you need and want in a job and what your basic philosophy is about your career. Remember the power of intention.

Before seeking employment, you should determine your needs and clarify your life goals and a philosophy that is consistent with them. Unfortunately, it is common for newly graduated massage therapists to accept the first job offer with little consideration given to how his or her philosophy coincides with the philosophy of the prospective employer. Carefully evaluate yourself, and establish some realistic goals. Ask yourself the following questions: Are my professional, moral, and social values compatible with those of my prospective employer? What do I want to be doing in 5 years or in 10 years? How important are salary, hours, and location?

After you have written down your philosophy of life and enumerated your goals, remind yourself that these goals will change over time. You will reevaluate your philosophy as you gain confidence from your new experiences.

After you have reviewed the various factors involved in job selection, decide your top five priorities for a job, and then rate each job offer. A decision-making grid such as the one shown in Table 18-1 may be helpful for this purpose. The job offers are listed in the left vertical column, and the priorities are listed across the top. Starting on the left, the priorities are given a point value based on your personal needs. Each job is evaluated, and the points totaled. If a tie occurs, other characteristics can be added.

You may need to do more than one or two interviews to find the job that satisfies your goals, needs, and priorities. It can take a while to find the best fit, but remain steadfast in your job search.

TABLE 18-1	Job Decision-Making Grid						
JOB OFFERS*	PRACTICE ENVIRONMENT (6)†	SALARY (5)	BENEFITS (4)	LOCATION (3)	CHALLENGE (2)	HOURS (1)	TOTAL (21)
Job offer no. 1							
Job offer no. 2							
Job offer no. 3							

*Instructions: Assess your priorities for each job offer by placing the point value you feel fits for each category. The totals in the last column will give you an idea about which job offer bests fits your priorities.

†Maximum possible point values are given in parentheses.

Determining Your Worth

What is worth? There are many definitions, but the ones most appropriate to this discussion are the *total value of something* and *to be deserving of something*. The concept of worth in business often translates into a service such as massage therapy or a product such as a self-massage tool being exchanged for money. Many determine their worth by how much money they make. Understand that your worth—your value—is much larger than what can be measured by money.

Some factors can limit the amount of money that can be earned by doing massage. For example, you cannot do more than 25 to 30 1-hour massage sessions per week on an ongoing basis without harming yourself. If you are being paid based on the number of massage sessions performed, then there will be a cap on income. Income can be increased by doing such a good job that the employer will increase the amount paid per massage or increase the hourly wage. The amount earned doing massage is determined by what the client base is willing or able to pay. A client base with an annual income of more than $100,000 is able to pay more for massage services than a client base with an average annual income of $30,000. When you understand these economic limitations, you can appreciate that you may never get paid what you are worth if money is your only measure. Fortunately, there are other measures of worth, such as knowing that you have made someone's pain easier to tolerate or helping someone have the mobility and strength to be able to take care of themselves. Knowing that a person can better endure chemotherapy for cancer treatment when receiving a massage, watching a young mother and father bond with their infant by using massage, and calming someone who is grieving cannot be measured in money, but it is a large part of a massage therapist's worth. Money earned is important, but it is not the only compensation for massage therapy.

Although many elements may be considered important in deciding whether to accept a job offer, for most people, salary and benefits need to be primary factors in job selection. However, money should not be the only determining factor. Working just for the money will not support the inner path of service most massage therapists desire. There needs to be a balance.

You do deserve to make an income that reflects your responsibilities and the value you bring to the business. The difficulty often arises when an employer asks you during an interview what salary you expect. You need to prepare yourself for this question and not say, "Oh, I don't know. What have you paid your other massage therapists?" You need to have a firm understanding of the cost of living in your area, the comparable salaries for similar responsibilities and educational attainment, the local and national salary data available for reference, and what you are worth in terms of your skills and knowledge. The following discussion provides ideas for formulating a benefits and salary package that could reasonably be suggested to a prospective employer. Box 18-3 lists several benefits that are commonly offered to employees.

Salary is often a difficult subject to bring up, but it must be discussed openly before you accept a job. You need to know the beginning salary, how salary increases are obtained, and when salary increases are awarded. An employer must expect to pay a fair salary that is based on education, experience, credentials, and merit performance. The salary should be competitive with other professionals who have equal responsibilities, but it should be cost-effective so that the employer can afford to pay the amount offered.

The economic factors of massage therapy vary widely across the country, depending on the specific position, the responsibilities, and the geographic location. Massage therapists who have a formal education, management skills, and appropriate credentials may receive significantly higher salaries. The U.S. Government Bureau of Labor Statistics is a reliable source of salary information (Box 18-4).

When salaries are discussed, care must be taken to determine that all factors related to the salaries compared are the same. Some dollar value must be given to each of the benefits to determine the total salary and benefits package. Determine whether the job responsibilities are equitable. Education, experience, credentials, and performance evaluations are factored into the salary. Some value is placed on job environment. No skilled massage therapist should be making a salary that does not reflect an honest respect for the individual's productivity.

It is wise to ask for a contract or an employment agreement that verifies in writing the conditions of employment. These conditions may include the salary scale, an explanation

SELF-REFLECTION

With each employment possibility, ask yourself the following questions:

Do I possess the skills needed to be productive?

Have I proved I have done this job elsewhere? If so, how successful was I at this job, and what problems did I encounter? Did those problems help me develop new skills and insight, or will they likely be stumbling blocks again?

If I have not already done this job elsewhere, is there enough evidence to suggest I have the necessary skills and that I am very likely to succeed in this job?

Even if I possess the skills, am I sufficiently motivated, and do I have the energy level and self-confidence to do the job? What evidence is there to support this?

Will I be dedicated, conscientious, fair, hard working, determined, and give 100%, or will I be distracted, drop the ball, be absent or late frequently, or otherwise not measure up to employability standards?

Am I sufficiently interested in this type of job to be motivated to do a good job and make a contribution?

Will I stay long enough to make a contribution after the expense and time that is invested in training me for the position?

Will I fit in and be a team player? Is there evidence to support this?

Will I be a positive influence on coworkers, or will I gossip, hurt morale, or talk down about others or the company?

Will I fit in with the environment—attitudes, values, personality, and personal style?

Will I be easy or difficult to manage? Is there evidence to support this?

Will I follow and support organizational policies and procedures?

How will I take direction?

Will I support organizational changes?

Will I fit in with the existing style of management?

Is the salary range of this job compatible with my salary history?

Is what I want to earn reasonable based on the ranges of salaries (low to high) paid in the massage profession?

BOX 18-3 | Potential Job Benefits

- Dress allowance
- Retirement plan
- Health insurance
- Profit sharing
- Child care
- Membership in professional organizations
- Travel and expenses for professional meetings
- Special bonuses for holidays or production achievement

---

heath care clinic. According to the Occupational Outlook Handbook, 2008-09 edition, from the U.S. Bureau of Labor and Statistics (http://www.bls.gov/oco/ocos295.htm), massage therapists work in an array of private and public settings, including private offices, spas, medical and physical therapy clinics, chiropractor's offices, hospitals, nursing homes, fitness centers, sports medicine facilities, airports, and shopping malls. They also travel to clients' homes or offices to provide a massage. It is not uncommon for full-time massage therapists to divide their time among several different settings, depending on the clients and locations scheduled.

Teaching massage is another career opportunity. Although you are not ready to teach immediately on graduation, teaching can be a future career goal. Numerous private massage schools, career schools, colleges, and universities have developed occupational educational programs that include massage therapy. Qualifications for teachers vary from state to state. The following are recommended qualifications that meet or exceed most state requirements:

- National certification by the National Certification Board for Therapeutic Massage and Bodywork or equivalent exam or licensure
- Completion of all legal requirements for practice in the jurisdiction
- Minimum of 2 years of professional experience, best defined by at least 2000 documented hours of professional massage experience; 5 years or 5000 hours is a better base of experience
- Professional affiliation with one of the professional organizations
- Teaching experience or active involvement in learning instructional strategies
- Ability to use and interpret the textbooks and present generic material (as opposed to teaching based only on personal style)
- Associate's or bachelor's degree in a related field

There are many more possibilities. Therapeutic massage is one of the careers paths that can be found in many environments. Unlike dental assistants, who must be employed with dentists, massage therapists are working in dental offices, gyms, and race tracks (horses and people); with midwives; for corporations; in wellness programs, at street fairs; with

---

of the merit performance evaluation, and the required probationary period.

EMPLOYMENT OPPORTUNITIES

The massage therapist can choose from myriad opportunities for potential employment, ranging from a small solo practice to a medium-sized spa to a large multidisciplinary

BOX 18-4	U.S. Bureau of Labor Statistics Occupational Employment and Wages for May 2007

31-9011 Massage Therapists
   Massage customers for hygienic or remedial purposes.
   Employment estimate and mean wage estimates for this occupation:

Employment (1)	Employment RSE (3) (% Error)	Mean Hourly Wage	Mean Annual Wage (2)	Wage RSE (3) (% Error)
45,920	3.2%	$19.39	$40,330	2.3%

Percentile wage estimates for this occupation:

Wages	10%	25%	50% (Median)	75%	90%
Hourly wage	$7.69	$11.18	$16.76	$24.74	$34.06
Annual wage (2)	$16,000	$23,240	$34,870	$51,460	$70,840

(1) Estimates for detailed occupations do not sum to the totals because the totals include occupations not shown separately. Estimates do not include self-employed workers.
(2) Annual wages have been calculated by multiplying the hourly mean wage by a "year-round, full-time" hours figure of 2080 hours; for those occupations in which there is not an hourly mean wage published, the annual wage has been directly calculated from the reported survey data.
(3) The relative standard error (RSE) is a measure of the reliability of a survey statistic. The smaller the relative standard error, the more precise the estimate.
From http://www.bls.gov/oes/current/oes319011.htm (accessed June 2009).

traveling musicians; and with athletes, babies, and veterans in rehabilitation.

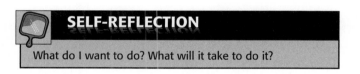

SELF-REFLECTION

What do I want to do? What will it take to do it?

Where do you begin to find employment opportunities? After surveying some of these potential areas of employment, where do you begin looking for the right job? Many prospects are available, and several different avenues may be used.

School Placement

The school placement office or faculty members often are notified of job opportunities in the area. Instructors frequently know employers who are interested in hiring new graduates, and they also know their students' qualifications and abilities. Most schools spend considerable time and effort obtaining information about potential job opportunities, and they take pride in placing their graduates.

Newspaper Advertisements

Local and out-of-area newspapers have classified sections of jobs available (Fig. 18-2). Advertisements in the classified section state the qualifications required and other details about the job. Many traditional newspapers now deliver the product online (Fig. 18-3).

In composing a letter of application and a resume to reply to an ad, remember that although first impressions are not

> Experienced Massage Therapist needed for a busy clinical office. Must be nationally certified with qualifying school credentials. Able to work flexible hours, days, and be able to multi-task. Call (123) 456-7890 or mail resume to: Luke Fritz, 204 E Nepessing Rd, Lapeer, MI 48446.

FIGURE 18-2. Job advertisement for a clinical massage therapist.

> SPA Massage Therapist: Interested in a position in a SPA working with other SPA professionals? Our SPA is growing and needing to hire another massage therapist with at least 2 years of experience, state certification, and massage insurance. Forward your resume to: PO Box 204, Lapeer, MI 48446

FIGURE 18-3. Blind ad for a spa massage therapist.

necessarily the most accurate, they often are the most influential. A little more initiative is required of the applicant to construct a resume than to pick up the telephone and call for an interview. The letter of application and the resume give the prospective employer an opportunity to evaluate the applicant's keyboarding skills, communication skills, and neatness.

Employment Agencies

Free and private employment agencies are available. Most states provide an employment service, and applicants may register with this service without charge.

Private employment agencies, which are service enterprises, provide many good job opportunities but charge a fee. Before registering with an employment agency, always check its reputation. This can be done locally or through the National Employment Association in Washington, DC. After selecting a reputable agency, the applicant should find out about testing and placement procedures.

Professional Organizations and Journals

Massage therapy professional organizations frequently maintain employment placement services. State and national professional journals usually have classified sections devoted to job offerings for massage therapists. Many of these jobs offer unique opportunities, possibly even relocation. State and local massage associations often allow new graduates to post their contact information in the association's newsletters or journals free of charge.

Internet and World Wide Web

The Internet is a group of computers connected all over the world that allows people to communicate with each other. For instance, on the Internet you can obtain information about companies that employ massage therapists worldwide.

Many Web sites are available (e.g., www.jobweb.com, www.monster.com, www.resumemachine.com, www.hotjobs.yahoo.com) that can provide information for your job search or allow you to post your resume. These links are annotated on the Evolve Web site (http://evolve.elsevier.com/Fritz/business).

Personal Networks

Networking is a process of identifying and establishing a group of acquaintances, friends, and relatives who can assist you in the job search process. This approach is one of the best strategies for finding a job. Some studies have shown that as many as 80% of jobs are obtained through some form of networking. Friends, relatives, business associates, local massage therapists, and schools offer myriad contacts that may lead to a job opportunity. If a friend is leaving a job and

knows you are interested in the same area of employment and are available for work, a good recommendation from your friend is always welcome.

How do you go about networking? If you have a part-time job or have had a clinical rotation in an office while a student, let the employer or other staff members know that you are ready for a full-time position. If these individuals know you are interested in a full-time job, they can talk with friends in the community about your skills and often can serve as an excellent reference for you. Contact your local Chamber of Commerce. The link is annotated on the Evolve Web site (http://evolve.elsevier.com/Fritz/Links).

GETTING THE JOB

Several steps must be taken between the determination of your goals and choice of employment and the time you begin work. The steps include career preparation planning, searching for job information, writing the letter of application, creating a personal resume, preparing for the interview, completing a job application, participating in the interview, touring the facility and meeting the staff, and following up on the interview (Fig. 18-4).

Preparing a Letter of Application

The *letter of application*, or cover letter, has three basic goals: to arouse interest, to describe your abilities, and to request an interview. The letter of application should be kept to a single page, including the date and the closing signature. Every effort must be made to customize this letter and to express your philosophy, motivations, and character in a less formal format than the resume. This letter may be the most important business letter you ever write (Fig. 18-5A).

AROUSE INTEREST

In the opening, introduce yourself to the prospective employer and include a brief description of your personal qualifications. This opening essentially gives you the

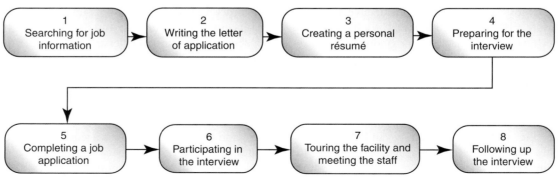

FIGURE 18-4. The career planning process. *(From Finkbeiner BL, Finkbeiner CA:* Practice Management for the Dental Team, *ed 6, St. Louis, 2006, Mosby.)*

opportunity to promote yourself. The letter should make the reader interested enough in your skills and abilities and to grant you an interview.

Example 1: "The position you have advertised in the Any Town News sounds challenging. My diploma in massage therapy and my credential as a national certified massage therapist have provided me the skills necessary to perform the job well."

Example 2: "Your employment announcement posted on my school bulletin board calls for a massage therapist who is interested in applying the latest concepts in the spa industry. My education at School XYZ has provided me with these skills."

Example 3: "Your employment announcement calls for a massage therapist who is interested in learning how to integrate massage into the chiropractic practice. My education at School XYZ for the past 2 years has provided me with these skills."

In each of these cases, the applicant lets the prospective employer know that she or he is interested in the position and believes that she or he has the skills needed for the job. Notice that each paragraph is reader oriented.

DESCRIBE YOUR SKILLS AND ABILITIES

The second paragraph of the letter should describe your skills in more detail. It should also call attention to your enclosed resume, curriculum vitae, or data sheet (discussed in the next section).

Example: "In August of this year, I will graduate from School XYZ. I will have completed courses in therapeutic massage, including specialized training in spa services and hospice care. I completed 300 hours of clinical practice in the local community. I had taken courses in accounting, management, business communications, and computers before entering the Massage Therapy Program. While in school, I worked part time as a receptionist in a day spa that offers massage."

This brief description includes an overview of basic skills. Further details about the skills and the dates of education and work experience are included in the attached resume.

REQUEST AN INTERVIEW

Because the purpose of a cover letter is to obtain an interview, you should ask for the interview directly.

Luke Fritz, MT, NCTMB
2050 Leisure Lane, Lapeer, MI 48446
(123) 456-7890 / leisurelymassage@hec.com

October 20, 20xx

Jana Larke
222 Relaxation Drive
Your Town, State 00000

Dear Ms Larke:

I am writing this letter in response to your need for an entry-level massage therapist. Given my excellent capabilities and training, I am confident you will find me an ideal candidate for this position. I would greatly appreciate your consideration. My resume is enclosed for your review.

I am trustworthy, competent, well-trained, and personable, and will dedicate myself to providing your clients with a quality massage experience. I also have advanced skills obtained from my clinical training. A graduate of the Health Enrichment School, I am currently working as a massage therapist at Sherri's Hair Salon in Lapeer. With my clinical education and relevant experience, I believe you will be very pleased with my performance.

I appreciate your time in reviewing my credentials and thank you in advance for your consideration. I look forward to speaking to you and setting up a time for an interview and demonstration of my skills. Please feel free to contact me anytime at (123) 456-7890.

Sincerely,

Luke Fritz, MT, NCTMB

A

FIGURE 18-5. **A,** Letter of application for an entry-level position as a massage therapist. ⊜ This letter template is posted on Evolve at http://evolve.elsevier.com/Fritz/business.

(Continued)

Quality Service
Customer Satisfaction
Welcoming and Friendly
☆☆☆☆☆

Luke Fritz, MT, NCTMB
2050 Leisure Lane, Lapeer, MI 48446
(123) 456-7890 / leisurelymassage@hec.com

Objective: To obtain a massage therapy position for an active massage practice that will enable me to use my skills and learn from others within the massage environment, while providing excellent patient care.

Professional Experience:

Sherri's Hair Salon, Lapeer, MI   Massage Therapist   June 2007 – Present

Perform chair massages on a diverse population focusing on neck and shoulder techniques. Conduct open therapeutic massages to promote and generate new business. Review calendars and schedule appointments for massage therapists and hair stylists according to availability.

Provide massage services to clients using safe, appropriate, and effective massage techniques. Perform client health history and update before each session; ascertain precautions/contraindications for massage before each session. Explain procedures and applied techniques appropriate to client needs and preferences. Observe client reaction to massage and modify as necessary. Solicit feedback and respond accordingly. Document all sessions performed according to established guidelines.

Other responsibilities include maintaining client confidentiality; maintaining sensitivity to age- and gender-related issues during all client interactions; reporting any unusual client interactions to supervisor immediately; scheduling and maintaining of appointments; assisting in collection of fees; consulting with appropriate treatment staff regarding treatment plans when necessary.

Detroit Marathon, Detroit, MI   Massage Therapist   October 2007 and 2008

Perform chair massages on a diverse population focusing on neck and shoulder techniques. Provided warm-up and cool-down massage for athletes competing in the Detroit Marathon. Assessed the needs of each athlete individually and selected the appropriate treatment. Invited to be the "Official Massage Coordinator" for future Detroit Marathon events.

Health Enrichment Center, Lapeer, MI   Student Massage Therapist   August 2006-June 2007

Performed chair massages, focusing on neck and shoulder techniques.

Education: Health Enrichment Center, Massage Therapy Diploma, 720 Credit Hours, June 2007

Certification: National Certification Board for Therapeutic Massage and Bodywork

B

FIGURE 18-5, cont'd B, Personal resume to accompany the letter applying for an entry-level position as a massage therapist. ⊜ This resume template is posted on Evolve at http://evolve.elsevier.com/Fritz/business.

Example: "Please give me an opportunity to discuss my qualifications with you. My telephone number is 616-999-2041."

Box 18-5 presents a list of action verbs that can be used to describe your activities. General guidelines for creating a cover letter are provided in Box 18-6. Figures 18-5 and 18-6 show letters of application submitted by two applicants with different backgrounds.

Contacting an Office by Telephone

If you have been informed of a job opening by an instructor or a friend, time may not allow you to write a letter of application; in such cases, a telephone call is required. This situation requires a different approach from writing a letter.

First, place a call to the office, and indicate to the individual receiving your call who you are and why you are calling. Second, explain how you learned about the position. Third, if the job is available, ask for an interview.

Whether you plan to send a letter of application or decide to contact the office by telephone, you must prepare a resume to enclose with the letter or to take with you to the interview.

Creating a Resume

A *resume*, personal data sheet, or personal history should be prepared to accompany the letter of application or to take with you to the interview. A resume is a marketing tool, and the product is you. The objective is to capture the attention

BOX 18-5   Action Verbs

Accomplish	Overcame
Achieve	Participate
Active in	Perfect
Assist	Perform
Attain	Persuade
Attend	Place
Brought about	Plan
Communicate	Prepare
Complete	Present
Conduct	Print
Contribute	Process
Cooperate	Produce
Coordinate	Program
Counsel	Propose
Create	Prove
Demonstrate	Provide
Design	Publicize
Generate	Realize
Form	Receive
Found	Recognize
Graduate	Recommend
Head	Recruit
Implement	Reevaluate
Improve	Refine
Increase	Regulate
Initiate	Represent
Install	Restore
Instruct	Review
Interview	Schedule
Kept	Secured
Lecture	Serve
Led	Set up
Maintain	Simplify
Manage	Sell
Mediate	Spearhead
Motivate	Staff
Observe	Streamline
Obtain	Substitute
Operate	Train
Order	Transform
Organize	Update
Originate	Validate

BOX 18-6   Guidelines for Writing a Letter of Application

1. Create a professional letterhead that includes vital data, including your full name, address, telephone numbers (i.e., home, cell, and fax), and your e-mail address if you have one.
2. Use standard business letter format.
3. Use personal stationery made of quality bond paper; do not use your current employer's stationery.
4. Make sure your spelling, grammar, punctuation, and capitalization are correct. If you are composing your letter on a computer, always use the spell checker.
5. Avoid opening with "My name is_____." Your name is on the letterhead and in the closing signature line.
6. Keep the letter short, usually three to four paragraphs. Put details in the resume.
7. Limit the letter to one page.
8. Address the letter to a specific person. Never address an application letter "To Whom It May Concern." Take time to find out the name of the employer. If it is not available, use "Dear Doctor" or, if the letter is going to a larger organization, "Dear Human Resources Manager."
9. Put the employer's needs first by making the letter "you" oriented; avoid "I" statements.
10. Send an original letter for each application. Do not send photocopies.
11. Do not copy a letter of application from a book. Make your letter representative of your personal characteristics.
12. Consider mailing your letter and resume in a large envelope so that it will stand out from the more commonly used no. 10 envelopes on the employer's desk.

From Finkbeiner BL, Finkbeiner CA: *Practice Management for the Dental Team*, ed 6, St. Louis, 2006, Mosby.

and then save it for future reference. Most software provides several optional templates that allow you to create a professional personal letterhead and a matching resume. You want to get the attention of the prospective employer when the person reads the letter, so take time to create an attractive, professional image through your stationery. After the letter has been completed, create several original copies. If this is not possible, try to obtain the finest quality copy possible from a commercial printer. You should keep a copy to take when going for an interview. Your resume should be designed with the following suggestions in mind:

■ Put yourself in the position of your prospective employer. Try to determine the qualities the person may be seeking and emphasize these qualifications.
■ Be as impressive as possible, but do not deviate from the truth. This is not the time to be shy and modest. You must tell the reader what you can do; no one else will do it for you.
■ Review the material carefully to make sure you did not forget anything. An overlooked item may be just the one the employer is seeking.

of the reader and maintain the person's interest. From the employer's point of view, the resume is a time saver because it gives a quick account of what you have done, what you can do, and what your goals are. A resume needs to be a brief, well-documented account of your qualifications. A simple resume is best suited for those who are entering the job market or who have limited work experience. Your objective is to be granted an interview; you therefore want to impress the reader with a resume that is a concise, positive presentation of your abilities and qualifications.

When preparing your resume, it is best to create the document in a word processing program on the computer

Marsha Schaffer, MT, NCTMB
2050 Leisure Lane
Lapeer, MI 48446
(123) 456-7890 / leisurelymassage@hec.com

October 20, 20xx
P O Box 2589
Grand Rapids, MI 49502

To Whom It May Concern:

Please accept my resume in response to your position advertised in the LA View News. This position is of great interest to me because you are seeking someone with experience and your position is within a growing spa business.

You will find me a qualified candidate who has successfully completed several spa technique courses, including Healing and Sacred Stone Massage and Spa and the Massage Therapist. I am also certified by the National Board.

I am trustworthy, competent, well-trained, and personable. My skill set includes the ability to provide deep tissue massage. A highly motivated individual, I am also very interested in increasing my knowledge in the field. The next class that I intend to take is Hydrotherapy for Spa Techniques.

I look forward to hearing from you concerning your available position and hope to arrange an interview in the near future. You may reach me by calling in the evening at (123) 456-7890. Thank you for your time and your consideration.

Sincerely,

Marsha Schaffer

Enclosure

Phone: (123) 456-7890

A

FIGURE 18-6. **A,** Letter of application in response to a blind advertisement for a spa massage therapist. This letter template is posted on Evolve at http://www.evolve.elsevier.com/Fritz/business.

Box 18-7 presents some hints for writing a resume. Every resume should have certain types of information, including career objective, personal data, qualifications, experience, and education. Optional areas may include objectives, affiliations, and references. The arrangement of and headings for this information can vary, depending on the person's work experience, education, and goals. It is wise to select a standard format and emphasize sections in which you have the greatest assets. Regardless of the format selected, there are do's and don'ts for creating an effective resume (Box 18-8).

PERSONAL DATA

Personal data include the following:
- Full name
- Address
- Telephone number
- Fax number and e-mail address (if you have one)

CAREER OBJECTIVE

The career objective section lets the reader know about your current career goals.

Example: "Career Objective: A position as a massage therapist with opportunities to use my clinical, technical, and human relations skills within the wellness setting."

You may also list your long-term goals in the objective:

Example: "Career Objective: A position as a massage therapist in a pain management clinic, with long-range goals of developing and managing a massage therapy department."

EDUCATION

Be sure to include relevant information about your educational background. List all colleges and universities attended and the date you graduated (list most recent schools first).

Marsha Schaffer, MT, NCTMB
2050 Leisure Lane, Lapeer, MI 48446
(123) 456-7890 / leisurelymassage@hec.com

Objective   To obtain a massage therapist position in a spa business that will utilize
my maturity, experience, and passion for the massage profession, as well as
encourage and motivate continuing education.

Experience	2007-present	Hillsdale Massage Clinic Massage Therapist	Hillsdale, MI
	2005-2007	Jordan Chiropractic Association Part-Time Massage Therapist	Grand Rapids, MI
	2004-2005	Road House Grill Dining Room Hostess	Grand Rapids, MI

Education	July 2006	Healing and Sacred Stone Massage Health Enrichment Center, Inc.	Lapeer, MI
	June 2006	Sports Massage Therapy Education Destinations, Sandy Fritz, Lecturer	Lapeer, MI
	2004-2005	Massage Therapy Program Health Enrichment Center, Inc.	Lapeer, MI

Credentials	NCTMB	National Certification Board
	ABMP	Associated Bodywork and Massage Professionals
	CPR	American Heart Association Certificate

References   Provided upon request.

B

FIGURE 18-6, cont'd **B,** Personal resume to accompany the letter applying for the spa massage therapist. ⊜This resume template is posted on Evolve at http://www.evolve.elsevier.com/Fritz/business.

List diplomas or degrees, awards, scholarships, and special achievements. Courses that you took when completing the massage therapist program may be listed (e.g., science, fundamental massage procedures, advanced massage procedures, adaptive massage application for outcome-based treatment plans within a clinical practice, professional etiquette).

WORK EXPERIENCE

A chronologic resume begins with your most recent job and includes dates of employment, name and address of employer, position held, and a brief description of the job. Summer and part-time jobs may be lumped in a single category; however, if work experiences have been limited, you may want to list them separately. Box 18-9 describes the advantages and disadvantages of a chronologic resume.

If your work experience is more recent than your education, the work experience should be listed before your education. At this point in your career, work experience is of greater value to a prospective employer than your education.

OPTIONAL AREAS

If you have participated in school or community activities or received awards or honors, this information could be valuable to the prospective employer, and it should be included. Activities and hobbies are optional but can indicate that you are a well-rounded individual and get along well with others. List professional and other affiliations.

References are provided on request and not before the personal interview. Be prepared with the names, addresses, and telephone numbers of at least two people who are willing to verify your abilities and skills and one person who can provide a character reference. If your work experience has been limited, list instructors or clinical supervisors who can evaluate your abilities. Always obtain the individual's permission to use his or her name as a reference and be sure that person is willing to give you a good recommendation.

Do not give information on the resume that may be detrimental to you. Details can be given when you are

BOX 18-7	Hints for Preparing a Resume

- Use all of the layout, formatting, and finishing techniques available to you.
- Use headings that allow the reader to find information easily.
- Be succinct.
- Use a spell checker.
- Make the resume easy to read (e.g., print size, font styles, arrangement of information).
- Put your education and experience information in chronologic order.
- Use sufficient white space to avoid a cluttered look.

BOX 18-8	Creating an Effective Resume

DO
- Emphasize your qualities and experience
- Substantiate your educational and experience qualifications to justify the abilities you claim
- Be clear and concise in your descriptions
- Choose a format that is easy to read
- Be consistent in using the format

DO NOT
- Include on the resume the date the resume was written
- Include a physical description of yourself (e.g., height, weight, age)
- Include race or religion
- Mention your health status
- Include salary information (unless specifically requested; then include it in the cover letter)
- Use abbreviations or acronyms that may not be understood

interviewed. At the interview, be prepared to discuss your weaknesses honestly, confidently, and in a way that puts you in the best light. Figures 18-5B and 18-6B show how resumes were designed to accompany the letters in Figures 18-5A and 18-6A, respectively.

Completing the Job Application Form

The type of therapeutic massage position for which you are applying determines the detail and complexity of the application form. The *job application* form is a series of questions requesting comprehensive data about you and your past education, work, and professional experience. It often may require you to complete a narrative statement about yourself and give the reasons you are seeking a particular job. You may have the opportunity to complete the application form before arriving for the interview, or you may be asked to complete the form when you arrive. Figure 18-7 presents an example of an application used for private practice.

Regardless of the job for which you are applying, you must keep several things in mind when completing the application form:

- If possible, try to obtain two forms, one to use as a working copy and the other to submit to the employer.
- Before entering data on the application form, read through the application thoroughly and avoid asking unnecessary questions. The application form often is used as the first employment test. It tests your ability to follow directions.
- The directions may indicate that the form can be typed or written. If you are required to complete the form in your own handwriting, it may be another test of neatness, and it gives the employer a sample of how well or poorly you write.
- Answer all the questions. If the question does not relate to you, write N/A (not applicable) or draw a line through the question. The employer then realizes you have read the question and have not overlooked it.

BOX 18-9	Advantages and Disadvantages of a Chronologic Resume

ADVANTAGES
- Highlights titles and company names, which is advantageous when the names or tiles are relevant or impressive
- Highlights consistent progress from one position to another
- Highlights length of time in each organization

DISADVANTAGES
- Readily shows gaps in the work history
- Shows frequent job changes
- Does not show the most impressive or relevant work experience first if it is not the most recent

- Be truthful when answering interview questions. Dates, names, and places need to be accurate. Make a list of your former addresses, schools, family names, and references to take along when going for the interview. It is better to have the information available even if it is not needed. Be sure that no discrepancies exist between your reported date of birth and your age. If you are residing at a temporary address, be sure to give a permanent address. Be particularly careful with spelling. A small pocket dictionary is a great item to take along as a handy reference.

LEARNING ACTIVITY

Obtain three different job applications. Request the forms from various business managers. Make sure to explain why you are asking for the forms. Then fill them out.

EMPLOYMENT APPLICATION
All information listed on this application will be considered and handled as personal and confidential.
Please write or print legibly.

AN EQUAL OPPORTUNITY EMPLOYER
This employer provides equal opportunity to all persons without regard to
handicap, race, color, religion, sex, age, or national origin.

Name:	Date of application:

Address:	City:	State:	Zip:

Home phone:	Cell phone:	Social security number:

GENERAL INFORMATION

Position applied for: _____

Available to work   ☐ Full-time   ☐ Part-time   ☐ Temporary

Date available to start work: _____

Are you over 18 years of age   ☐ Yes   ☐ No   Will transportation be a problem for you?   ☐ Yes   ☐ No

If you are not a U.S. Citizen, do you have the right to work in the United States?   ☐ Yes   ☐ No

Have you ever been convicted of a felony?   ☐ Yes   ☐ No

   (A conviction is not an automatic bar to employment. Each case will be considered on its own merits.)

Does body odor bother you?   ☐ Yes   ☐ No

EDUCATION

	Name and address of school	Major/degree/ certification(s)	Number of years completed	Did you graduate?
High school				
Community college				
4 Year institution				
Vocational				
Other (specify)				
Describe specialized training, apprenticeship, skills, seminars, courses, extra-curricular activities				

FIGURE 18-7. Application form for employment.

(Continued)

The Interview

PREPARING FOR THE PERSONAL INTERVIEW

The day you receive a response from a prospective employer, you will be elated to know that someone is interested in your qualifications after reviewing the resume and now wishes to meet you in person. This elation is immediately followed by a feeling of fear—fear of the unknown. You may or may not know anything about the prospective position, but you do know yourself. The following suggestions can be used to prepare for an interview.

Learn about the employer. After you have identified business to which you are interested in applying, spend time learning more about the office or clinic, its mission, and its

SKILLS

Task	Circle One		Task	Circle One
Keyboarding WPM	Yes No		Stone Massage	Yes No
Bookkeeping	Yes No		Craniosacral Therapy	Yes No
Computer Operations	Yes No		Reflexology	Yes No
Handling Group Insurance	Yes No		Essential Oil Therapy	Yes No
Have you used insurance software?	Yes No		Pregnancy Massage	Yes No
Other(s): Describe				

EMPLOYMENT RECORD

Beginning with your current employer, please list your work experience over the past 10 years.
You may include pertinent volunteer activities.

Name of Employer		Start Date	End Date
Address	Phone	Start Salary	End Salary
Job Title	Supervisor	Phone	
Duties			
Reason for Leaving			

Name of Employer		Start Date	End Date
Address	Phone	Start Salary	End Salary
Job Title	Supervisor	Phone	
Duties			
Reason for Leaving			

Name of Employer		Start Date	End Date
Address	Phone	Start Salary	End Salary
Job Title	Supervisor	Phone	
Duties			
Reason for Leaving			

FIGURE 18-7, cont'd

vision. Find out about its reputation and how it treats its employees. This can be done in several ways:

- Ask friends, relatives, and acquaintances what they know about this business.
- Check the office or clinic Web site if one is available.
- Search Web sites to identify professional memberships.

- If you are a student, consult with local professional contacts or school faculty.

For the interview, wear something that looks business-like. You may have a new outfit that you would like to wear but cannot decide whether it is the proper choice. If you question whether an outfit is right, do not wear it. Wash

REFERENCES

Name	Address	Phone

EMERGENCY CONTACT

Name	Relationship	
Address	Phone	Alt. Phone

DUTY PERFORMANCE

Are you able to perform the essential duties of the position for which you are applying, either with or without reasonable accommodations?   ☐ Yes   ☐ No

If yes, please indicate what type(s) of reasonable accommodations are needed:

In this course of making an employment decision, this employer makes it a practice to verify with previous employers information such as dates of employment, description of job duties, attendance records, reason for leaving, etc. If there are any employers you do not want us to contact, please indicate their names below and reasons why:

_____

_____

_____

_____

I understand that if I am employed and if any statement herein is not true, I may be released immediately, I will be paid only through the day of release, and this employer may cancel any rights to accrued benefits.

_____   _____
Date   Signature

FIGURE 18-7, cont'd

your hair, and style it so that it feels comfortable and looks good on you. A light amount of makeup can be worn, but do not wear a perfume. Personal appearance is an important part of the interview, and it is prudent to follow the old adage: First appearances are lasting ones. You may know all the answers and have a lot of skill, but you must win the approval of the employer before you will have an opportunity to display your skills. Take your professional uniform, and be prepared to give a massage if requested. This is a common practice when interviewing for massage positions.

The day you receive the call for the interview, write down the time, place, and name of the interviewer. Prepare the materials to take with you to the interview. These should include a ballpoint pen, a pencil, an eraser, a small spiral notebook, a pocket dictionary, and a copy of your school transcripts and your resume. In the notebook, list many of your outstanding characteristics that you wish to bring to the attention of the employer, a list of questions you hope to cover during the interview, and the names, addresses, and telephone numbers or e-mail addresses of your references.

It is common for a massage therapist to provide a sample massage session. This can occur at the time of the interview or be scheduled later. Be prepared by having your massage table, supplies, and uniform available. You do not want to say that you are not able to do the massage.

Depending on the type of job for which you are applying, you may want to take a *portfolio*, which is a compilation of samples of your experience. If you are applying for a massage therapist position, a portfolio can include the following:

- Letters you have written, which show your writing style
- Copies of diplomas and certificates from education
- Pictures of you providing massage

Preparing a portfolio and presenting it during the job interview allows you to show what you can do rather than merely talk about it.

NAVIGATING THE PERSONAL INTERVIEW

Plan to arrive a few minutes early at the office. Your first contact may be with the office manager. The office manager plays an important role in the office, and it is important to be friendly and courteous to this person. You may want to introduce yourself by saying, "Good morning, I am Jennifer Ellis (use your own name!), and I have a 10:30 appointment for an interview with Ms. Randle." The office manager will acknowledge you and may ask you to complete an application form similar to that shown in Figure 18-7. After the form is completed, the office manager may review your resume and application and will escort you to meet Ms. Randle. If you are not introduced, take the time to introduce yourself by saying, "Good morning, Ms. Randle, I am Jennifer Ellis." At this point, you will be asked to be seated, and the interview will begin. Look directly at the interviewer, and respond to the questions clearly and distinctly; do not be evasive. An evasive answer leaves doubt in the interviewer's mind.

The applicant should be responsive and answer in complete sentences. Box 18-10 provides suggestions about things to avoid during an interview. Box 18-11 provides a series of commonly asked interview questions.

After the series of questions, salary and job responsibilities are discussed. If the salary the employer offers you is lower than you are willing to accept, you may reply that you had hoped to start at a higher salary but that you are willing to accept an opportunity to demonstrate your ability and value to the practice. This undoubtedly will result in further discussion, and you should be prepared to give firm answers about what you will accept. You should inquire whether any benefits are included that can offset the lower salary.

After an interview that included many of the questions in Box 18-11, an applicant, Jennifer Ellis, was offered an acceptable salary, although it was lower than her initial request. She replied, "I feel I have the skills you need, and it is going to save you a great deal of time in not having to teach me about all the technical skills. I would be willing to start at the lower salary if you will explain to me what the total salary scale is and how I will be evaluated for salary raises. I would like the opportunity to advance by merit or production, because I am certain you will be pleased with my ability and production in your office." Ms. Randle explained the numerous benefits and outlined the salary system to Jennifer. Salary is not the primary aspect of the job, but you must be

| BOX 18-10 | Missteps to Avoid in a Job Interview |

- Being too aggressive
- Talking about salary and hours immediately
- Chewing gum
- Lacking enthusiasm
- Lacking a neat appearance
- Using little or no eye contact
- Appearing preoccupied
- Using poor grammar
- Being vague
- Wearing too much makeup
- Lacking curiosity

| BOX 18-11 | Commonly Asked Interview Questions |

INITIAL QUESTIONS
- How did you learn about this position?
- Are you familiar with our office?
- Why are you interested in this practice?
- How would you describe yourself?
- Why do you think you are qualified for this position?

INTEREST IN THE JOB
- Are you currently employed? If so, does your current employer know you are seeking a new position?
- Why do you want to change jobs?
- What do you consider the ideal job for you?
- What are your long-range and short-range goals?

EDUCATION
- What formal education have you had?
- Why did you choose to study massage therapy?
- What was your academic average when you were in school?
- What do you consider your greatest strength? Your greatest weakness?

EXPERIENCE
- Have you ever been fired or asked to resign from a position?
- Why did you leave your previous job?
- Which duties performed in the past have you liked the best? The least? Why?
- Why should I hire you?
- What salary do you expect?

able to earn enough to support yourself and not eliminate some of the more enjoyable things in life. The benefits of a job often outweigh the basic salary, so do not overlook this aspect in your assessment of the offer.

OTHER FORMATS FOR INTERVIEWING

Some employers like to have team interviews, in which several members of the staff who will work with you participate in the interview. A team interview in a private practice setting involves three or four people. Although this type of interview may sound intimidating, it may not be. Pay attention to the individuals' names as they are introduced so that you can later refer to them by name. Listen carefully, and answer questions succinctly, giving your attention to the individual who asked the question. Make eye contact with all participants if the question or statement is meant for the group.

Working Interview

An employer may use the working interview format to assess an applicant. The employer will invite you for a day of work at the office, for which some form of compensation is prearranged. This is an opportunity to observe the office activity, and it can give you a sense of how well the office is organized.

Virtual Interview

Virtual interviews are not common in small massage practices, but some situations may warrant them. For example, if you are applying for a job in Torrance, California, at a large spa, and you live in Biltmore, New Jersey, it may be feasible to conduct a virtual interview. Rather than having you fly to California for the interview, the spa staff conducting the interview makes arrangements for you to go to a facility that has a teleconferencing center. This allows the interviewer from California to see you, and you can see the interviewer.

Careful planning must be done in advance of the virtual interview. Many people become nervous when they are going to be videotaped, but a virtual interview is a two-way system that allows you to communicate with the other person as if you were in the same room. You still greet the interviewer warmly and with a smile, just as you would in person. Sit in the chair provided, and avoid nervous habits. Try to forget that the camera is present, and concentrate on the interviewer and the questions. Avoid wearing black, gray, or white, because they do not come across well on camera. Avoid wearing jewelry that is distracting or that makes noise.

INTERVIEWING THE INTERVIEWER

During interviews, you are collecting information to help you decide which position to take. Practice integrating questions into a dialog so that the questions appear information based and conversational. Asking intelligent and relevant questions demonstrates that you are aware of the importance of understanding the position being sought. Consider asking employers the following questions:

- Please describe the duties of the job for me.
- What kinds of assignments may I expect the first 6 months on the job?
- Are salary adjustments geared to the cost of living or job performance?
- Does your company encourage further education?
- How often are performance reviews given?
- What services are in the development stage now?
- Do you have plans for expansion?
- What are your growth projections for next year?
- Have you cut your staff in the past 3 years?
- How do you feel about creativity and individuality?
- Do you offer flextime?

- Is your company environmentally conscious? In what ways?
- In what ways is a career with your company better than one with your competitors?
- Is this a new position, or am I replacing someone?
- What is the largest single problem facing your staff (department) now?
- May I talk with the last person who held this position?
- What is the usual promotional time frame?
- Does your company offer single or dual career-track programs?
- What do you like best about your job (company)?
- After the probation period is completed, how much authority will I have over decisions?
- Has there been much turnover in this job area?
- Do you fill positions from the outside or promote from within first?
- What qualities are you looking for in the candidate who fills this position?
- What skills are especially important for someone in this position?
- What characteristics do the achievers in this company seem to share?
- Is there a lot of team or project work?
- Will I have the opportunity to work on special projects?
- Where does this position fit into the organizational structure?
- How much travel is involved in this position?
- What is the next course of action? When should I expect to hear from you, or should I contact you?

CONCLUDING THE INTERVIEW

An interview is not a lengthy process, and it often is terminated with a tour of the office. Do not be overly flattering to the staff, but thank them for their time before you leave. You may not receive a job offer during the interview, because the employer may have other applicants to interview. However, you may inquire about when the employer anticipates arriving at a decision. Do not be discouraged if you do not get the job. Each interview is a learning experience, regardless of whether it produces a job offer.

FOLLOWING UP THE INTERVIEW

A follow-up letter (Fig. 18-8) should be written 1 or 2 days after the interview. This is an indication to the interviewer that you are interested in the position, and it may make you a priority applicant.

The follow-up letter does not have to be long. It restates your interest in the job and mentions some of the facts that interested you about the position.

Another type of follow-up may be necessary if you have not had a reply from the prospective employer. If the job is still available and you are interested, it is permissible to call the interviewer 1 or 2 days after the interview. A telephone call lets the interviewer know of your continued interest; however, too many telephone calls can be annoying.

Luke Fritz, MT, NCTMB
2050 Leisure Lane, Lapeer, MI 48446
(123) 456-7890 / leisurelymassage@hec.com

October 20, 20xx

Jana Larke
222 Relaxation Drive
Your Town, State 00000

Dear Ms Larke:

Thank you for taking the time to talk with me yesterday and for allowing me to demonstrate my massage abilities. It was a privilege to experience such a well-rounded, organized clinic. I appreciate your time and consideration.

After speaking with you and your office staff, I believe that I would be a perfect candidate for your available position. I can offer my top-notch clinical training and education, quick learning, and adaptability, which is often needed in a practice with so many diverse clients.

In addition to my enthusiasm, I will bring the technical and analytical skills necessary to not only maintain but also increase your excellent client base.

I am very interested in working at Massage Today and look forward to hearing from you. Please feel free to contact me anytime if further information is needed. My cell phone number is (123) 456-7890.

Thank you again for your time and consideration.

Sincerely,

Luke Fritz

FIGURE 18-8. Follow-up letter. ⊜ This letter template is posted on Evolve at http://www.evolve.elsevier.com/Fritz/business.

If you decide later that you are not interested in the position, you should send a letter explaining your decision. This is thoughtful, and a time may come when you find yourself in a position to go back to this employer.

If you are called and offered the position and you accepted the offer, you should send a letter to formalize your acceptance (Fig. 18-9). Be sure to include your understanding of important details such as starting salary and start date.

KEEPING THE JOB

Regular self-evaluation is necessary to retain your position and clients. Client retention is a key to success. People often carefully evaluate themselves before they are hired but may become careless after working for a time.

Do not become negligent about evaluating yourself. You are constantly in the public eye and must maintain a good image in your employer's office. After you have obtained the position, you must maintain your skills and acquire new ones. You should promptly join a professional organization for massage therapists, which offer information about educational activities in relevant techniques.

SELF-REFLECTION

How do I behave when I am interviewed? Do I get nervous or defensive? Do I become shy and withdrawn, or am I comfortable? How would I feel if I had to interview someone? Do I act like an interrogator? Friend? Boss? Peer?

LEARNING ACTIVITY

Go to the local Chamber of Commerce, and ask if there are managers who would interview you for a nonspecific job. Do the same thing with some cooperative local business owners and managers. You can find these individuals at service organizations such as the Lions Club or Kiwanis. Practice interviewing or being interviewed by a fellow student or friend.

Professional Etiquette

Learning and remembering the names of your immediate associates should not be difficult. If the staff is large, learning the names of those not in your immediate department may be more difficult. Learn the names as quickly as possible.

Luke Fritz, MT, NCTMB
2050 Leisure Lane, Lapeer, MI 48446
(123) 456-7890 / leisurelymassage@hec.com

October 20, 20xx

Jana Larke
222 Relaxation Drive
Your Town, State 00000

Dear Ms Larke:

I am very pleased to accept your offer for the position of entry-level massage therapist. Thank you for the opportunity! I am eager to make a positive contribution to your practice and to work with everyone on the Massage Today team.

As we discussed, my starting salary will be $32,000. I understand that health and life insurance benefits will be provided after 90 days of employment.

I look forward to becoming a part of the team on December 1, 2008. If there is any additional information or paperwork you need before then, please let me know.

Again, thank you for the opportunity.

Sincerely,

Luke Fritz, MT, NCBTMB

FIGURE 18-9. Acceptance letter. ◎ This letter template is posted on Evolve at http://www.evolve.elsevier.com/Fritz/business.

It may be wise to maintain a list of names and the position of each employee until you are able to remember them.

Listen attentively. You will be eager to learn as much as possible about your new position as quickly as possible. Listen carefully to directions, and avoid talking persistently. If you relax and listen well, the questions you are eager to ask often will be answered. If not, do not hesitate to ask for clarification of a procedure.

Establish meaningful social friendships. Most employers do not object if employees develop personal friendships with other employees. However, many traps can develop in your first days on a new job. One of these is developing a close relationship with one or two people too quickly, which can cost you friendship with others at a later time. Office cliques frequently create rivalry. Although you must have a friendly attitude toward other employees in the office, you do not need to participate in all the social activities or interests the others have. However, you should avoid a superior attitude that can be interpreted as snobbish.

Use a notebook and calendar to record important activities and procedures. When you begin your new job, many unfamiliar rules and regulations and other information will be given to you. To avoid misunderstandings or neglecting important information, develop the "notebook habit" and write down each bit of information. It is surprising how many successful people use this system.

Observe office hours. In most cases, the office hours have been determined before your arrival. The efficiency of an office depends on your being prompt at all times. Your tardiness delays the work process for which you are responsible. You should ensure your means of transportation at all times. It is your responsibility to anticipate inclement weather and compensate for any potential delay. It is better to be 20 minutes early for work than 2 minutes late. The employer will not be interested in your excuses.

Use judgment in working overtime and taking breaks. Employees sometimes try to impress their employer by working extra hours or skipping lunch hours or breaks. However, you should avoid continual overtime and loss of lunch hours because it may cause friction with other employees. Your actions may be misinterpreted, and other employees may make life miserable for you. This does not mean you cannot use your discretion on days that are extra busy.

Do not flaunt your education and abilities. Nothing is more irritating than a new employee who constantly informs other employees of his or her exceptional abilities. It is better to prove your ability through your work than to tell everyone about your great potential. Your coworkers may have had many years of experience, and you may learn something from them if you give them a chance to help you. Offer to show others how to do some method they may comment on.

BOX 18-12	Hints for Success in a New Job

- Learn the names of staff members.
- Listen attentively.
- Establish meaningful social friendships.
- Use a notebook and calendar to record important activities and procedures.
- Use judgment in working overtime and taking breaks.
- Do not flaunt your education and abilities.
- Seek honest evaluations.
- Maintain office policies.
- Observe office hours.
- Be yourself.

Share your knowledge freely when asked, and ask others to teach you (Box 18-12).

Clean up after yourself. You should maintain high standards of sanitation in the massage area. However, that is not the only place you will be. Wipe down counters in the break area or restroom after using. Dispose of all refuse you create. Pick up clutter even if you did not generate it. Do not leave food in the refrigerator or break area. Hang your coat up. Empty full trash baskets and so forth. If we all left an area in better condition than when we entered it, just think how nice the environment would be. It takes less energy to clean up a mess than to complain about it.

Seek honest performance evaluations. Most employees want to learn about their performance. Before accepting the new job, you should have asked how and when your performance would be evaluated. As time passes, periodic reviews of your performance should be obtained from the employer, and you should have an opportunity to discuss the performance evaluation. Determine ways in which you are performing satisfactorily and areas that need improvement. Figure 18-10 shows an example of a performance evaluation form. Such forms are reviewed periodically with you to evaluate your day-to-day performance. It is wise to use this evaluation form first as a self-evaluation, before your employer completes it.

Maintain office policies. Most offices have established policies for grooming and uniform styles. You should carefully review the office policy and adhere to it. You should take home any other handbooks the office uses for its employees and read them carefully so that you will be well informed. If you do not understand a policy, ask for clarification to avoid making an embarrassing mistake.

Be yourself. As you make your first impression in the office, it is wise to be yourself. Temper this with context appropriate behavior. It may be okay to laugh loudly at a party but not in the office. You may admire characteristics in another person, but you cannot be that person. If you attempt to be someone else, you will destroy the finer parts of your character. Be yourself, and you will be a happier person.

Asking for a Raise

Pay increments may be discussed when you begin work, and you may find that raises are given after 6 months or 1 year of successful employment. To avoid any misunderstanding, determine how and when these raises can be obtained before accepting the job. Few employers would consider performing extensive treatment on patients before informing them of the anticipated fees. Similarly, you should not be working unless you are aware of your potential salary and anticipated promotions. It is wise to obtain written verification of employment conditions and responsibilities and a salary scale before beginning work. This can be accomplished in an office procedures manual (see Chapter 2). However, if pay increments have not been discussed and you have completed a year of employment, you might wonder when and how the subject can be raised.

Before approaching the employer about a raise, you should do a self-evaluation to determine that you are justified in making such a request. The questions listed in Box 18-13 can be considered in the evaluation. A salary conference should be a two-way discussion that allows you to identify your assets for the job and explain your performance success and that allows the employer to relate the performance to a monetary amount that will reward your performance and inspire increased productivity.

If you have given serious thought to the factors mentioned previously, and you feel you deserve a raise, how do you approach the employer? Select an opportunity when the work schedule allows enough time for a discussion of the subject. Do not wait until the end of the day, when the employer is tired and ready to leave the office. It also is not wise to start the day by asking for a raise, especially if the schedule is rather heavy.

Let the employer know why you believe you deserve a raise. If he or she asks why you should have one, be prepared to answer. For example, cite the rising cost of living, transportation costs, insurance, increased business production because of your efforts, or compensation for good performance.

Employees often do not assert themselves enough to make the employer aware that a raise should be given. If you become passive and content with a salary, naturally you will continue to be paid at this rate; however, if your professional skills are an asset and because of these skills the employer is realizing a profit, you should be given a raise. If the employer cannot raise your salary, consider the benefits as alternatives to a salary increase.

If you are unsuccessful in getting a raise, express your appreciation for the employer's understanding and consideration, and consider your alternatives. If you receive a raise, be sure to thank the responsible person.

Salary matters should be treated confidentially and are not discussed with other members of the team. Salary problems destroy positive attitudes and productivity and should be resolved as quickly as possible.

Performance Evaluation Form

Employee Name _____

Job Title _____

Supervisor _____

EVALUATION

4   Excellent performance that demonstrates consistent and important contributions that meet and frequently surpass expectations of the position.
3   Performs with a very acceptable degree of skill that demonstrates the expectations of the position.
2   Performance has not met satisfactory level. Makes mistakes but usually corrects errors after further instruction. Improved performance is needed to achieve defined expectations of this position.
1   Performance indicates deficiencies that seriously interfere with attainment of the defined expectations of the position.

Attendance   **Evaluation**
Adheres to scheduled work hours.   4   3   2   1
Uses leave appropriately.   4   3   2   1
Adjusts work schedule to office needs.   4   3   2   1

Job Knowledge
Uses required job skills.   4   3   2   1
Updates skills periodically.   4   3   2   1
Demonstrates knowledge of procedures needed to perform the job.   4   3   2   1

Organizational Skills
Prioritizes tasks.   4   3   2   1
Plans steps in advance to accomplish tasks.   4   3   2   1
Meets deadlines.   4   3   2   1

Work Quality
Performs work accurately.   4   3   2   1
Demonstrates thoroughness and attention to detail.   4   3   2   1
Demonstrates neatness.   4   3   2   1

Human Relations/Communications
Demonstrates a sense of humor.   4   3   2   1
Demonstrates good listening skills.   4   3   2   1
Maintains eye contact when speaking to another person.   4   3   2   1
Displays good manners and professional etiquette.   4   3   2   1
Conveys ideas effectively.   4   3   2   1
Responds to ideas conveyed by others.   4   3   2   1
Demonstrates sensitivity to diverse staff and patients. 4   3   2   1

Problem Solving Skills
Remains calm in stressful situations.   4   3   2   1
Demonstrates ability to identify the problem.   4   3   2   1
Demonstrates ability to select the best solution.   4   3   2   1
Takes action to prevent future problems.   4   3   2   1
Does not require supervision to accomplish routine tasks. 4   3   2   1
Follows through on chosen solution.   4   3   2   1
Gives constructive criticism in a positive manner.   4   3   2   1
Responds to supervision in a positive manner.   4   3   2   1

Cooperation
Respects responsibilities of others.   4   3   2   1
Provides assistance and guidance to others.   4   3   2   1
Accepts guidance from supervisor/employer.   4   3   2   1
Works as a team member.   4   3   2   1

Initiative
Seeks work that needs to be done.   4   3   2   1
Seeks new methods and ideas to improve work.   4   3   2   1
Exhibits self-motivation to achieve team goals.   4   3   2   1

Integrity
Respects other people and their property.   4   3   2   1
Maintains confidentiality.   4   3   2   1
Can be trusted with money that belongs to the office.   4   3   2   1
Refrains from gossip.   4   3   2   1
Is truthful regardless of potential consequences.   4   3   2   1

Supervisor/Employer Comments _____

Employee Comments _____

Employee's Signature_____   **Date**_____

Supervisor/Employer Signature _____   **Date**_____

FIGURE 18-10. Performance appraisal form. *(From Finkbeiner BL, Finkbeiner CA:* Practice Management for the Dental Team, *ed 6, St. Louis, 2006, Mosby.)*

BOX 18-13	Questions to Consider before Asking for a Raise

- Have I performed my duties well enough to deserve a raise?
- Have I improved or advanced my skills since beginning the job?
- Have I been cooperative with other members of the team?
- Have I continued to maintain good client management skills?
- Can I verify that my attendance and punctuality have been above average?
- Have I continually maintained professional ethics, safe practice, and quality standards?
- Can I verify that the practice's productivity has increased because of my performance?
- Do economic factors in the practice and in the economy warrant a raise?

JOB TERMINATION

Three things can occur where you are leaving an employment position. You can leave, you can be fired, or you can be laid off. If you leave, it is on your terms, and you should plan in advance. If you are fired, you should have known that your job performance was problematic because employers are required to inform the employee with a series of warnings and interventions. If you are laid off, there typically is some sort of downsizing of the business, usually due to lack of business. If you are an employee and are laid off due to no fault on your part, you are eligible for unemployment.

Resignation

Terminating a job can be an obstacle for some individuals, especially when the job change is from one massage practice to another in the same general locale. When you change jobs, make sure the change is to your advantage. Circumstances over which you have no control may be the reason for a change in jobs. However, a massage therapist who frequently changes jobs with inadequate notification or reason soon gains a poor professional reputation. Whatever the reason for terminating the job, do it ethically.

- Give the reason for leaving the job.
- Give sufficient notice, at least 2 weeks or longer if your job requires an extensive training period for a new massage therapist.
- Write a letter of resignation as a follow-up to your verbal resignation.
- Do not discuss the termination of your job with other members of the team until you are ready to inform the employer that you will be leaving. The grapevine is a poor method of informing.

- If you terminate a job where serious conflicts exist, it is best to leave these conflicts where they originated and not carry the feelings to another job. When beginning a new position, you should not make negative comments about a former employer. This is simply good ethics.
- Determine what is ethical for clients who wish to follow you to a different location. Discuss this topic openly with the employer.

According to the U.S. Department of Labor (http://www.ctdol.state.ct.us/progsupt/unemplt/new-faqui.htm), the general rule is that a person, who voluntarily leaves suitable work without good cause, attributable to the employer, is not eligible for benefits. For good cause to be attributable to the employer, it must relate to the wages, hours, or working conditions of the job. A change in conditions created by your employer or a breach of your employment agreement that is substantial and adversely affects you may be good cause to quit. If the job itself adversely affects your health or aggravates or worsens a medical condition, it may be good cause to quit.

Regardless of the cause, in most cases, a good cause attributable to the employer may be found only if you took reasonable steps to inform your employer of your dissatisfaction and sought to remedy the problem before you left. If you quit, it is your burden to prove that there was good cause for leaving. When applying for benefits after quitting a job, you will be scheduled to attend a predetermination hearing to establish whether you had good cause for leaving. Your employer will be notified of this hearing and will be invited to attend or to send a written statement.

Being Fired

There had to be a reason. It is important to evaluate what happened so that the employee–employer relationship failed. Be honest with yourself. What did you do or not do that created the problem? Learn from the experience, and be determined to not make the same mistakes again. According to the U.S. Department of Labor, if you are fired or suspended, you may be disqualified for benefits if the employer can prove one of the following:

- Willful misconduct in the course of your employment. The term *willful misconduct* means deliberate misconduct in willful disregard of the employer's interest or a single knowing violation of a reasonable and uniformly enforced rule or policy of the employer, when reasonably applied, provided such violation is not a result of the employee's incompetence. In the case of absence from work, an employee must be absent without notice or good cause on three separate instances within a 12-month period.
- Conduct that is a felony under the law and occurred in the course of your employment
- Larceny of property or service whose value exceeds $25 in the course of your employment

- Participation in a strike that is illegal under law or regulations
- You were sentenced to a term of imprisonment of 30 days or longer and had begun serving that sentence.
- You were discharged or suspended because you were disqualified by law from performing the job for which you were hired as a result of a drug- or alcohol-testing program mandated by law.

If you are discharged, it is the employer's burden to prove that there was willful misconduct. When applying for benefits after being discharged or suspended from a job, you will be scheduled to attend a predetermination hearing to determine eligibility. Your employer will be notified of this hearing and will be invited to attend or to send in a written statement.

SELF-REFLECTION

Have I ever been fired or laid off? Did I quit a job? What do I remember about the experience? How did if react? What would I do if I was the employer and had to fire or lay off someone? If one of my employees were about to quit working for me, how would I want him or her to quit?

Being Laid Off

If you are laid off, it is likely because the business was not producing enough income to justify your salary. This is a difficult situation for the employee and employer. There are times when no matter how hard someone works and even when they are doing all the correct things to support a productive business, larger issues such as an economic downturn may occur.

Be supportive of the employer. If business improves, it is likely that you will be called back to work. There may even be some sort of contribution you can make to increase business, especially if you enjoy the people you work with and believe in the business. When employers have to lay off employees, they usually provide positive letters of recommendation and offer references for employees who get other jobs. If laid off, you are likely eligible for unemployment benefits.

According to the U.S. Department of Labor (http://www.ctdol.state.ct.us/progsupt/unemplt/new-faqui.htm), the basic eligibility requirements to qualify for unemployment are as follows:

- Be fully or partially unemployed.
- Be unemployed through no fault of your own (the law imposes disqualifications for certain types of separations from employment).
- Be physically and mentally able to work full time. Individuals who cannot work because of a physical or mental

BOX 18-14	U.S. Department of Labor Employment and Training Administration Basic Eligibility Requirements

You can receive benefits if you meet a series of legal eligibility requirements:
- You must be monetarily eligible.
- You must be totally or partially unemployed.
- You must have an approvable job separation; the law imposes a disqualification for certain types of separations.
- You must meet certain weekly legal requirements; weekly requirements include being physically and mentally able to work, being available for and seeking work, and filing your weekly claim for benefits on a timely basis.
- If you are identified as likely to exhaust unemployment benefits and are enrolled in the worker profiling and reemployment services program, you must fully participate in all assessment interviews, orientation, and referred reemployment services.

More information on this subject can be found at www.doleta.gov

impairment that is chronic or expected to be long term or permanent may qualify for benefits if they are available for suitable part-time work (Box 18-14).
- Be actively seeking work by making reasonable efforts to find employment each week.
- Participate in selected reemployment services if you are identified as a dislocated worker by the profiling system.
- File your weekly claims as directed.

STARTING AND MAINTAINING YOUR OWN BUSINESS

You should first ask yourself whether you have the skills and qualities required to become an entrepreneur and maintain the business structure. The answer requires some reflection and self-analysis. Use this checklist for self-evaluation:

Management: Confident, leading, planning, problem solving, target setting, reflective

Marketing: Understanding markets and people, winning customers and their confidence

Communication: Verbal and written using different media; networking and establishing relationships

Administration: Keeping accounts and organizing data

Creativity: Innovative in identifying new "original" business; adapting to new circumstances

Commercial skills: Financial awareness of grants, funding, accounts, and sources of competition

Self-motivation: Drive to succeed; tenacity and self-discipline

If you do not have all the skills, do not worry; they often develop as you are running a business or spend time working for other or while you are taking classes. An even better approach is to combine all of these and add a mentor to the mix. The U.S. Small Business Administration (SBA) SCORE program can help you.

Have you thoroughly considered the risk? Not all new businesses succeed at first. Many have setbacks, but learn from these, and with support, you can eventually succeed. Henry Ford said, "Failure is the opportunity to begin again, more intelligently."

Are you aware that eventually other people may also have a say in your business venture? It is unlikely that you will succeed alone. Help, support, and professional skills will be required from many sources, not just family and friends. In your quest to nurture a secure business, advisers, bank managers, accountants, landlords, and clients will become involved. You may need to adapt and change direction with your business ideas after considering their differing advice and demands.

According to the SBA, there are two core questions prospective business owners need to ask themselves: What service or product does my business provide, and what needs does it fill? Who are the potential customers for my product or service, and why will they purchase it from me?

If you are considering starting a massage therapy business, you need to consider many points of general business practice. For an employee, it is enough to be a great massage therapist and team member. If you are the business owner and the massage therapist, you have to understand how to do everything. Those who have decided to pursue a career as employees need to realize that it is still important to understand what is involved in business operations to support the employer.

After you have generated your ideas and begin to identify a range of opportunities for your future enterprise, you need to evaluate the opportunity. Who will buy, where is the office located, how will the business be run, and will it be profitable?

EXPERT Outlook

Tucson Touch Therapies
3903 E. Pima Street
Tucson, AZ 85712
www.tucsontouchtherapies.com
Owners: David K. Anderson, LMT, NCTMB and Sandra K. Anderson, BA, LMT, NCTMB

Tucson Touch Therapies is a ten-room treatment center located in central Tucson. We opened it in 2001 as a small, three-room office in a different location, and moved to our current location in 2004. Thirty practitioners, including ourselves, provide treatments and everyone is an independent contractor. Because of the many skills of all our practitioners, Tucson Touch Therapies offers fifteen different types of treatments, which we have divided into three categories: Integrated Massage Therapies (therapeutic massage, Neuromuscular Therapy, hot and cold stone treatments, and so forth), Asian Bodywork Therapies (shiatsu, Thai massage, and so forth) and Energy Therapies (Healing Touch, craniosacral therapy and Reiki).

Our treatment center is located in a 3,000 square foot space which, besides the ten treatment rooms, has a spacious reception area, a retail area with massage and bodywork products, art by local artists and gift items, a large break room for our practitioners, and two bathrooms. Each fully furnished treatment room is at least ten feet by twelve feet, with two rooms measuring ten feet by sixteen feet. We have a music CD library, two hydrocollators, and numerous props and bolsters available for practitioner use. Practitioners supply their own linens and lubricants, and each has a storage cabinet for their personal use.

Three part-time employees staff the reception desk. They answer the phone, schedule treatments, and perform other administrative duties that support Tucson Touch Therapies' day-to-day operations. As independent contractors, practitioners set their own schedules but they interact with the reception desk staff to ensure that client booking goes smoothly.

Tucson Touch Therapies offers practitioners a choice of three shift lengths: 8 hours, 5½ hours, and 3 hours. Practitioners must commit to at least one 8 hour shift or two 5½ hour shifts weekly. They pay rent for all the shifts they have committed to each month by the first day of the month. Practitioners are then paid directly by their clients unless the client pays by credit card or has a package with Tucson Touch Therapies. A package is a group of four discounted treatments that the client has paid for all at once. Credit card and package payments are disbursed to practitioners on a bimonthly basis.

The independent contractor business model works quite well for practitioners because they have the potential for earning more than they would as an employee. Once they've paid their monthly rent to Tucson Touch Therapies, they keep all treatment fees from their clients. On the other hand, we do not guarantee practitioners that they will be booked, and even if they are not booked, they are required to pay their rental fee.

Because of this, we let all prospective practitioners know that in order to be successful in our treatment center, they need to either have their own clientele they bring with them, or the drive and ambition to build one. Tucson Touch Therapies has a well-known name in the community and a reputation for excellent client care and skilled practitioners. We are located on a busy intersection and have prominent signage, and we have a large telephone book ad. Because of all of this, many prospective clients call wanting treatments, so those practitioners who have not yet established a clientele have the opportunity to do so with clients who do not request a specific practitioner. The blend of experienced and new practitioners works very well for us. Several practitioners who have joined us right out of school have done very well because they have been willing to work hard.

Tucson Touch Therapies has a very stable roster of practitioners. Practitioners do not leave very often, and many of our practitioners have been with us either since we opened in 2001 or moved and expanded in 2004. We also have a reputation for fair treatment of practitioners, resulting in a waiting list of those who want to work in our center. This is because they know they can preserve their independence but still have the advantages of a group practice. Practitioners benefit from each others' knowledge and experiences,

Like all businesses, we need to be cautious about who we let work at Tucson Touch Therapies. Not everyone is a good fit. Practitioners must be comfortable with not necessarily having a steady income, but one that can fluctuate at times. They need to be able to work without supervision, and they need to have excellent hands-on and communication skills. We require practitioners to have at least 1000 hours of education, either from their primary bodywork program or from a combination of their primary program and continuing education courses. They also need to be licensed and carry liability insurance.

When we decided to open Tucson Touch Therapies, we drew on our years of experience, both within the bodywork profession and in our previous careers. Sandy had worked for 10 years and David had worked for 7 years as professional bodywork practitioners at another Tucson treatment center where we were independent contractors, and both had built steady clientele. Sandy was also an instructor at the Desert Institute of the Healing Arts in Tucson where she ultimately taught for 12 years in topics such as anatomy and physiology and massage therapy and shiatsu theory and techniques. Prior to becoming a bodyworker in 1991, Sandy received a BA in biology from Ithaca College in Ithaca, NY and worked as a research lab technician and data analyst. David worked as a diesel mechanic, independent grain farmer, and parts salesman for tractor trailers.

What we brought with us into this profession is common sense, a willingness to work very hard, and passion for finally finding our life's work. We chose not to have investors to fund our startup because we did not want to be beholden to others. Instead, we funded it ourselves and formed an LLC to protect our private property. We were also able to save a lot of costs because we have the skills to design, build and decorate our infrastructure. For example, David built our reception desk, filing cabinet, and storage cabinets. Sandy sewed curtains, made

some of the artwork, and has written the text for the brochures and Web site.

We think that the reason Tucson Touch Therapies is successful is because we incorporate our personal philosophies into our business philosophies. For example, we chose the independent contractor business model because it is worthwhile for everyone involved, not just us. Both of us perform treatments as well as run the business so we know exactly what it is like to be practitioners.

We do not believe that a bodywork business "owns" the clients who come for treatments. Most people see practitioners they are comfortable with and from whom they receive effective treatments, and they will see them in whatever setting they are located. Therefore, if practitioners leave Tucson Touch Therapies, they can take their clientele with them. We believe this engenders a spirit of networking, not competition, which makes a healthier environment for bodywork.

We like working with friends and colleagues. In fact, when we decided to open Tucson Touch Therapies, we did not have to look much further than within our network to find practitioners to work with us. Because of Sandy's length of time teaching at the Desert Institute, she knows many graduates who are now professional practitioners in the area. Because of the time spent working at the previous treatment center, David and Sandy have gotten to know quite a few other practitioners as well. When we opened our office, many of these practitioners became quite interested in working with us and moved their clientele to Tucson Touch Therapies.

We have, of course, faced challenges. One of the drawbacks of the independent contractor business model is that cost-to-profit ratio is narrow because we rely on rental income from practitioners. If we were taking a percentage of each treatment, then our income would be higher. However, we have never wanted to be employers of bodywork practitioners because we see that business model as having more headaches then rewards. Instead, with our type of business model, because we've built a really good name in Tucson, we have stable month to month rental income and a brand name that will be sellable one day.

Because we cannot and choose not to treat our independent contractors like employees, we have had to learn how to filter comments, suggestions, and complaints from thirty people while honoring and respecting their feelings and opinions. This can be overwhelming at times. Just as an example, we recently decided to paint our reception area and retail space, and we chose three shades of green. Needless to say, we heard thirty different opinions about the colors.

We sincerely believe that that we have not made very many mistakes in our business. There have been some people that we regretted inviting to join Tucson Touch Therapies and had to ask to leave. Other than that, we have made good business decisions and are pleased with our success. We think it is

(Continued)

EXPERT
Outlook

because we have paid attention to details, observed what has worked and not worked in other businesses, and used what we have learned from our past experiences.

The words of advice we give anyone in the bodywork profession or thinking of entering the profession are:

■ Be willing and able to work very hard, long hours. It will be worth it because nothing beats being your own boss.

■ Be patient. Work at your business every day, but do not be discouraged if you do not always see immediate results.

Anything worthwhile usually takes time and effort to build.

■ Use common sense. Most businesses fail because of lack of common sense. Plan your steps, and figure out the most cost-effective methods to achieve each one. For example, do not spend a lot of money you do not have on an interior decorator for your business; rely on your own good taste. Make sure you have the client base to support all your financial decisions.

The Business Plan

LEARNING ACTIVITY

As you proceed through this section, make a list of what you would include in a business plan. Complete this activity regardless of whether you have decided to seek employment, because it will help you appreciate the responsibility of any business owner. At the end of the chapter, you will be asked to write an actual business plan.

The most important tool to assess the likelihood of new business success is the *business plan*, a summary of your business and the objectives and activities needed for it to succeed. A business plan is a written document that describes the future path of a business. A good business plan explains the business concept, summarizes the objectives of the business, identifies the resources (money and people) that will be needed by the business, describes how those resources will be obtained, and explains why the business will succeed. The Evolve Web site (http://evolve.elsevier.com/Fritz/Links) provides a sample business plan. The SBA links to and cooperates with the Canadian Business Resource Center in British Columbia, which has a step-by-step business planning tool for new or existing businesses (Box 18-15).

The following components typically make up a business plan:

■ Executive summary that summarizes key points of the business plan in one or two pages

■ Overview, which introduces the reader to the business

■ Company summary that describes the products and services

■ Overview of the industry in which the business will compete

■ Marketing strategy that summarizes the service or product, promotion, pricing, and distribution strategies of the business

■ Description of the management and staff personnel

■ Implementation plan, which includes a financial plan

BOX 18-15	Writing a Business Plan

A written guide to starting and running your business successfully is essential. The business plan can encourage loans, promote growth, and provide a map for you to follow. All of the following topics are explored at Strategic planning http://www.sba.gov.

Learn to strategize for your business to succeed: Essential Elements of a Good Business Plan For Growing Companies

Outlines how to write your plan: Writing The Business Plan

Detailed, step-by-step explanation to help write your plan: Business Plan Workshop

An online workshop to help start and improve your business plan: Using The Business Plan

How to get the most out of your plan: Finding a Niche

A small, steady corner of the market could be your success story: Business Planning FAQs

Answers to the most popular business plan questions: A Business Plan: The Roadmap To Success

The SBA's guide to developing a comprehensive business plan: Interactive Business Planner

This information is based on guidelines from the Small Business Administration Program Office (www.sba.gov).

A financial plan includes balance sheets, income statements, and cash flow statements. A balance sheet compares what your business owns with what it owes. A cash flow statement compares how much money will be coming in with how much you will be spending. An income statement compares your revenues with your expenses to see if you are going to make money.

Business plans can vary in length from a few pages to more than 100 pages. Although there are no rules, many sources recommend that business plans should be between 10 and 25 pages long. A business plan is a summary; you can always provide more information if asked, or you can attach more detailed background documents to your business plan. The Good Stuff from the Government section at the end of this chapter provides access to a template to help you complete a business plan.

Producing a business plan has certain benefits. The process of preparing a business plan will force you to think about your business, research some options, recognize opportunities and risks, and test some of your expectations. It can help you identify the cash needs of your business, and a business plan can be used to obtain financing from banks and from investors. The plan can be used to tell employees, investors, and others about your plans and strategies, and it provides a benchmark against which to compare the progress and performance of your business.

It is a good idea for all businesses to prepare and regularly update their business plans. However, small businesses are most likely to prepare a business plan when they are just starting up or when a major change in their business is occurring—often when additional investment or a loan is needed.

When preparing a good business plan, consider who is going to read the plan and what do you want them to do, such as loan money, to help you decide how much emphasis to put on various sections of the business plan. A business plan is only as good as the research that went into producing it. You will have to research your industry, your potential customers, your potential competitors, and your potential sales and costs. Take your time. Show drafts of your business plan to others. It can be very useful to get feedback on your draft business plan from various people, including people associated with the business and others.

Write your own business plan. One common mistake made by entrepreneurs is to copy too much information from a sample business plan and change the names and some of the numbers. A good business plan should flow together like a good story, with the sections working together to demonstrate why the business will be successful. Most importantly, it must be your story.

Outline the key points, and review your outline to ensure that your sections are consistent with each other, that there is no duplication, and that all the key issues have been covered. Make sure your financial projections are realistic. A good financial plan indicates that you thoroughly understand your business.

Write the executive summary last. It can be the most important section of your business plan because people will read it first, and it may be the only section they read. A good executive summary should be short (two pages at most), should highlight what is important in your plan, and should get the reader excited about your business.

The Business Structure

What type of business do you want? There are so many possibilities in the massage therapy profession. Are you interested in having a small office location where only you work or finding shared space with another health professional? Do you want to take to the road with a massage-on-wheels program in a specially designed van or motor home in which the massage is provided? What about a home-based business or going to others' homes? Do you want to create

space for others to work or even invest in one of the new massage franchises? The possibilities are limitless. You also need to consider whether your business structure will be sole proprietor, corporation, independent contractor, or another form.

START-UP COSTS

Start-up costs are the initial expenses required to begin a business. In addition to these start-up costs, you should have a minimum cash reserve equal to the amount of money needed to cover basic business and personal living expenses for 6 months to 1 year. Many people begin a business without these cash reserves and do fine. Others give up the business venture because they do not have enough money to pay bills. This situation forces them to find other jobs. Keeping a cash reserve allows you to focus on developing your business with less financial worry.

In giving a massage, the student is taught to keep it simple and to go slowly. The same ideas apply to business. A person beginning a massage business does not need a suite of offices. For self-employed individuals, the least expensive way to do business is to develop an on-site massage business for private homes or offices and have the business office in the home.

Starting small, with the bare essentials, keeps start-up costs at about $4000. A basic portable table should not cost more than $500. Business cards and a simple brochure are needed, as are client-practitioner statements, policy and procedure booklets, receipt books, and client information forms. The total cost for these is about $500. It is a good idea to have a separate telephone and answering system, which together cost about $300. Membership in one of the professional organizations also provides liability insurance; the membership and insurance usually cost less than $300. Linens and supplies should cost about $300, and opening a bank account plus miscellaneous expenses takes about $500. An expenditure of $1000 for initial advertising is reasonable.

Renting a small office can push up the start-up cost to about $6000. This includes the expenses detailed previously plus office costs, such as rent (about $1000, because renting office space often requires payment of the first and last months' rent) and office furniture and utility hook-ups (another $1000).

SELF-EMPLOYMENT

The self-employed massage professional typically becomes affiliated with an established business (e.g., a health club, chiropractor, full-service cosmetology business) by renting a room in that business establishment. Any agreement of this type must be written in contractual form and reviewed by an attorney.

A pitfall in this type of arrangement develops when the owner or manager of the business wants the massage practitioner to function as an employee but to be classified as self-employed for payment and tax purposes. With this arrangement, the business owner does not have to pay matching payroll taxes or benefits. For true self-employment status, the professional essentially is renting space from the owner. The massage business is completely independent in the way business is conducted. The business owner cannot direct the massage practitioner regarding what hours to work, what kind of work to do, or what to wear.

The owner of the existing business can be paid in one of two ways. One arrangement is to pay the owner a percentage of every massage performed. This percentage varies from 10% to 50% (the average is 30%). With this arrangement, the business owner profits from every massage done and may be more likely to support your business with word-of-mouth advertising and referrals. The two businesses commonly advertise together.

Under the other type of agreement, the practitioner pays the owner a monthly rent. Rental fees depend on the business location and the area of the country. Most rooms in established businesses can be rented for $200 to $600 per month. One formula for figuring rent involves calculating the percentage of the total square footage of the space. For example, if the room you want to rent is 12 feet by 12 feet (144 square feet) and the business occupies 2000 square feet, room is about 7% of the total available space. The owner pays $2800 per month for rent ($14 per square foot); 7% of $2800 is $196. The business owner needs to make some money to apply the business principle of making a reasonable profit. A 50% return is normal; 50% of $196 is $98. The rent for the space would be $196 plus $98, or $294 per month.

The better choice at first may be to pay a percentage for each massage. If the practitioner has a slow week or gives very few massages, he or she is not obligated to pay a monthly bill. As the business builds, the practitioner commonly ends up paying more per month with a percentage agreement than with a flat fee. If a mutually beneficial relationship is desired, a compromise can be negotiated, such as an upper limit cap on monthly rent. This is the type of information that must be included in a written legal agreement, or contract.

THE TARGET MARKET

In developing a business, it is important to know the market. Many opportunities are open for the massage business, ranging from the service approaches of stress reduction massage to the allied health opportunities of working in clinical settings. The future for massage is bright. Research has provided the long-awaited verification of the benefits of massage. Educational standards continue to improve, and the profession is becoming standardized and formalized. These developments should achieve a broader acceptance of therapeutic massage and bodywork methods. As a result, more people will consider using massage as part of a health maintenance program.

Massage probably will assume a larger role in corporate stress reduction programs. Athletes will use the services of a massage practitioner more often. Pain control clinics will see its value. Both elderly and young persons can benefit from the nurturing touch of the massage therapist. Opportunities for the development of the massage business will be even greater after people understand the benefits of massage, and the need for consistently well-trained practitioners will increase.

There is no typical massage business. Successful massage professionals can be found practicing in many different formats. Massage professionals may be full-time employees of a chiropractor or may work part time out of their homes. A business can be developed entirely at one location or in three or four locations. A massage therapist may work one day at a local manufacturing business for the employees and the next day may do on-site visits for local business people. The third day may be spent teaching a self-help massage class for the local community education program. On the fourth day, the therapist may see clients at a full-service cosmetology establishment in the morning and, in the evening, provide on-site massage for a local support group dealing with stress.

With all the available possibilities, it is wise to narrow the focus to one, two, or three specific markets to keep advertising and promotional activities manageable. Answering the following questions begins the process of narrowing and developing a target market for a therapeutic massage business:

- Where do you plan to work?
- What potential client groups or populations are available within a half-hour drive of the location?
- What type of massage or bodywork do you enjoy giving?
- What group or type of people do you want to help most?
- How are you going to reach those potential clients?
- When do you want to be available to do massage?

By the fifth year of business, the practitioner usually has established a solid focus, a narrow target market, and a consistent clientele.

MARKETING

Marketing encompasses the advertising and other promotional activities required to sell a product or service (see Chapter 12). Advertising is a necessity when starting a new business, and many forms of advertising are very costly. For massage, some types of advertising work better than others.

It is not enough to have a great service at a great price that meets a true need. For your new business to be a success, you need to let people know about the business. Here are some approaches to do just that:

Business cards: A quality business card is essential. Hand them out wherever you go. Be sure to include a logo, what your business does, and contact information.

Web site: Every business today needs a professional-looking and well-designed Web site. You want client and others to be able to learn about your business and just what products and services you have to offer. The professional organizations serving the massage industry offer help in creating Web sites.

Postcard marketing: Nothing beats postcard marketing for cost and readability. Use postcards as an effective way to generate sales leads, promote special offers or coupons, drive traffic to your Web site, or introduce new products or services.

Hold a grand opening: A well-thought-out and successfully executed grand opening can greatly assist with your ultimate goal: matching your business's products and services to the people in your community who would most need and benefit from them and increasing your profits along the way.

Join groups: Become a part of your local business and civic community. Join your local Chamber of Commerce and a service organization like the Kiwanis or Lions Club. Attend meetings and become involved in your community.

Public speaking: Identify opportunities to educate the public about massage. Speak at service organizations, social clubs, support groups, and schools, and spread the word about your massage business.

Press releases: You have a new business with a great innovative concept. Get the word out, and your customers will come. Send out a well-written press release detailing your new business and what makes it special. The media is always looking for stories on hot new businesses and trends; why not let it be about yours?

Judicious advertising: Budget an affordable amount for advertising. This may include advertising in the Yellow Pages, local newspapers, business directories, and similar places on the Internet. Do not overspend on these forms of advertising.

Most clients are found through a direct meeting, an educational program, networking, and word of mouth. Word of mouth is the best advertising. Meeting people and talking with them is far more effective than placing an ad in a newspaper. Having satisfied clients who tell other potential clients about you is even better. In the beginning, the massage practitioner must talk with many people to develop a client base. Building a business takes time. It is important not to become discouraged, because if you want to succeed, quitting is not an option.

The massage practitioner should persist in handing out business cards and brochures and giving demonstrations until the clients are found. Placing an ad and then sitting in an office waiting for clients to call does not work. Success comes by arranging to speak at service clubs and churches in the area or by volunteering to work at races and local events. Businesses may want to offer a stress management class. Local school districts often have adult education classes, and short classes that teach simple massage routines are

popular. Charitable organizations often have auctions, which are wonderful opportunities to give away gift certificates for massage. The Evolve Web site (http://evolve.elsevier.com/Fritz/business) presents an interactive activity for creating a business card.

Being visible in the community helps to generate business. A regular base clientele of about 100 is sufficient to support a thriving therapeutic massage business. Some clients will have weekly standing appointments, others biweekly appointments, and the rest will visit monthly or occasionally. It may be necessary to talk to 2000 people to find 100 clients.

The main marketing obstacles for personal service wellness massage are convincing the public that regular massage is beneficial to a lifestyle program that focuses on managing stress and striving for wellness and helping would-be clients justify the fees for massage. A wellness massage business is built on clients who receive therapeutic massage regularly. Clients who get a massage on a weekly, bimonthly, or monthly basis are the mainstay of a personal service massage business. A successful business of this type depends on quality; consistent, personal attention to the client; and affordable fees. Clients who are happy with the work are the best source of word-of-mouth advertising.

The Brochure

The brochure is the primary tool for educating the public and potential clients about the services offered. It should give specific information about the following (and a template for your use is provided on Evolve):

Nature of the services offered: The brochure should explain clearly that therapeutic massage is a general health service. It should state that no specific treatment of any kind is given for preexisting physical or mental problems. It also should make clear that all specific problems of a medical, structural, psychological, or dietary nature will be referred to the appropriate licensed professional. Written permission and supervision by the medical professional or other licensed health professional will be required for the massage practitioner to work with any conditions that fall within that specific scope of practice.

Description of the services offered: The brochure should give a simple explanation of the process of a massage. It should include a full description of the types of services offered and the procedures followed in rendering those services. It should explain that the client may remain dressed and will always be properly draped. It should clearly state that the client may stop the session at any time and may choose not to have any area of the body touched or to have any particular technique used.

Qualifications of the practitioner: The massage professional's credentials, documenting his or her education, training, and experience, should be outlined in a manner that allows potential clients to verify the practitioner's competence. A valid organization that issues the credentials, such as a school or continuing education provider, must have a record of the practitioner having completed the course.

Client's financial and time investment: The brochure must provide a realistic statement of costs and fees. It should emphasize that the effects of massage are temporary and that massage is best used as a maintenance system. The brochure should state that the massage practitioner could teach self-help to the client if requested. It also should make clear that the best results from massage are maintained when treatment is given on a weekly or biweekly basis and that therapeutic massage, when used only occasionally, provides only temporary effects.

Client's role in health care: The brochure should address the importance of the client's responsibility for his or her personal health care. It is important that the client realize that the massage practitioner is a facilitator in the wellness process.

The Evolve Web site (http://evolve.elsevier.com/Fritz/business) provides various brochures and a brochure-writing activity.

The Media

Local newspapers often run stories about new and unusual businesses. A word of caution about newspapers: The massage professional should write the story to avoid embarrassing mistakes. Including a black and white photograph of the professional giving a massage is a great idea. It is also beneficial to provide the writer with copies of other good news stories about therapeutic massage.

Media advertising (i.e., newspaper, radio, and television) is very expensive and not the best idea initially. The clientele developed most likely will be located within a 30-mile radius of the business location. Direct mailing to a specific area is more effective than newspaper advertising. Web sites and Internet advertising are rapidly expanding the concept of advertising.

Before advertising in the Yellow Pages of the telephone book, which is expensive, the massage professional must be sure that the business location will not change for at least a year. The advertisement will be locked in for a year after the phone book has been distributed, and the contract must be paid even if the business moves. The trend for the phone book to be delivered electronically will provide more flexibility for changes.

A much more cost-effective method is to use media advertising the way automotive companies do: A group of massage professionals in the area can advertise together. When the cost is split, newspaper, radio, Internet, and television advertising becomes affordable. Whenever a cooperative venture such as group advertising is formed, the professionals involved must get the agreement in writing with the help of an attorney. Never make oral contracts or agreements. When you develop any written material or advertising, make sure you provide potential clients with the answers to these basic questions:

- Who? (you)
- What? (therapeutic massage)
- Where? (address and phone number)
- When? (appointment times)
- How? (phone, e-mail, or Web page)

This information also should be provided on your business card. The card should be simple and direct and should not list all your credentials. It is convenient to put the information about the next appointment date on the back of the card.

MANAGEMENT

Management consists of all the activities required to maintain a business, particularly record keeping, and financial disbursement. The KISS principle (keep it simple and specific) is an excellent concept to help organize the details of business practices. A business operation can be set up in many ways. A business consultant and an attorney usually are the best advisers. The simplest business arrangement, the sole proprietorship, is detailed in this textbook. The steps in setting up this arrangement are as follows:

1. Obtain all necessary licenses.
2. Choose a business location.
3. Determine the legal structure of the business.
4. Register the name of the business.
5. Register for tax purposes.
6. Arrange for insurance.
7. Open business banking accounts.
8. Set up investments.
9. Keep records.
10. Develop a client-practitioner agreement and policy statement.

Obtaining Licenses

Massage professionals usually deal with two types of licenses: professional and business. A professional license shows that you have achieved the skills to practice your profession. It may be issued by the state or by a local governmental body and may be required for all who practice massage. For a massage practice, difficulties occasionally arise with local licensing if state licensing is not in place. If this problem is encountered, it is important to organize a group of massage professionals and other supporters in the local community and work to change any local control that does not support massage as a profession.

If a state licenses massage practitioners, the professional usually must show proof of a certain level of education and pass some sort of licensing test. The best way to find out about licensing in any state is to contact the Department of Licensing and Regulation in the state capital. The licensing department for massage usually is in the Occupational License Department. This agency can provide the necessary information. Most states now license massage therapists or are in the process of developing licensure. The Evolve Web site (http://evolve.elsevier.com/Fritz/Links) provides a list of states that license massage therapists.

A business license, which is obtained from the local government, allows that governmental body to regulate the type and location of business operations. If a profession is licensed, the professional may need to show a copy of the professional license to obtain a business license. Any required forms should be filled out carefully.

Choosing a Business Location

When deciding where to locate your business, remember that each community has specific zoning regulations. These regulations protect the investment of those who own property. Without zoning, someone could put a junkyard next to a home. A massage business requires general office or commercial zoning. Because of difficulties with local ordinance control of massage establishments, some restrictions may apply to locations for a massage business. To obtain this information, the practitioner should visit local government offices and ask to see the zoning ordinances.

A permit or business license may be needed. The business owner should develop a good working relationship with government officials. These officials usually have a sincere concern for their communities, and the massage professional must respect this. Occasionally, these officials need to be educated about therapeutic massage. As with a massage, go slowly and be gentle and understanding.

Difficulty with massage parlor ordinances has diminished substantiality over the past 5 years, but the problem still exists. Growing public awareness about therapeutic massage eventually should resolve this problem.

Home-Based Business

Working at home is not new, but more and more people are trying it. The home is being called the new workplace. Home-based businesses (HBBs) have begun to gain credibility, longevity, stability, and financial success. People often have personal reasons for choosing to begin a business in their home.

HBBs vary from part-time to full-time employment. For some owners, the business provides the sole household income, whereas for others, the business provides money for extras. Some HBBs are operated by an individual, others are a family venture, and some employ people other than family members. The possibilities for an HBB are as limitless as the owner's creativity. Various types of HBBs include manufacturing, service, consulting, mail order, and sales. Massage therapy lends itself to an HBB.

Because laws vary by city or county, knowing what is legal for your locale will help to prevent problems and allow you to adapt your business accordingly. You should contact your local government or zoning office or consult with lawyers, insurance agents, and accountants, who will be able to advise you.

SELF-REFLECTION

Will I be an effective business owner? How have I determined the answer to this question? If I answered yes, what are my strengths, challenges, and weaknesses as a business owner? If I answered no, what aspects of self-employment do I not want to deal with? Have I changed my mind about how to develop my massage career after completing this textbook? What changed?

There are many pros and cons for having a business in your home. You must be able to operate a business in your home legally. You may have unlimited ideas and plans for your business, but what you can do is controlled by laws. Because your business occurs in your home, local regulations may limit activities that can affect the residential character and quality of your neighborhood. For example, you may not be able to manufacture certain products, may have to install specialized equipment or modify facilities, may be limited in the use of employees, or may be restricted on other issues, such as parking, signs, or noise. Examples of laws or regulations that may limit your HBB include zoning, restrictive covenants in your deed, homeowners' association covenants, and local ordinances. Your homeowner's insurance will likely be affected, and you need to consider issues such as liability.

After the legal concerns are addressed, other factors may be considered:

- What will the business demand from the home space?
- What does the family need from the space in the home?
- How can you develop a management plan for household space use that best accommodates your family and your business?
- How is having your business in your home affecting your family?
- Do you have a plan for integrating family and business space needs?

The work environment is important to the success of any business. For the HBB, the work environment is unique because it is also a home. The use of space in the home changes when an HBB is begun. By definition, an HBB introduces a business activity into residential space, your home. The needs of the business and the needs of the family members are different, and conflict can result. This conflict threatens the success of the business and family harmony.

The primary cause of conflict is the lack of a clean division of space for business use. Effective management of the home space is needed to reduce conflict. Specific examples of conflict include clutter from the business in family space, lack of adequate space for both business and family activities, need to move business activities to accommodate family activities, increased household work due to the business, and business clients' lack of respect for the home space.

In a typical situation, beginning an HBB involves bringing a business into what was previously considered family space. By definition, an HBB takes up space in the home, and before the business starts, the home is seen as family space. After the business starts, family space must be given up to the business. The family and the HBB must be integrated into the same structure. Because of this, a plan for integrating a business into the home space includes an evaluation by each family member of when and where it is acceptable for the business to intrude on family space.

There are other issues in changing the perceptions of space and access in the home. The use of a space is changed by the presence of the business. For example, a dining room may double as a space for consulting with a client, or the kitchen may be shared at lunchtime. The activities that can take place in a home are altered by the presence of a business. For example, TV watching may be banned during business hours due to noise. Control of space used by a business may eliminate space formerly used by the family; for instance, a guest room may become an office. The question of maintenance arises when areas are used by the family and the business. Who is responsible for the upkeep of common areas such as the entry and stairs?

The perception of the workplace is important. A home is normally a private place, and a business is public. Outsiders see the HBB as a business, a public space, whereas the family may still perceive the business as home space and regard outsiders as showing a lack of respect. How would your family react?

An HBB is not for everyone. For many people, it will provide a supplemental income source for retirement or extra income for the family. Only 46% of HBB and micro-business owners surveyed cited that making lots of money was a motivation for starting their own business. Seventy-eight percent of business owners stated that having more control over their lives was an important reason, and 90% said they would go into business again. Even though you may not get rich from such an endeavor, it may be worth the effort to see if your idea can be successful. Entrepreneurs may not see a profit right away; it depends on the type of business.

Several facets should be considered when starting an HBB. Determine if there will be a market for your products or services and whether such an endeavor is possible. This is crucial before a large amount of money is spent. The business may not be feasible. Too many businesses fail because people do not test their market plan and manage the business properly.

Operating an HBB has several advantages:

- Can start as a part-time business
- More flexible lifestyle and more integrated with the family
- Lower start-up and operating costs
- Cost-savings on child and adult care
- No commuting
- Flexible work hours
- Satisfaction of being own boss
- Increased tax benefits and write-offs
- Outlet for creative or unique talents
- Employment of family members by the business

Operating an HBB also has disadvantages:

- Space may be cramped, limiting growth potential and family use.
- Personal and family lifestyle patterns may be disturbed.
- Business and family privacy may be disrupted.
- Long work hours and time away from family
- Lack of fringe benefits
- Lack of informal social contacts or opportunities to network
- Stress due to inability to balance family and business needs
- Family members, friends, and neighbors may demand more of you when you are home all day.
- Business activities may cause problems with neighbors.
- Discipline is required to establish steady work patterns and manage home responsibilities.

DETERMINING THE LEGAL STRUCTURE OF THE BUSINESS

A sole proprietorship (one-owner business) is the simplest way to set up a business. Partnerships and corporations are complicated business structures, and the need for them should be discussed with an attorney.

SELF-REFLECTION

Consider the space in your home for your business. What are the positive aspects of being in business at home? What are the negative aspects or disadvantages? It is important to take a realistic look at both aspects. List your thoughts below.

ADVANTAGES OF A HOME BUSINESS	DISADVANTAGES OF A HOME BUSINESS

Registering the Name of the Business

Registering the name of your business is known as obtaining a DBA (i.e., doing business as). When choosing a business name, the public's interpretation must be considered. One person chose BODY-WORKS and received calls about automotive body repair. The fee to register the name of your business is about $20, and it usually is done at the county clerk's office. The clerk will check to see whether anyone else in the county is using the name and then issue the DBA. This document may be needed to open a business checking account.

Registering for Tax Purposes

Federal, state, and local taxes must be paid. A sales tax identification number may be needed. Information about federal taxes can be provided by the Internal Revenue Service (IRS) at 1-800-829-1040. State tax information can be obtained from the Department of the Treasury in any state. Information about local taxes can be obtained from the county and local government offices. The IRS has many publications and counseling services that can explain the payment of business taxes. The business owner is strongly urged to seek the advice of a business attorney or certified public accountant regarding tax requirements.

One third of the gross income of a business usually is needed to cover various taxes. This money must be set aside every month and left untouched. One of the biggest problems new business owners have is nonpayment of taxes because the tax money was spent on overhead expenses. The best protection is to pay the government first, because the penalties are high and tax laws are difficult. A professional tax preparer can help with the management of your taxes.

ARRANGING FOR INSURANCE

All massage therapists need professional liability insurance, often called malpractice insurance. The term *malpractice* refers to professional negligence or malfeasance. Negligence is an unintentional wrong. A negligent person fails to act in a reasonable and careful manner and consequently causes harm. Malfeasance is causing deliberate harm. Clients expect a certain level of professional education, standards of practice, and responsibility for conduct. Unfortunately, in our highly litigious climate, the best protection against a lawsuit is insurance. Insurance reduces the risk of having a liability claim filed against you personally. To advertise this, however, only invites a lawsuit. Accurate, comprehensive records are the next best protection; anything that seems even slightly important must be documented.

The best place to obtain liability insurance is through the professional organizations. Those that have been in existence for many years are the Associated Bodywork and Massage Professionals (ABMP) and the American Massage Therapy Association (AMTA). The addresses and phone numbers of these organizations can be found on the Evolve Web site (http://evolve.elsevier.com/Fritz/business). Other professional organizations for massage and bodywork professionals have been established, and careful investigation of their insurance plans is recommended. The insurance costs usually are part of the dues structure of these organizations, an arrangement that makes insurance available at a reasonable cost. Obtaining insurance from private companies is very expensive.

Premise liability insurance is needed; this is often called "trip and fall" insurance. It can be obtained through professional organizations or from a local insurance agent. Because home business offices are not covered under a homeowner's policy, additional coverage in the form of a business rider is needed. The insurance agent also can discuss fire and damage insurance for equipment.

The more complicated a business, the more comprehensive the insurance coverage must be. Sale of products requires product liability insurance. Independent contractor liability insurance protects the contractor against third-party claims from hired independent contractors. The insurance agent and the insurance representative of the professional organization can provide additional information.

OPENING BUSINESS BANKING ACCOUNTS

A business account can be opened at a local bank. The DBA usually is required to use a business name. All income from the business is deposited in the business account, which serves as a record of gross income. All expenses are paid from this checking account, which provides a record of business deductions. What is left over is the net income.

If the massage professional is disciplined enough to pay off a charge card every month, a business credit card is a good idea. The monthly statement provides a record of business expenses.

Taxes are paid quarterly on the net income. A wise professional will contact a good bookkeeper or accountant to help set up the payment schedule for taxes.

After all business expenses and taxes have been covered, the massage professional may write himself or herself a paycheck, called a draw check. This money should be deposited in a personal account, and personal expenses can be paid from this account. Personal and business money must not be mixed.

SETTING UP INVESTMENTS

All massage professionals, whether self-employed or employed by others, should set up an individual retirement plan. After taxes are paid, 10% of income could be invested in a long-term growth investment. A local bank or insurance company may have access to stable mutual funds. Individual retirement accounts (IRAs) also are available. Some employers offer investment plans. Money can be invested in compound interest–bearing accounts in many ways. This takes discipline, but we inevitably get older, and planning for that time is important.

KEEPING RECORDS

Record keeping likely seems like an overdiscussed topic at this point. However, much of the nuts and bolts of business involves record keeping. All business receipts must be saved and filed. Copies of all important documents should be stored in a location other than that of the originals. Everything must be dated, and no oral contracts should be made. Information should be organized monthly on a spreadsheet so that when it is time for the tax preparer to do the business and personal taxes, everything can be verified. This so-called paper trail is very important for a properly run business, and it must be established.

Comprehensive client files must be kept in order. Payment records are also kept in the paper or electronic client files. Note whether payment was made by cash, credit card, or check; if a check is used, note the check number. If cash is paid, note the receipt number. If a monthly billing system is used, post the date the bill was sent and the date the check was received, along with the check number. Any credit card information should be taken and recorded. Records must be kept current. If you must use professional liability insurance or if you are billed by a client's insurance company, the first thing the company will request is the client's records.

Anyone who wants to manage his or her own business is advised to take some classes in small business management at a community college or to attend workshops offered by the local Chamber of Commerce. For the self-employed, the need to keep accurate records is unavoidable. Many commercial record-keeping systems are available. A wise course is to choose one and use it consistently. All massage professionals, whether employees or self-employed, must keep accurate, comprehensive client files. The success of your professional life depends on it. The current trend toward electronic data storage and various types of user-friendly software supports this process.

There are many pros and cons to being self-employed and of owning and operating a business. It can become even more complex if you have employees. One of the first areas discussed in this textbook is the application of intention, intuition, and inspiration. Even with the best business plan, it is the intention to be self-employed, the intuition to make important decisions, and inspiration to proceed with ideas regardless of risks that will support your success.

LEARNING ACTIVITY

Using your outline and the knowledge gained from this text, write a comprehensive business plan. You can use one of the templates identified in the Good Stuff from the Government segment.

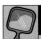

SELF-REFLECTION

Review all the self-reflection questions, starting in Chapter 1. Ask yourself the same questions again. What has changed?
- I am the same in what ways?
- Why do I understand others better?
- Why am I more organized?
- Why am I more aware of the nature of business function?
- In what ways am I different?
- What subjects do I need to learn more about?
- How will I be more successful in my career?
- What is my dream for my career?
- What is my plan to reach my dream?
- What motivates me to be successful?
- What am I still nervous about?
- Who will help me?
- What is my vision for my future?
- What is my source of motivation for persistence in attaining my goals?
- What is my source of inspiration?
- What does my intuition tell me my plan is?
- What is my intention for being a massage therapist?
- What is my path of service?
- What is my greatest strength?
- What is the most important thing I have to give?
- What am I most thankful for?
- What is the basis of my hope, faith, and energy for success?
- Why am I confident?

Good Stuff from the Government

BUSINESS PLAN TEMPLATE

Consult the Small Business Association's business plan template (http://web.sba.gov/busplantemplate/GenRpt. cfm). Here are five important tips before you start:

1. The business plan should tell a compelling story about your business, explaining who, what, when, where, how, and why.
2. Your plan should be focused and clear. It is not about the number of pages or style of the cover.
3. The plan should define specific business objectives and goals with general parameters to guide the organization.
4. Writing a business plan should force logic and discipline into a business.
5. A good business plan is a living document. It should be updated regularly.

This template is designed to help you build a business plan. Review and complete each section of the template. At the end of the program, you will be able to generate and save a formatted business plan, which can later be further modified or presented as a final product. Completing this plan is a first step to building a successful business. There is also a free online course called How to Prepare a Business Plan (http://web.sba.gov/sbtn/registration/index.cfm? courseid=27).

massage is found in many environments. Massage therapists also have the option of having our own small business. Although there are many career options, the ultimate determinant for your success is your commitment to professional and business skills, your massage therapy skills and expertise, and your professional focus on serving your clients.

Your career journey begins. This textbook, your instructors, peers, mentors, and good stuff from the government can offer ongoing support. Intention, intuition, and inspiration will serve you well if you spend the time to pay attention. Be deliberate and persistent. Do not be fearful, but it is okay to be realistic. Be optimistic, not pessimistic. Work hard and smart. Be committed and joyful. You will grow and mature as your career progresses.

Be kind to yourself, and be kind to others. Focus on the big picture, but also attend to the details. Massage is considered valuable because it is low tech, but maybe our ability to touch in a compassionate and effective way to meet the needs of our clients is the most sophisticated application of all.

Row, row, row your boat gently down the stream. Merrily, merrily, merrily, merrily, life is but a dream. Row steadily and with focus on your career path. While you are doing so, learn to make the flow work for you instead of fighting against it. Make compassion your goal, enjoy yourself, and remember that your life is the manifestation of your dream. Go for it!

Bibliography

Fulton JPG: *General Office Procedures for Colleges*, ed 12, Cincinnati, OH, 2003, South-Western.

Locker KO: *Business and Administrative Communication*, ed 6, New York, 2003, McGraw-Hill/Irwin.

Sabin WA: *The Gregg Reference Manual*, ed 10, New York, 2004, McGraw-Hill/Irwin.

SUMMARY

Massage therapy is a fantastic, rewarding career with many opportunities for success. Unlike many professions that have a narrow career path because of restricted environments (e.g., veterinary assistant, medical assistant, cosmetologist),

Workbook

1. Write your career philosophy in which you describe who you are, where you are going, and what you hope to accomplish. This philosophy should include your goals for life, your basic values, and your strengths and weaknesses.

_____

_____

_____

_____

_____

2. List six areas of potential employment and explain briefly the benefits of each.

_____

_____

_____

_____

3. Choose one of the advertisements in Figure 18-2 or 18-3. Respond to the advertisement by writing a letter of application for the position. Prepare a resume to accompany the letter.

4. Make a copy of the letter and the resume for your personal files. Assume that you have been interviewed for the position mentioned in question 3, and write an appropriate follow-up letter.

5. List five of your assets that would attract the favorable attention of a future employer.

_____

_____

_____

6. Give five ways an application form may attract unfavorable attention. List 10 questions that you may be asked during an interview.

_____

_____

_____

_____

_____

_____

_____

_____

_____

_____

_____

7. Complete the application form in Figure 18-7.

8. For your personal use, review the performance evaluation form in Figure 18-10.

9. With two people assuming the roles of interviewer and applicant, answer the questions in Box 18-9. Discuss six suggestions for success on the job.

_____

_____

_____

_____

_____

_____

_____

_____

_____

_____

10. Discuss the procedures for the following: asking for a raise and terminating a job.

_____

_____

_____

_____

_____

_____

_____

_____

_____

Index

Note: Page numbers followed by f refer to figures; page numbers followed by t refer to tables.